Trauma and Grief Assessment and Intervention

With clarity and eloquence, *Trauma and Grief Assessment and Intervention* comprehensively captures the nuance and complexity involved in counseling bereaved and traumatically bereaved persons in all stages of the life cycle.

Integrating the various models of grief with the authors' strengths-based framework of grief and loss, chapters combine the latest research in evidence-based practice with expertise derived from years of psychotherapy with grieving individuals. The book walks readers through the main theories of grief counseling, from rapport building to assessment to intervention. Each chapter concludes with lengthy case scenarios that closely resemble actual counseling sessions to help readers apply their understanding of the chapter's content. In the support material on the book's website, instructors will find a sample syllabus, PowerPoint slides, and lists of resources that can be used as student assignments or to enhance classroom learning.

Trauma and Grief Assessment and Intervention equips students with the knowledge and skills they need to work effectively with clients experiencing trauma and loss.

Renée Bradford Garcia has over 25 years of experience providing psychotherapy to children, adolescents, and adults. Her specialties include loss, trauma, anxiety, and depression as well as leadership and organizational development.

Elizabeth C. Pomeroy is notable for her distinguished teaching and her prolific research on the effectiveness of mental health interventions for adults, children, and families.

Trauma and Grief Assessment and Intervention

Building on Strengths

Renée Bradford Garcia and
Elizabeth C. Pomeroy

Routledge
Taylor & Francis Group
NEW YORK AND LONDON

First published 2022
by Routledge
605 Third Avenue, New York, NY 10158

and by Routledge
2 Park Square, Milton Park, Abingdon, Oxon, OX14 4RN

Routledge is an imprint of the Taylor & Francis Group, an informa business

Library of Congress Cataloging-in-Publication Data
A catalog record for this book has been requested

ISBN: 978-0-367-11215-8 (hbk)
ISBN: 978-0-367-11216-5 (pbk)
ISBN: 978-0-429-05363-4 (ebk)

DOI: 10.4324/9780429053634

Typeset in Sabon
by Apex CoVantage, LLC

Access the Support Material: www.routledge.com/9780367112165

We dedicate this book to all first responders, peacekeepers, justice seekers, and healers.

Contents

List of Illustrations

FIGURE

TABLES

BOXES

Author Bios

Renée Bradford Garcia, MSW, LCSW-S is a licensed clinical social worker with a private practice near Austin, Texas. She has over 25 years of experience providing psychotherapy to individuals and families, including children, adolescents, and adults. Renée's specialties include grief and loss, anxiety, depression, trauma, relationships, parenting, and life transitions. She has taught at the University of Texas at Austin School of Social Work as an adjunct professor and provides presentations and training to both professional and lay people. Renée is co-author with Elizabeth C. Pomeroy of the *Grief Assessment and Intervention Workbook: A Strengths Perspective* (Cengage, 2009), *Children and Loss: A Practical Handbook for Professionals* (Lyceum, 2011), and *Direct Practice Skills for Evidence-Based Social Work: A Strengths-Based Text and Workbook* (Springer, 2018). She also co-authored *Don't Look at Me in That Tone of Voice: Tween Discipline for Busy Parents* (2013). In addition, she provides business and organizational consulting as co-founder of G2 Solutions: Organizational Change Consulting. You can learn more about Renée at www.garciareneeb.com.

Elizabeth C. Pomeroy, PhD, LCSW is the Bert Kruger Smith Professor of Aging and Mental Health at the School of Social Work, University of Texas at Austin. She teaches in the undergraduate and graduate social work program. Her research has focused on the effectiveness of mental health interventions for adults, children, and families. She has published over 100 journal articles and has also conducted numerous presentations and workshops on the *DSM-5*, grief and loss issues, and social work values and ethics. Dr. Pomeroy has authored numerous articles on the effectiveness of group interventions using experimental and quasi-experimental research designs. She is a member of the Academy of Distinguished Professors and a UT Regents' Outstanding Teaching Professor. She has published four textbooks, *The Clinical Assessment Workbook: Balancing Strengths and Differential Diagnosis* (1st edition, Cengage, 2003), *The Clinical Assessment Workbook: Balancing Strengths and Differential Diagnosis* (2nd edition, Cengage, 2015), and has co-authored three texts with Renée Bradford Garcia titled *The Grief Assessment and Intervention Workbook: A Strengths Perspective* (Cengage, 2009), *Children and Loss: A Practical Handbook for Professionals* (Lyceum, 2011), and *Direct Practice Skills for Evidence-Based Social Work: A Strengths-Based Text and Workbook* (Springer, 2018).

Preface

Students and professionals in a wide variety of helping professions will inevitably be faced with the task of helping persons who have experienced the death of a loved one, often in traumatic circumstances. As this manuscript goes to publication, the world is battling the life-threatening pandemic of COVID-19. At the time of this writing (November 2020), the coronavirus has taken the lives of well over a million people, and the numbers continue to climb, with marginalized communities, communities of color, and the elderly being hit the hardest. Restrictions put in place to prevent further spread of the virus resulted in families being separated from their loved ones in their final days. Additionally, mourning rituals have had to be dramatically altered, scaled down, and attended remotely instead of in person. These vast changes from how we traditionally say goodbye, memorialize our beloved, and comfort each other represent additional losses for those grieving the death of a loved one. While it is too early to know the long-term effects of how these circumstances impact the bereavement process, it is our hope that this book will equip practitioners with a fundamental understanding of grief and traumatic grief so that they can effectively respond to those who have experienced so much loss within loss.

Understanding how to conduct assessments and intervene with bereaved children, adolescents, adults, and families are important skills for professionals working in the fields of social work, nursing, school and pastoral counseling, psychology, and other helping professions. This text was designed for use as a text in courses that teach assessment and practice methods, grief and loss, counseling, as well as other practice-related courses. In our experience teaching these types of courses, we have found that students have limited knowledge of and experience with grief and loss concepts. Furthermore, they often have difficulty applying some of these concepts to clients that they encounter in practice.

Previous books about grief that are commonly used for classroom instruction are often written from one specific theoretical framework, are not generally designed to be used in a classroom, and provide very short case examples that provide little information to form an assessment. Furthermore, many such books were written for the general public and do not provide the type of information necessary for becoming an astute counselor. In addition, while there are many scholarly works that provide in-depth information about grief and loss issues most do not provide any practical information for using this knowledge in practice situations.

This book was written to fill this gap. It will not only enhance a student's understanding of grief, but also improve their confidence and ability to practice effectively with clients who are grieving.

This book begins with a review of various theories of grief that have been fundamental to contemporary understanding of the bereavement experience. From these traditional models, we developed a strengths-based framework of grief and loss that emphasizes a person's coping abilities and environmental resources. This framework is used throughout the text and is the basis for the assessment and intervention skills that are presented. Grief as it relates to societal values, cultural perspectives, and family dynamics is also discussed.

The text then explores the relationship between grief and trauma, fields that have long been regarded separately, though there is considerable overlap between the two. It includes a foundational overview of trauma, the ways that loss and trauma often intersect, in addition to what this means for working with traumatically bereaved clients.

Discussion about the interplay of grief on the cognitive, emotional, behavioral, physical, spiritual, and cultural experiences of a person in mourning is presented. A review of relevant assessment techniques and instruments is included along with strengths-based intervention skills. Due to space limitations, we limit our focus to grief resulting from death and provide brief overviews of other relevant topics with the expectation that this will spur additional learning.

Since the research on grief originated with adult populations, the authors begin the skills portion of the book with adults. Theories related to specific populations such as children, adolescents, and older adults grew out of this earlier research and thus are presented later in the text. Grief as it relates to special populations and circumstances is also included. Specifically, we discuss bereavement for persons with developmental disabilities, LGBTQ persons, anticipatory grief associated with terminal illness, parents grieving the death of a child, refugees, military veterans, ambiguous loss, and pet loss.

The primary purpose of this book is to enhance skill development through practice cases by which readers can learn interviewing, assessment, and intervention methods for working with a variety of populations who are bereaved or traumatically bereaved. The cases focus on skills that are used at the direct practice level after the crisis of learning about the death of a loved one has subsided and are followed by questions for reflection. Instructors can use these case questions as homework assignments or test questions. This method enables students to attain a more comprehensive understanding of assessment and intervention planning by practicing the application of their knowledge to scenarios that closely resemble actual interactions. Feedback from students indicates that this type of learning experience is invaluable. The cases also allow for richer class discussions about sensitive emotional issues that can be otherwise hard to discuss.

The relevance of culture to the grief experience is discussed throughout the book. The importance of practicing cultural humility is emphasized, as is enhancing practitioner awareness of social justice issues related to grief and loss. In addition, text boxes dispersed throughout the text provide information about death and grief as they relate to specific value and cultural orientations. These are not intended to replace more in-depth understanding about a group or individual nor are they to be generalized to all members of a particular group. Rather, they are there to remind the reader of the vast diversity that exists in views and practices related to death and mourning. Issues of culture and social justice merit a great deal of discussion, and readers are encouraged to continually pursue knowledge and practice skills in this area.

The book concludes with a chapter discussing implications for the practitioner, including the risk of developing vicarious trauma and highlighting the need for self-awareness, self-care, supervision, and continuing education. In addition, we have included additional websites and student activities to augment the reader's learning experience. These activities are also suitable for instructors to use as classroom assignments.

The authors relied heavily on their clinical experiences in devising case scenarios for this book. However, any resemblance between actual clients and those presented herein is completely coincidental. The cases were developed from aggregations of experiences with clients in various practice settings. Great care was exercised in obscuring any identifying information related to the clients upon whom a specific case scenario was based.

As with any large project, the authors are indebted to a number of others for their assistance and support in the process. We are grateful for the assistance of Anna Moore and Katherine Tsamparlis for their support and expertise in the completion of this publication. Our thanks to Abigail Stanley, production editor, Emily Boyd, copy-editor, Graham Frankland, proofreader, and Rosie Wood, indexer for shepherding this project through the production process. Much appreciation goes to Ian Woodroffe for allowing us to share his Invisible Suitcase analogy and to Cheve Garcia for his graphic design of the P-I-E Perspective of the Grief Experience.

We would also like to thank the University of Texas, Steve Hicks School of Social Work whose support throughout this project was invaluable. We are fortunate to be associated with such an energetic and collegial faculty.

Immense gratitude also goes to Chloe Scarborough, who kept this enormous project flowing. This book would not have come to fruition without her administrative talents, tenacious resourcefulness, and keen eye for detail.

Finally, this book would not be possible without the continual encouragement and unfailing support of friends and family members. Renée gives special thanks to Daniel, Tilo, and Cheve for graciously sacrificing family time to make room for this work. Also, to Wanda Bradford, who modeled compassionate care for others from day one. Beth would like to thank siblings Nancy Togar, Peggy Higginbotham, and Bill Pomeroy for their immeasurable support both personally and professionally throughout the years. We are exceedingly grateful to the many others who cheered us on along the way.

CHAPTER 1

Understanding Grief and Loss – An Introduction

Loss is a universal experience that everyone encounters at one time or another. Though an expected aspect of being human, the death of a loved one can fundamentally upend the lives of survivors and leave them casting about for a way to continue living without their beloved. The turmoil caused by a significant loss disrupts a person's functioning both internally (physically, emotionally, cognitively, and spiritually) and externally (socially and occupationally). When loss is coupled with elements of trauma, it can give rise to additional complications in physical and emotional well-being and sometimes have lasting implications for how the bereaved survivors move through their lives and experience the world. A recent survey related to grief, loss, and spirituality reveals that helping professionals receive little in-depth education or training in grief and end of life care prior to entering the field (Pomeroy et al., 2019). Though there are numerous theories of grief and loss that have been postulated by experts, there are fewer that address trauma and grief combined, though the two are intricately linked more often than not. As interest and demand for grief and loss services increase, there is a need for an understanding of the grief process that considers individuals within the context of the environments in which they function, rather than just examining their intrapsychic experiences. This chapter will provide a brief overview of prominent theories and models of grief and loss. Readers are encouraged to explore the extensive body of literature that exists on these theoretical frameworks for more in-depth explanations. This chapter will also present the authors' framework of grief that encompasses a person-in-environment and strengths-based perspective. Trauma, and the ways that trauma and grief intersect, will be discussed in Chapter 2.

THEORIES OF GRIEF AND LOSS

Freudian Theory of Loss

In the early 20th century, Freud provided a theory of "mourning and melancholia" that distinguished between "normal" and "pathological" mourning. He suggested that relinquishing emotional ties with the object of attachment involved obsessive remembering followed by a complete severance of emotion to the loved one and re-attaching that emotion to another person. While this other person is only a substitute for the lost

DOI: 10.4324/9780429053634-1

loved one, the mourner eventually internalizes the reality of the loss, extinguishes the emotional energy expended on the lost loved one, and, in turn, frees it to be directed toward another. Freud also believed that the psychological identification with the lost person is internalized so that aspects of that person become part of the mourner's psychological make-up thus making the grief process challenging yet survivable (Berzoff, 2004; Freud, 1917).

Freud also distinguished healthy mourning from pathological mourning and differentiated between "mourning and melancholia." In both cases, the emotional experience is similar; however, with melancholia the mourner has a lack of self-esteem, is self-critical, and eventually develops pathological melancholia (depression) or grief. Freud postulated that this prolonged depression that accompanied the grief process was due to unconscious conflicts with the person who died which led to a more complicated mourning period. Threads of Freud's theory of mourning can be found in more recent theories and frameworks that guide current practice. Clearly, Freud's theory furthered our understanding of the grief process; however, his focus on the intrapsychic and unconscious elements of a person's psyche failed to account for environmental influences that impact the mourner's coping capacities.

Erich Lindemann and Crisis Theory

Following in the footsteps of Freud's theory of mourning, Erich Lindemann's research following the 1944 Cocoanut Grove Night Club disaster in which over 500 people were killed advanced ideas about the grief process (Parkes, 1964, 1970, 1972). Lindemann coined the term "grief work" with his suggestion that resolution of grief required the completion of three specific tasks. First, mourners must relinquish the attachment to their loved one. Second, they must re-adapt to life without the presence of the deceased. Finally, they must establish new relationships with others. Based on interviews with survivors of the nightclub fire, Lindemann named six characteristics of "acute" grief: 1) physical distress; 2) ruminations about the deceased; 3) survival guilt; 4) angry reactions to others; 5) decline in functioning; and 6) tendency to internalize characteristics of the deceased (Parkes & Weiss, 1983). This work also contributed to crisis intervention theory and understanding how mourners respond to traumatic grief experiences.

Bowlby's Theory of Attachment

John Bowlby's theory of attachment developed from his early research on infants separated from their mothers and the emotional, cognitive, developmental, and biological consequences of attachment versus separation. Attachment refers to the innate tendency for humans to develop close affectionate bonds with others who are central to their lives. When the attachment bonds are threatened or broken, emotional distress ensues. According to Bowlby, life span development of attachment involves the formation of a bond (i.e. falling in love), maintenance of the attachment (i.e. loving someone), and disruption (i.e. grief and mourning) (Bowlby, 1980). He wrote extensively on his theory over the course of three volumes about how attachment behaviors maintain the affectional bond and, therefore, a state of homeostasis or balance. When loss of the attachment figure occurs and the bond is disrupted, the person experiences distress, fear, and insecurity as represented by crying, clinging, and angry behaviors in an attempt to regain the connection. When these behaviors are repeatedly unsuccessful they gradually diminish but do not stop completely.

Bowlby (1980) hypothesized that the grief process is a reflection of this basic attachment dynamic. He further described the psychological reorganization that must take place following a loss as involving four phases. The first phase entails a period during which the mourner experiences numbness and denial that serves to deflect the anguish and despair accompanying the loss. This phase can be periodically disrupted by extreme and physically exhausting emotions. The second phase is characterized by yearning and searching as the mourner begins to confront the loss. Common behaviors during this phase include interpreting events as signs from the loved one and seeking out evidence of the loved one's presence. When these activities are unsuccessful, anger and frustration ensue. The third phase is predominated by feelings of disorganization and desolation. The realization that the attachment bond has been severed and the activities of prior phases have failed is integrated by the mourner. The person experiences a depletion of energy and a sense of being overwhelmed. This prompts a re-evaluation of the mourner's identity and self-concept which can lead to massive psychological upheaval. The final phase, according to Bowlby, involves gradual movement toward reorganization. There is growing acceptance of the permanence of the separation and the need to construct a life despite the absence of the loved one. These phases may be experienced multiple times during the grieving process and may take days, months, or years.

In conclusion, Bowlby's theory of attachment and loss lends itself to modern understanding and interventions currently used in practice. Bowlby's thorough examination of attachment provides us with insight into the nature of behaviors associated with separation and loss and has been foundational to our understanding of grief and the mourning process. The advanced understanding of interpersonal neuroscience has added scientific validity to attachment theory (Cozolino, 2014; Montgomery, 2013; Siegel, 2012). The result is a growing awareness of how attachment styles that originated in childhood influence the course of bereavement later in life including the support seeking strategies that mourners use. For example, individuals with an anxious attachment style are likely to grieve in a manner that is highly emotional with lots of crying, wailing, and other outward expressions of inner pain. Individuals with an avoidant attachment style are more reserved. They are uncomfortable expressing emotions, often insisting they are all right. This knowledge may help explain why some mourners navigate significant loss more successfully than others and provides guidance on how to best help mourners with varying attachment styles (Kosminsky & Jordan, 2016). Knowledge of attachment theory adds an additional lens for viewing other models of grief and provides greater understanding of complicated grief. It allows practitioners to tailor their interventions according to the individual attachment style of the mourner. Kosminsky and Jordan (2016) provide an excellent discussion of grief from an attachment perspective in their book, *Attachment-Informed Grief Therapy: The Clinician's Guide to Foundations and Applications*. Attachment theory also plays a role in understanding interpersonal trauma and will be discussed further in subsequent chapters.

Kübler-Ross and Stages of Grief

Although Lindemann was a pioneer in crisis intervention, death and dying were still taboo subjects when the United States was forced to confront the mass destruction of the Vietnam War. It was the 1960s and 70s, and America was a "society bent on ignoring or avoiding death" (Kübler-Ross, 1969, p. 25) despite the fact that death and trauma were occurring on a monumental scale due to the Vietnam War, the Kennedy assassinations, the assassination of Martin Luther King, Jr., and the Kent State student protest and shootings. Elisabeth Kübler-Ross's work was revolutionary in that it opened the doors to discussion about death and dying as well as grief and loss – subjects that were stigmatized in American culture during the middle of the 20th century. Originating from her experiences as a physician of terminally ill persons, her first book, *On Death and Dying* (1969), included a stage model of the psychological coping process experienced by those who were terminally ill. Later, this model was applied to the grief experience and was the accepted paradigm for many years. Kübler-Ross's model included five stages of grief: 1) denial and isolation, 2) anger, 3) bargaining, 4) depression, and 5) acceptance.

During the stage of denial and isolation, the person has difficulty comprehending the loss and the reality that death is imminent. The person could be considered to be in a state of shock – numb to the emotional ramifications of loss. Isolation or withdrawal was noted as a common behavioral component of this initial reaction to a terminal diagnosis (Kübler-Ross, 1969).

In the second stage, denial fades as anger and rage over the terminal prognosis take over. Often the person feels as if the terminal diagnosis is unfair or a cruel turn of fate. At times, this experience may take on irrational proportions and be difficult for others to comprehend. The anger then yields to the third stage called "bargaining" (Kübler-Ross, 1969).

During the bargaining phase, the person attempts to "strike a deal" with a higher being for a postponement of the inevitable death. For example, the person may secretly promise to be "good" in exchange for more time on Earth. Bargaining eventually leads to the fourth stage, "depression" (Kübler-Ross, 1969).

Kübler-Ross (1969) says depression is experienced as "a sense of great loss" (p. 97) and suggests that there are two types of depression: reactive and preparatory. In reactive depression, the person experiences the multiple losses resulting from the terminal illness (e.g. financial, employment, family roles, physical deterioration). In preparatory depression, the person grieves the impending losses associated with the knowledge that death is imminent. Loss of significant others, loss of physical self, loss of the material world, and the final separation from others are all components of preparatory depression. In this sense, Kübler-Ross links depression and grief as similar emotional experiences.

The final stage of this model is "acceptance," during which the person resolves their feelings of anger and sadness. While not necessarily content, they await their death with "quiet expectation" (Kübler-Ross, 1969, p. 124). She suggests that during this stage, the person may experience an absence of emotion and be "void of feelings" (Kübler-Ross, 1969, p. 124).

Though introduced as a model to assist health professionals in understanding their dying patients, Kübler-Ross's work has been applied to the experience of bereaved persons after the death of a loved one. Her framework has been considered the hallmark for understanding death and dying and many elements of her conceptualization are still used by professionals today. The primary criticism of this model was the fixed and sequential aspect of the stages.

David Kessler, a renowned expert on grief and collaborator with Kübler-Ross, added a sixth stage to the model: finding meaning (2019). This can take many forms such as advocating for a cause connected to the loved one, recalling memories of them, doing things they enjoyed, or helping others in honor of the deceased. Kessler explains that this process involves "finding a way to sustain your love for the person after their death while you're moving forward with your life" (Kessler, 2019, p. 6). By finding something positive that can come out of the tragedy, the suffering is mitigated.

Rando's Theoretical Framework of the Grief Process

Building on Kübler-Ross's work, Therese Rando suggested that mourning involves six tasks, often referred to as the six R's, that must be completed for a healthy resolution of grief. The tasks are grouped into three phases. During the first phase, "avoidance," the mourner's task is to "recognize" the reality of the loss. During the second phase, "confrontation," the mourner "reacts" to the loss as they experience and express the emotions prompted by their grief reaction. The next task is to "recollect and re-experience" memories of the deceased, both good and bad. This is followed by the subsequent task of "relinquishing" the attachment to the loved one. The final phase, "accommodation," involves a "readjustment" to the world without the deceased and a "reinvestment" of energy into current and future relationships (Humphrey & Zimpfer, 1996; Rando, 1993).

Worden's Task-Oriented Framework of Mourning

Worden (2018) developed a task-oriented, practice framework based on Bowlby's theory of attachment that emphasizes the continuum of grief as moving from the pain of separation to the adjustment of new relationships. He describes four basic tasks that must be completed for mourning to be resolved. He emphasizes the fact that these tasks are not necessarily sequential in nature and a person can move back and forth from one task to another. All of the tasks, according to Worden, involve effort by the bereaved person. The four basic tasks are:

1. To accept the reality of the loss
2. To process the pain of grief
3. To adjust to a world without the deceased
4. To find a way to remember the deceased while embarking on the rest of one's journey through life.

Worden's practice model emphasizes the need for assessment and distinguishes between uncomplicated and complicated grief. It has been a useful guide for practitioners in the field because the tasks indicate an active approach toward grief resolution unlike other models in which phases are passively endured by the mourner.

Two Track Model of Bereavement

Freud's theory of bereavement and loss was a cornerstone underlying grief work for several decades. However, in the late 1970s and early 1980s a biological conceptualization of bereavement centering on the cognitive and emotional levels of functioning and an emphasis on the importance of separating from the deceased began to be challenged by more empirically based theories of crisis, trauma, and stress. Researchers began to examine a biopsychosocial approach to attachment and loss, and in 1981, the Two Track Model of Bereavement (TTM) was developed and published by Simon Shimshon Rubin based on his empirical observations of parents coping with the loss of a child. The first track in this model indicates the bereaved person's biopsychosocial functioning before and after the loss. For example, it addresses the individual's functioning from a cognitive, emotional, social, physical, spiritual, and occupational standpoint. The second track involves the individual's relationship with the deceased and their investment in maintaining and changing that relationship. This can include wishes and experiences involving connection with the loved one, being preoccupied with matters regarding the death, experiencing conflict regarding the loss or the deceased, and establishing an altered relationship with the loved one.

Both tracks are important in obtaining a clear picture of the individual's current functioning and how they can be helped to navigate the loss. Rubin et al. (2012) emphasize that this is not a "stage" approach and that both tracks need to be examined simultaneously. The TTM outlines ten areas of biopsychosocial and relational functioning that should be considered when assessing a person's loss experience (Rubin et al., 2012). The assessment developed by the authors and outlined in Chapter 3 includes these domains.

Grief and the Constructivist Framework

Another popular view of grief originates from a constructivist framework which views the bereavement experience as one in which the mourner actively searches for a way to understand the loss, their changed life following the loss, and to attach some symbolic significance to the loss and its influence on their "new" life. The extent to which a mourner is able to "make meaning" of the loss is believed to influence their transition to life without the deceased. This conceptualization may be especially relevant to those who are grieving a traumatic loss (Neimeyer et al., 2002). Research on traumatic grief suggests that bereaved persons who search and find some meaning in the loss as well as those who feel no need to look for significance in the death may have better psychological outcomes compared with those who search but cannot find meaning (Neimeyer, 2000).

According to this viewpoint, the process of re-constructing one's life after losing a loved one is grounded in sociological, cultural, and community influences that regulate norms around grief and bereavement. As mourners interface with their environment, their grieving experience is affirmed, enabling their efforts to "relearn the self" and "relearn the world" (Attig, 1996).

Additionally, bereaved persons also interact with an internal psychological component as they attempt to adjust their life to the loss. Such adjustments include attempts to integrate the loss into the "personal narrative" of their life and fit it into a "meaningful plot structure" (Neimeyer et al., 2002).

The construction of meaning around the death of a loved one is a very personal endeavor that varies with each individual. Often mourners will engage in activities or begin projects or organizations in memory of their loved one. Their hope is that some good, such as helping others, can come from their pain. The non-profit, bereavement support organization "The Christi Center" is one such example. This organization was founded by parents whose daughter was killed by a drunk driver and found little support available to help them with their trauma and grief. It provides community-based grief groups for adults, children, and families. As another example, many family members of persons who died by suicide become engaged in advocacy and prevention education to raise awareness about the warning signs of suicide and how to help someone who is at risk. For other mourners, making meaning of the loss may take the form of significant changes in their priorities and how they live, such as attending to one's health, staying in closer touch with family and friends, and working less in order to spend more time relaxing or with family.

Continuing Bonds Framework of Grief

The Continuing Bonds (CB) perspective of grief builds on Bowlby's framework of attachment and loss. Unlike other models that focus on detaching from the deceased, the CB approach gives attention to the mourner's connection with the deceased post-death. Rather than severing the relationship, the mourner maintains an internal and psychological attachment to the deceased. In its early development, the CB approach suggested that it is not pathological to have a continuing relationship with the deceased and that it, in fact, may be healthy to do so (Klass et al., 1996). Additional research suggests that there are different types of CBs with some being adaptive and others being maladaptive. Externalized CBs may be present when mourners are unable to grasp the finality of their loved ones' death and experience the deceased as still being alive which can block adaptation to the loss. Field and Filanosky (2009) described this kind of continuing relationship with the deceased as a quasi-perceptual experience that may involve hallucinations of the dead loved one. These externalized CB expressions are believed to indicate that the mourner has not fully integrated the knowledge that their loved one has died (Field & Filanosky, 2009; Field et al., 2013; Yu et al., 2016). There is evidence to suggest that externalized CB expressions are more common among bereaved who had insecure attachments to the deceased as well as with losses that were violent in nature (Field & Filanosky, 2009; Meier et al., 2013; Yu et al., 2016). Externalized CBs share symptoms similar to Post-Traumatic Stress Disorder (PTSD) in that the mourner attempts to avoid reminders of the loved one or the mode of death to the extent that they may become dissociated (Field & Filanosky, 2009). PTSD will be discussed in greater depth in Chapter 2.

In contrast, Field and Filanosky (2009) referred to internalized CB expressions as those in which the bereaved carries a mental, emotional, or spiritual connection with the deceased that functions as a secure attachment to the loved one while also grasping the reality that the loved one is dead. This internal connection allows the mourner a secure base from which to build a new life without the deceased and is thus indicative of healthy adaptation. For example, a widower may talk to a picture of his partner every day. When faced with a dilemma, a child may think of his deceased mother and imagine the guidance she would give him. In some cases, mourners integrate aspects of the deceased into their personality and in that sense are always maintaining a connection with them. Such was the case with an adolescent who internalized the positive attributes of her deceased father and describes her drive to become a successful professional as rooted in his optimistic attitude toward her career goals. In this sense, the young woman's development encompassed her father's belief system and shaped her identity as a competent and goal-oriented individual who could succeed in her college education and career. While externalized CB expression is more typical during the early and more intense grieving process, internalized CB expression is often seen in the later phases of grief as the mourner learns to adapt to life without their loved one (Scholtes & Browne, 2015).

Distinguishing the different types of CBs can help practitioners in knowing whether or not mourners should be encouraged to establish and enhance CBs with the deceased. They will want to consider the kind of loss, the relationship the mourner had with the deceased prior to death, and the form that the continuing relationship takes.

Dual Process Model

The Dual Process Model of Bereavement (DPM) was developed by Stroebe and Schut (1999, 2010) and provides a more nuanced approach to understanding what constitutes effective coping with grief. This model identifies two types of stressors that mourners encounter: those that are oriented to the loss and those oriented to restoration. Loss orientation involves experiences of the mourner that focus on the absence of the loved one, the yearning for that person, the process of grieving the loss, and the painful feelings commonly associated with grief. Restoration orientation centers on the difficult endeavor of learning to adapt to a world in the absence of the loved one. This additionally involves adjusting to secondary losses that occur as a result of the loss, such as being a single parent, losing the role of caregiver, or becoming the family breadwinner (Stroebe & Schut, 2010). According to the DPM, it is the mourner's oscillation between these two facets of grieving, at times facing elements of the loss and at times avoiding them, that leads to adaptive coping. Grief becomes stalled or complicated when mourners are unable to shift between loss orientation and restoration orientation, becoming extremely preoccupied with either confronting the loss or avoiding it. The practitioner's role is to walk with mourners as they move between loss orientation and restoration orientation, helping them participate in the portion of the loss experience that gives them the greatest difficulty (Kosminsky & Jordan, 2016). This model acknowledges that grieving requires effort and is not merely a passive process that happens to mourners. It also recognizes that grieving is an arduous endeavor and that mourners can benefit from taking breaks from dealing with the loss (Stroebe & Schut, 2010).

A STRENGTHS-BASED FRAMEWORK OF GRIEF AND LOSS

The early conceptualizations of the grief process contribute to the notion that grief is a negative, painful, and disruptive experience for the mourner which must be treated as an illness or disorder to overcome. As a result, practitioners may deemphasize the mourner's strengths and resiliencies that can be brought to bear on their unique experience of loss. The strengths-based framework of grief developed by the authors assists practitioners in building on the inherent strengths of the individual while they navigate the grieving process. The strengths-based approach empowers bereaved persons to use their coping abilities and environmental resources. In this conceptualization, grief in response to the death of a loved one is a natural, expectable, and potentially health-producing process that aids the individual in adjusting to the absence of the loved one.

The strengths perspective of social work practice developed by Saleebey (2006) and Rapp (1998) views all persons as having assets and resources that enhance their ability to cope with life events. People have both individual strengths and environmental strengths. Individual strengths include aspirations, competencies, and confidence (Rapp, 1998). Aspirations include goals, dreams, hopes for the future, ambitions, and positive motivation to achieve and grow. Competencies are manifested by one's unique ability to utilize talents, skills, and intellect. Confidence refers to a person's positive self-regard, their belief and tenacity in achieving goals, and feelings of being worthy of positive life events. While strengths are present in every individual, some people appear able to capitalize on their strengths more than others. This phenomenon may be due to a combination of biological, psychological, and social factors.

Environmental strengths include resources, social relations, and opportunities. Resources include financial support, access to services, access to information, and other tangible assets. Social relations encompass friends, family, co-workers, neighbors, and others with whom one has interactions. Opportunities refer to openings in one's life that are receptive to change. They represent positive events that potentially have life-altering consequences.

The classification of an individual characteristic or environmental condition as a strength passes through the filter of the surrounding culture. For example, a young man who rejects opportunities to advance his career so that he may remain in the town in which he grew up may be judged differently depending on the beliefs and views of the broader society in which he lives. In a culture that places a high value on individual achievement, family loyalty may not be regarded as a strength, although in many cultures it is.

In addition, a person maintains specific niches in life, e.g. habitation, job, friends, and leisure activities. According to Rapp (1998), "The quality of the niches for any individual is a function of that person's aspirations, competencies, confidence, and the environmental resources, opportunities, and people available to the person" (p. 42). Together, a person's individual and environmental strengths influence their sense of well-being, empowerment, and life satisfaction (Rapp, 1998).

For clients who are grieving, the strengths perspective is a particularly salient framework. It builds on previous theories of grief with an added emphasis on the health-producing aspects that are intrinsic to the mourner and the process of grief. Focusing on client strengths rather than deficits provides the practitioner with a valuable tool that can aid in assessment and intervention. It effectively highlights aspects of the person and their environment that can be enhanced and utilized to assist in the grieving process and promote positive growth. The integration of this perspective leads to a non-medicalized understanding of the grief process and new insights into grief-related interventions, as outlined in the following tenets. The basic tenets of our strengths-based framework of grief are as follows:

1. Grief in response to the death of a loved one is a natural, expectable, and potentially health-producing process that aids the individual in adjusting to the absence of the loved one.
2. The symptoms, emotions, and behaviors associated with expected grief reactions represent a process of healthy adaptation as defined by one's culture and are not inherently pathological.
3. Mourners benefit by knowing that life-enhancing grief reactions facilitate healing within the mourner and are productive and beneficial.
4. All persons have individual and environmental strengths that can assist them as they experience grief. The mourner benefits from the reinforcement of those strengths and the encouragement to consciously employ them during the grief process.
5. Environmental conditions can either help or hinder the mourner's ability to adapt to the loss and enhance the person's life.
6. Many symptoms of grief, though they may be uncomfortable, represent healthy coping mechanisms in that they facilitate the process of separation, adaptation to change, and integration of the loss.
7. Life-enhancing grief reactions to loss facilitate the process of adaptation and psychological separation from the deceased.
8. Life-enhancing grief symptoms should not be discouraged. Rather, they should be allowed expression so long as they remain helpful to the mourner's process of adaptation.
9. Grief may be considered life-depleting when the symptoms it produces significantly interfere with the mourner's aspirations, competencies, and confidence. Life-depleting grief reactions are those responses and circumstances which act as impediments to the expected grieving process and interfere with the mourner's ability to live a fulfilling life.
10. Life-depleting grief reactions thwart the process of adaptation and lead to entropy.
11. Life-enhancing and life-depleting grief reactions exist on a continuum of intensity.
12. The experience of grief evolves over a person's lifetime and is experienced with varying levels of conscious awareness.
13. The process of grief is fertile ground for communal or personal growth and the development or enhancement of the mourner's strengths.

(Pomeroy & Garcia, 2009)

BOX 1.1 STRENGTHS AND RESILIENCE

Students of the strengths-based approach to practice will also benefit by studying the literature on resiliency. Although the terms are often used interchangeably, resilience refers to "the human capacity to face, deal with, overcome, and be strengthened by or transformed by experiences of adversity" (Grotberg, 2005, p. 1). However, a strength is a "beneficial quality or attribute of a person" (McKean, 2005, p. 1676). Therefore, a combination of strengths that are utilized during times of difficulty creates resiliency within a person. One can possess several strengths but not be resilient, that is, "bounce back," if those strengths are not actively applied to the situation.

By understanding different theories of grief, practitioners enhance their ability to implement interventions that will benefit their clients. The unique issues facing each client may determine the theoretical underpinning for interventions chosen. Throughout this book, the strengths-based framework of grief will be emphasized but can be used in conjunction with the other models presented in this chapter.

PRIMARY AND SECONDARY LOSSES

Primary loss can be defined as the initial loss that forms the foundation for the grief experience. The death of a loved one is the most obvious example of a primary loss. Primary losses are often the presenting issue and focal point when clients initially seek assistance from a counselor. The onset of grief occurs the moment the mourner becomes aware of the loss. The initial emotions of extreme sadness, loneliness, emptiness, and tearfulness are usually attributed to the primary loss. While these experiences tend to capture the attention of counselors, it is important that secondary losses be considered as well.

Secondary losses are defined as those losses that occur as a result of the primary loss. Examples of secondary losses include changes in financial status, social status, familial roles, personal identity, and family structure. Each of these presents specific and unique changes to which the mourner must adapt. Clients are often surprised as they become aware of all the secondary losses that have occurred as a result of the death of a loved one. By giving attention to secondary losses, both the client and practitioner become attuned to the full impact of the loss. They uncover the meanings associated with the loss and the strategies the client is using as they try to adapt. They also bring to light client strengths and barriers that impede adjustment (Shallcross, 2012).

Both primary and secondary losses can trigger memories and feelings of distress that are associated with previous losses, particularly if those losses were unresolved. The accumulation of loss over time can significantly impact a person's ability to cope with the current disruption in their life. In such cases, it may be more difficult for a person to recognize and utilize their individual and environmental strengths. Practitioners will want to explore previous losses with their client as discussed in Chapter 3 on assessment.

BOX 1.2 SECONDARY LOSSES ARE CULTURALLY SPECIFIC

The secondary losses that mourners experience are influenced by the broader societal and cultural context. In many cultures, the death of a husband also brings about greatly diminished respect for the widow and affects her social, political, and economic status. Older women, in particular, may have difficulty being independent both financially and socially (Boerner et al., 2015). In some areas of Pakistan, for example, widows may be more vulnerable to extortion and sexual assault. In addition, they are often shunned at social gatherings and religious celebrations due to the belief that they bring bad luck (Ahmad et al., 2020).

FAMILY SYSTEMS AND THE GRIEF PROCESS

Family systems theory is particularly relevant for understanding the grief process both for individuals and the family as a unit. Nathan Ackerman (as cited in Freeman, 2005) describes the family system as a dynamic, organic whole that is influenced by changes in the internal and external environment. Repeated family transactions form the basis of rules by which family members communicate and behave. The death of a family member can disrupt these patterns of interaction and cause a state of disequilibrium. In order to regain homeostasis and continue functioning, the family must establish new rules and redefine members' roles. Sometimes families can do this with relative ease and revise previous rules and members' responsibilities to accommodate the changes resulting from the death. A state of equilibrium is established as the family integrates and adapts to the loss, and, in essence, a new family emerges (Freeman, 2005).

For other families, accommodating the death of a family member is fraught with confusion, tension, and disagreement about how family rules and roles should change. Additionally, there may be differing views and comfort levels regarding how grief should be expressed (openly versus privately, discussed often versus not mentioned, etc.). Navigating these challenges is especially difficult while individuals are also struggling to manage their individual reactions to the loss. Their ability to listen empathically to each other is hindered and can prevent the family from re-establishing new boundaries and rules, assuming new roles, and developing healthy communication patterns (Rosenblatt, 2017). These families can often benefit from outside intervention in order to effectively assimilate the loss and develop life-enhancing ways of operating as a family unit.

The strengths-based perspective can be particularly useful in helping families navigate these changes. Helping family members recognize, value, and utilize the individual strengths of each other can foster understanding and appreciation. When families learn to leverage their collective strengths, a new familial identity can begin to evolve. The period of adjustment for families may take a few months to a few years. As family development occurs with children growing up, getting married, and having children of their own, the grief over the loss may be revisited periodically and the need for additional intervention may arise.

SOCIETAL RESPONSE TO GRIEF AND LOSS

In general, the majority of Americans are intensely fearful of death. This fear permeates society, viewing death as an adversary that must be overcome. Millions of dollars are spent on products and services that promote youth, health, beauty, and pleasure in attempts to circumvent death and distract us from its inevitability. This phenomenon is often credited to advances in technology that have extended the average life span. Indeed, it is not unusual to find middle-aged individuals in grief counseling for their first significant loss. Additionally, the typical death no longer occurs in the home, but in the hospital, and is thus removed from common experience.

At the same time, the 24-hour news cycle supplies continual exposure to death by violence, natural disasters, accidents, and strained healthcare systems. The constant bombardment of information and images related to such events has led to a desensitization from the true impact of death (King, 2020). Thus, even while exposure to the reality of death is increasing, it remains largely an abstract concept with little personal resonance.

It is important for clinicians to understand the mourner's social climate surrounding issues of dying, death, and bereavement because this influences how they perceive themselves and their grief process. Due to society's tendency to avoid the topic of death and the dearth of accurate education and information about grief, many bereaved persons find themselves feeling inadequate in how they are managing their loss. Statements such as, "I don't know why I'm having such a hard time" and "I know I should be over it by now" are indicators that these societal beliefs are playing a role in mourners' expectations about how they are coping with the loss (Granek, 2016). While there are differences among cultures, some of the dominant society's beliefs about grief suggest the following:

- One should "get over the loss and move on with life" as quickly as possible.
- A person should not talk about their grief in social situations.
- Grief is depressing and thus should be avoided.
- There is something "wrong" with someone who emotes extensively in response to loss.
- It is best to avoid or ignore feelings of grief.
- There is a prescribed script of emotions that everyone should follow when experiencing grief.
- Grief is a time-limited experience with a definite endpoint.

Unfortunately, many bereaved individuals accept these societal norms as valid notions of the "right" way to grieve and, therefore, experience their grief in life-depleting ways. They may refuse offers of support or counseling due to their belief that asking for help would indicate personal weakness or conversely, seek counseling because they assume that continued pain over the loss means there is something wrong with them. Mourners often experience immense relief when practitioners point out the fallacy of these expectations and normalize the reality of their experience. Practitioners can also reframe these expected and understandable responses to grief as strengths: asking for support is a life-enhancing coping mechanism and feeling the pain of the loss merely exemplifies their love for the deceased.

In addition, certain types of death, such as suicide, homicide, or drug overdose, are highly stigmatized by society, making it even more difficult for mourners to find support for their loss. For example, if a woman's partner dies by suicide, she will likely not feel comfortable explaining to others how her partner died, much less discussing the subject in detail. Even her close friends may behave awkwardly when providing support to her. This unfortunate, but common experience sets the stage for isolation, intense feelings of loneliness, rejection, and shame.

As a product of society's ineffectiveness in grief-related matters, there are compelling reasons for a person in mourning to isolate themselves and repress their emotional experiences. Therefore, it is incumbent upon practitioners to educate the public about the process of death, dying, grief, and loss.

CULTURAL RESPONSES TO GRIEF AND LOSS

It is important to remember that the knowledge and understanding that have been accumulated about grief have been filtered through a cultural lens. Therefore, theories, diagnoses, and ideas about what is considered normal, customary, and healthy while grieving are implicitly tainted with bias. It should not be assumed that the dominant culture's views on grief are the standard against which cultural and individual differences should be compared, measured, or judged. For example, the mainstream view of grief often regards the high degree of emotionality exhibited by bereaved African Americans as different or inappropriate. Many African Americans, however, perceive white people in mourning as holding in their sorrow or as feeling less pain when a loved one dies (Rosenblatt & Wallace, 2005a, 2005b). From this standpoint, what is inappropriate is the dulled expression of emotion exhibited by many European Americans (Rosenblatt, 2017).

In addition to great variance in the more observable mores, customs, and rituals surrounding death and bereavement among diverse groups, the internal grief experience is implicitly influenced by culture as well as social justice issues. American people of color disproportionately have poorer health due to structural racism that limits their access to nutritious food, clean water, safe housing, and adequate healthcare. They are also at higher risk for being harmed and killed by hate crimes and government authorities. The grief experience of mourners, including the narratives and unique meanings they make of the loss, are constructed against these backdrops of society. When bereaved persons of color believe racism caused or contributed to their loved one's death, additional reactions of anger, bitterness, and indignation are understandable and expected reactions. If practitioners limit their conceptualization of grief to that which is promoted by the dominant culture, they run the risk of misunderstanding and diminishing their clients' grief experiences and thereby not providing them with the services they deserve.

Practitioners should continually expose themselves to education and experiences that inform and expand their cultural knowledge base, a practice often referred to as cultural competence. It is, however, a mistake to make assumptions about a client based solely on this knowledge. Rather, it should be assumed that every person has a unique expression of their culture that can only be learned by listening to them. This approach reflects the embodiment of cultural humility, a concept first coined by Tervalon and Murray-García (1998). For example, relying solely on textbook information might cause a practitioner to conclude that an Asian client would be uncomfortable expressing intense emotions. Until that has been determined to be true for the client with whom they are working, it would be misguided to interact with the client according to textbook knowledge.

In addition, practitioners must consider all of the facets that comprise the client's cultural and social identity, including their personal experiences and how they have been impacted by structures of power and privilege in society (Garran & Werkmeister Rozas, 2013). For example, a Puerto Rican American who is lesbian and works as a police officer will have multiple layers of identities. How she experiences a death in the family may be influenced by any one or all of these identities and this may be further dependent on the social context she is in at any given moment. Practitioners cannot be expected to fully understand how these variables influence the client's experience except by attentive listening, an openness to learning from the client, and a willingness to acknowledge what they do not know. Cultural humility implies collaboration with clients, regarding each person as the expert on themselves. By being humble enough to surrender the role of expert and being willing to learn from clients, practitioners are freed from having to know everything about every client's culture, an impossible task. The practice of cultural humility also involves a simultaneous and life-long commitment to acquiring additional knowledge about other cultures and thus does not exclude the need for cultural competence (Greene-Moton & Minkler, 2020).

Self-reflection along with awareness of power differentials and inherent privilege are required elements of cultural humility, particularly for practitioners who belong to privileged groups. Without this they can easily presume that their knowledge and experience encompass all there is to know which can result in behaviors that are oppressive and controlling (Rosenblatt, 2016). As Rosenblatt (2016), who has done extensive studies of grief in different cultures, eloquently explains,

> I try to have humility as I relate to people dealing with grief and loss. Partly it is a matter of being respectful and ethical, and partly it is a matter of knowing that however much I know I do not know enough. Thus, in humility I have to be open to what they provide as we interact. I have to learn from them.
>
> (p. 70)

The importance of self-awareness and reflection will be discussed further in Chapter 8.

In addition, culturally based perspectives, values, traditions, and mores can be a potent source of strength for individuals and communities. When these strengths are honored and utilized, they can positively impact a client's journey with grief.

Practitioners are better able to discover and activate these strengths when adopting a learner's stance as they work with their clients. Thus, the authors regard cultural humility as an inherent component of the strengths-based framework of grief and loss. Cultural issues related to grief and loss will be addressed in more detail in subsequent chapters.

CASES

CASE 1.1

Identifying Information:

Client Name: Irene Bennett
Age: 67 years old
Race/Ethnicity: African American
Marital Status: Widowed with two grown children
Education Level: Some college
Occupation: Retired administrative assistant

Intake Information:

Irene's daughter, Leyanne, called the counseling center and requested an appointment for her mother whose husband of 45 years died three months ago.

Initial Interview:

Irene arrives for her appointment at the scheduled time and responds cordially to your greeting. Her demeanor and dress are somewhat formal, and she sits on the couch in your office holding her back up straight, her purse in her lap, and a look of expectation for you to begin the session.

"How can I help you, Mrs. Bennett?" you ask.

"Well, I'm here for grief counseling. My daughter thought I should come," she replies professionally.

"Okay," you respond. "I understand you lost your husband, is that correct?"

"Yes." Irene pauses. "He died about three months ago." She seems reluctant to continue. You suspect that she is feeling self-conscious and unsure of how to behave in this setting. You decide to address this with an inquiry about her presence in counseling.

"So, you said your daughter wanted you to come for counseling? Do you know why she believed that you needed this?" you ask.

Irene answers, "I'm not sure. I think she is worried about me. My husband and I were together for over 45 years. I think it is hard for her to see me alone in the house. It's the same house she grew up in. I think it's especially hard right now because she's six months pregnant and her father's death hit her pretty hard."

"Forty-five years is a long time. It must be very strange for you to not have him around," you venture.

"Yes, it is very strange." She pauses, then continues. "Every time I go into the living room, I expect to see him sitting in his chair. The house feels so empty. I find that I just walk around, not really doing anything – just going from room to room. It's kind of like I'm looking for him." Her posture relaxes a bit and she looks at her hands, which are still holding her purse. "Yes, it's very strange," she adds.

"What was your husband's name?" you ask gently.

"Ray," she answers. "Ray Bennett."

"How did Ray die?" you inquire.

Irene takes a deep breath. "He was on a fishing trip. The friend that was with him said he had been real quiet and when he looked over at Ray, he noticed that he was bent over. Fred said that he could tell something was wrong. He got him in the car and drove him to the hospital, but he died shortly after getting there." Irene's voice is level, but she speaks slowly and with little energy. "It seems he had a heart attack."

"So you had no warning that this was going to happen," you say.

Irene looks at you. "No. No, I didn't. One minute he was here, talking about putting a deck in the backyard and the next minute he's gone." Her eyebrows furrow and you see the sadness in her eyes. "I wasn't ready for this. I don't really know what to do with myself."

"It must be very hard to adjust to losing someone who has been in your life for such a long time. I would expect that you would feel pretty disoriented," you empathize.

"Well, I do. Very disoriented. I feel like I've lost my right arm." She looks at her lap for a few moments and then looks at you as if wondering what she is to do next.

"It sounds like this loss has been quite debilitating for you," you say. Irene nods. You pause, but she remains silent. "Perhaps you could tell me more about Ray and your relationship with him. What was he like?"

She looks out the window and you notice that her eyes soften a bit. "He was a good man – a good husband, a good father, a good provider for his family. He had a quiet and gentle spirit. I rarely saw him angry. He just didn't let himself get ruffled up about stuff. He kept life simple. Everyone remembers him fondly. I don't think he had any enemies. He was a really good man." She pauses. "He loved to be outdoors. I'm glad he was outdoors for his last moments, but..." her voice trails off. You wait patiently. After a few moments she tearfully continues, "I wish I could have been there with him to at least say goodbye."

"Yes, I'm sure you do," you respond softly.

She sighs deeply, "I hate waking up in the morning and realizing he is gone. I keep hoping it is just a dream."

"It's a reality you don't want to face," you reflect.

Mrs. Bennett nods silently.

"Do you have any support with this or are you mostly trying to manage on your own?"

"My daughter has been very supportive. She comes over a lot. She has offered to let me move in with her, but I don't really want to. And I've had some invitations to go out to eat with some of the people from church but I don't want to have to pretend I'm happy. I just don't feel like I have the energy for that."

"I can understand that," you respond. "The grief itself is exhausting. Have you been able to sleep?"

"No," she answers. "Nights are the worst time for me. I feel so tired during the day but when I lay down, suddenly my mind starts churning and I can't turn it off. I toss and turn and lay awake for hours. The bed feels so empty without him lying next to me. My doctor gave me some medication to help me sleep but I don't want to use it too often."

"Well, I'm not surprised to hear that you are having trouble sleeping. That is a very common response to loss," you say.

"Then I guess I'm normal," she says.

"Yes, I think it's quite normal to be feeling lonely and sad when you've lost your husband, and nighttime can be especially difficult. Have there been nights when you have been able to sleep?"

"Sometimes, yes. And I feel quite a bit better the next day, now that you mentioned it."

"On days when you've gotten enough sleep and you're feeling better, how do you spend your day?" you ask.

"I used to like to get outside and take a walk. Ray and I used to take long walks after dinner and I know all my neighbors because we would stop and chat with anyone who was outside."

"Are you still getting out and walking?" you query.

"Sometimes, I do. I always feel better afterwards. Kind of lifts my spirits, at least for a little while," Irene replies.

"Are there other things you like to do that lift your spirits?" you ask.

"Well, I'm pretty connected to my church, and Ray and I always enjoyed having lunch with friends after church," she replies. "Sometimes we'd go out as a group to the cafeteria, and the pastor and a big group of us always showed up. We'd spend two or three hours just gabbing away. When the weather was good, we'd meet at someone's house and have a Sunday potluck dinner in the yard. You wouldn't believe the spread that friends brought to share. We ate really good on those days! Oh, gosh that was our big outing for the week. But I haven't done that lately. I don't seem to feel hungry these days."

"It sounds like that was a good time! I'm wondering if there's anything else you enjoy doing?" you ask.

"Well, I've been helping my daughter get ready for the baby. It will be my first grandchild!" You notice a hint of light in Irene's eyes. "She just found out that she's having a girl and we've been poring over the baby books for a name that she and her husband like. I must say, when we are doing things for the baby, I actually feel good for a few moments."

"That must be very exciting. I'm glad you have something to look forward to," you say.

"As a matter of fact, I really do. It's just been hard to get going lately."

"And that's completely understandable and to be expected. But you're here today and that's a big step you've taken." After a brief pause, you ask, "How is it for you to be here, talking about this to someone you don't know?" you ask.

"It's a little strange, to be honest. I don't mean any disrespect to you but I'm not sure how this is supposed to help," she admits.

"I don't feel any disrespect by that comment and I appreciate your honesty. It helps me to know how you are feeling, and it is my hope that you will feel comfortable here to say what is on your mind. People use grief counseling in different ways," you explain. "For some it is to learn more about the grief process and what to expect. It can also be a place for you to talk about your loved one and your experience missing him without having to pretend to be happy or okay. It may also be a place where you can get some help problem solving the new challenges that you face now that your husband is gone, such as how to deal with social invitations." You pause to gauge her reaction.

"Well, that does sound kind of useful," she concedes. "I've lost both of my parents and that was real hard, but this feels completely different."

"Yes, each loss is unique and the loss of a spouse is one of the hardest. You had a very special relationship with Ray."

"Yes," she agrees.

You continue conversing with Mrs. Bennett so that you can learn more about her and also help her feel at ease with you. Towards the end of the session you say, "However you use this space, people often find strength by knowing they are not so alone, that there is someone in their corner to walk with them as they go through the grief. And I hope you'll let me know if I get something wrong that's not a part of your experience. This is a team effort and it's about how the grief feels to you that is important. Does that sound okay with you?"

"Well, that seems to make sense. I suppose I'll try it," Irene says.

"I admire you for trying something new, Mrs. Bennett. We'll go at this in a way and at a pace that feels comfortable for you. As we spend more time together, I hope you'll feel free to give me any feedback about me or the process so that I can best meet your needs. I hope you will continue to be honest with me, as you were today."

"That sounds good. I feel comfortable with that," Irene responds.

"Okay. Let's find a time when you can come in again. And if you would like, maybe you could bring some pictures of Ray to show me."

"Okay. I'll do that," agrees Irene.

1.1-1. Using the strengths-based framework of grief and loss, summarize Irene's current experiences with the loss of her husband.

1.1-2. How would you summarize Irene's situation, using the Dual Process Model of grief?

1.1-3. How would Bowlby's theory of attachment apply to Irene's experience?

1.1-4. Using the strengths-based framework of grief and loss, how would you use the pictures Irene brings of Ray in your next session?

1.1-5. Do you think the Continuing Bonds approach could be helpful as Irene navigates her grief? Why or why not?

1.1-6. Provide two questions that you might ask Irene about her culture with regards to grief.

CASE 1.2

Identifying Information:

Client Name: Sarah Seinfeld
Age: 43 years old
Race/Ethnicity: Jewish
Marital Status: Divorced
Education Level: Doctoral degree
Occupation: English professor

Intake Information:

Sarah called the counseling center to inquire about grief support services. She told the intake worker that her mother passed away a month ago and she has since had problems coping with family situations. She specifically asked to meet with someone who has expertise in grief counseling.

Initial Interview:

Sarah arrives on time for her first appointment. You meet her in the waiting room and note that she is on her cell phone speaking in short, terse sentences and appears agitated. When she sees you standing at the door, she quickly ends the conversation and greets you.

"Are you the grief counselor?" she asks.

You say "yes" and introduce yourself.

"Well, am I glad to see you! I just got off the phone with my sister and WHOA!" She rolls her eyes and at the same time grabs your outstretched hand.

"I'm pleased to meet you, Sarah! Are you ready to head back to my office?" you invite.

"Am I ready? Yes! I've been waiting for four days to talk to somebody who understands what I'm going through."

As you lead Sarah down the hall to your office, she continues talking about how her cell phone has been ringing "off the hook" with calls from her family.

"You know, these cell phones are a blessing and a curse. I can't get away from them!" You suggest that Sarah turn off her phone during your session so that you will have some uninterrupted time to talk with her. As she enters your office she points to the box of tissues on the couch and says, "I guess I sit by the tissues?"

You nod and you both chuckle. She sits down and sighs.

You begin, "It sounds like there is a lot going on, Sarah."

"Oh! You wouldn't believe! My family puts the 'F' in dysfunctional! I haven't had a moment of peace since my mother died. I'm almost at the end of my rope and don't know how to handle it."

"Oh no! Tell me what's going on," you suggest.

"Well," she sighs, "I have four brothers and sisters. My father is 85 years old and living in a retirement community. My entire family never thought my father would outlive my mother. We're the type of Jewish family where Mom is the 'glue' that holds all of us together. Since she passed, we can't agree on anything and lately everyone has been so hostile."

"Tell me a little bit about your brothers and sisters," you prompt. "Where are you in the birth order?"

"I'm number four out of five children. I have a 55-year-old sister who thinks she knows everything because she is a lawyer. My brother, Sam, is 50 years old, gay, and owns his own restaurant. He and my sister can really go after each other because both of them are highly opinionated. Then there's my 47-year-old sister, Leah, who is a soccer mom with four children of her own and who never stops moving for a minute. And then there's my baby brother, Michael. He's a financial guy who wants to control Mom's estate."

"Okay. I think I have a sense of your family composition. Tell me about yourself," you suggest.

"Well, I'm single. I got divorced two years ago after ten years of fighting with my ex. I teach English at the university here. My former husband was also teaching at the university until he had an affair with a student and didn't get tenured," Sarah explains.

"So you've been through a lot in the last few years. Can you tell me what occurred after your mother's death that is creating so much hostility?" you ask.

Sarah explains to you that for the past month the family has been continually arguing about the needs of their father and the division of possessions from their mother's home.

"First of all, we have to make a decision about where Dad is going to live now that Mother is gone. Dad is 85 years old and Mom was his caretaker. He needs more assistance than he can get living by himself. Secondly, we need to sell their house and that means going through everything and dividing it up. We keep going around in circles and can't seem to get anywhere with any of this. We just sit around and yell at each other and no one seems to hear what anyone else is saying."

"Those are some big decisions and large tasks. I can see how difficult it might be to work all of those things out so shortly after your mother died," you respond.

"I think that's part of the problem," Sarah says. "We were all very close to Mother. In fact, she did such a good job that we all have commented that we each felt like we were her favorite."

"So all of you have been experiencing a lot of grief while you are trying to work out these issues," you state.

"Yes. Before Mother died we generally got along really well. We like each other and we respect the diversity in our family. My sister married a Roman Catholic, one of my brother's married a Baptist, another sister married a Muslim. My other brother is gay and married an agnostic and I bowed to the conventional religion of my parents and practice Judaism. In fact, we often joke about being so different that it makes us compatible."

"So, when you first came in and said that your family was dysfunctional," you quip, "does that 'F' stand for frustration right now?"

Sarah laughs softly and says, "Absolutely. Most of the time we get along, and what is so distressing is that Mom would be so upset if she knew how we are treating each other right now."

"You know, Sarah, we like to believe that when a family member dies, everyone will come together and support each other. Unfortunately, it often doesn't happen that way. Many times family members get hostile with each other because they are racked with grief. Family members can seem like a safe target. Do you think maybe all this conflict with your siblings is a reflection on how everyone is feeling about your mom being gone?"

Sarah's eyes tear up and she nods her head knowingly. "I think you're right. I hadn't really thought about that. We've been so immersed in all these details that it's almost as if we have forgotten to talk about how we are all feeling. I'll admit that sometimes these details keep my mind off of how much I miss Mom."

"Yes. And that's not unusual. It can feel a little better to focus on some things we can control than to feel the pain of the loss." After a pause, you add, "One thing that could be helpful is to have you all come in as a group and have a session together. Do you think your brothers and sisters would be willing to do that?"

"I think it's possible. Therapy is not foreign to my family. I can definitely ask them," Sarah says.

"I think it might be a good place to start and it could prevent a lot of hard feelings between you all in the future. You are obviously a very accomplished group of people who care very much for your parents."

You and Sarah talk more about what she would hope to get out of family counseling sessions in addition to the impact that the conflict and her mother's death is having on her. She leaves your office with several possible appointment times so that she can coordinate a session with her siblings.

1.2-1. What are the strengths of this family?

1.2-2. What are the primary and secondary losses Sarah's family is experiencing?

1.2-3. Using the family systems approach, summarize how this family is being affected by the mother's death.

1.2-4. How might the broader society's views on grief and mourning be influencing this family?

1.2-5. Choose two theories of grief and loss from the chapter and write about how they might apply to Sarah's family.

1.2-6. Find an academic article on grief in families and summarize the findings.

REFERENCES

Ahmad, I., Alam, I., Hakim, A. U., & Yousaf, F. (2020). Psychological deprivation among widows and its effects on their quality of life in Malakand Division. *Pakistan Journal of Society, Education and Language*, *6*(1), 71–80.

Attig, T. (1996). *How we grieve: Relearning the world*. Oxford University Press.

Berzoff, J. (2004). Psychodynamic theories in grief and bereavement. In J. Berzoff & P. Silverman (Eds.), *Living with dying* (pp. 242–262). Columbia University Press.

Boerner, K., Stroebe, M., Schut, H., & Wortman C. B. (2015). Theories of grief and bereavement. In N. Pachana (Ed.), *Encyclopedia of geropsychology*. Springer, Singapore. https://doi.org/10.1007/978-981-287-080-3_133-1

Bowlby, J. (1980). *Attachment and loss: Loss, sadness, and depression* (Vol. 3). Basic Books.

Cozolino, L. J. (2014). *The neuroscience of human relationships: Attachment and the developing social brain* (2nd ed.). W.W. Norton & Company.

Field, N. P., & Filanosky, C. (2009). Continuing bonds, risk factors for complicated grief, and adjustment to bereavement. *Death Studies*, *34*(1), 1–29. https://doi.org/10.1080/07481180903372269

Field, N. P., Packman, W., Ronen, R., Pries, A., Davies, B., & Kramer, R. (2013). Type of continuing bonds expression and its comforting versus distressing nature: Implications for adjustment among bereaved mothers. *Death Studies*, *37*(10), 889–912. https://doi.org/10.1080/07481187.2012.692458

Freeman, S. J. (2005). *Grief and loss: Understanding the journey*. Brooks/Cole.

Freud, S. (1917). Mourning and melancholia. *Standard Edition*, *14*, 243–258.

Garran, A. M., & Werkmeister Rozas, L. (2013). Cultural competence revisited. *Journal of Ethnic and Cultural Diversity in Social Work*, *22*(2), 97–111. https://doi.org/10.1080/15313204.2013.785337

Granek, L. (2016). Medicalizing grief. In D. L. Harris & T. C. Bordere (Eds.), *Handbook of social justice in loss and grief: Exploring diversity, equity, and inclusion* (pp. 111–124). Routledge.

Greene-Moton, E., & Minkler, M. (2020). Cultural competence or cultural humility? Moving beyond the debate. *Health Promotion Practice*, *21*(1), 142–145. https://doi.org/10.1177/1524839919884912

Grotberg, E. (2005). *Resilience for tomorrow* [Paper Presentation]. The International Council of Psychologists Convention 2005, Iguazu, Brazil.

Humphrey, G. M., & Zimpfer, D. G. (1996). *Counselling for grief and bereavement*. Sage.

Kessler, D. (2019). *Finding meaning: The sixth stage of grief*. Simon & Schuster.

King, S. (2020, May 21). Are we becoming desensitised to death in light of Covid-19? *CapeTalk*. www.capetalk.co.za/features/380/covid-19-coronavirus-explained/384403/are-we-becoming-desensitised-to-death-in-light-of-covid-19

Klass, D., Silverman, P. R., Nickman, S. L., & Nickman, S. (1996). *Continuing bonds: New understandings of grief*. Taylor & Francis.

Kosminsky, P. S., & Jordan, J. R. (2016). *Attachment-informed grief therapy: The clinician's guide to foundations and applications*. Routledge.

Kübler-Ross, E. (1969). *On death and dying*. Touchstone.

McKean, E. (Ed.) (2005). *The new Oxford American dictionary* (2nd ed.). Oxford University Press.

Meier, A. M., Carr, D. R., Currier, J. M., & Neimeyer, R. A. (2013). Attachment anxiety and avoidance in coping with bereavement: Two studies. *Journal of Social and Clinical Psychology*, *32*(3), 315–334. https://doi.org/10.1521/jscp.2013.32.3.315

Montgomery, A. (2013). *Neurobiology essentials for clinicians: What every therapist needs to know* (Norton Series on Interpersonal Neurobiology). W. W. Norton & Company.

Neimeyer, R. A. (2000). Searching for the meaning of meaning: Grief therapy and the process of reconstruction. *Death Studies*, *24*(6), 541–558.

Neimeyer, R. A., Prigerson, H. G., & Davies, B. (2002). Mourning and meaning. *American Behavioral Scientist*, *46*(2), 235–251.

Parkes, C. (1964). Recent bereavement as a cause of mental illness. *British Journal of Psychiatry*, *110*, 198–204.

Parkes, C. (1970). Seeking and finding a lost object: Evidence for recent studies to bereavement. *Social Science and Medicine*, *4*, 187–201.

Parkes, C. (1972). Health after bereavement: A controlled study of young Boston widows and widowers. *Psychosomatic Medicine*, *34*(5), 449–461.

Parkes, C., & Weiss, R. (1983). *Recovery from bereavement*. Basic Books.

Pomeroy, E. C., & Garcia, R. B. (2009). *The grief assessment and intervention workbook: A strengths perspective*. Brooks/Cole.

Pomeroy, E. C., Hai, A. H., & Cole, A. H. (2019). Social work practitioners' educational needs in developing spiritual competency in end-of-life care and grief. *Journal of Social Work Education*, 1–23. https://doi.org/10.1080/10437797.2019.1670306

Rando, T. A. (1993). *Treatment of complicated mourning*. Research Press.

Rapp, C. A. (1998). *The strengths model: Case management with people suffering from severe and persistent mental illness*. Oxford University Press.

Rosenblatt, P. (2016). Cultural competence and humility. In D. L. Harris & T. C. Bordere (Eds.), *Handbook of social justice in loss and grief: Exploring diversity, equity, and inclusion* (pp. 67–74). Routledge.

Rosenblatt, P. C. (2017). Researching grief: Cultural, relational, and individual possibilities. *Journal of Loss and Trauma*, *22*(8), 617–630. https://doi.org/10.1080/15325024.2017.1388347

Rosenblatt, P. C., & Wallace, B. R. (2005a). *African American grief*. Routledge.

Rosenblatt, P. C., & Wallace, B. R. (2005b). Narratives of grieving African-Americans about racism in the lives of deceased family members. *Death Studies*, *29*, 217–235. https://doi.org/10.1080/07481180590916353

Rubin, S. S., Malkinson, R., & Witztum, E. (2012). *Working with the bereaved: Multiple lenses on loss and mourning*. Taylor & Francis.

Saleebey, D. (2006). *The strengths perspective in social work practice* (4th ed.). Pearson Education.

Scholtes, D., & Browne, M. (2015). Internalized and externalized continuing bonds in bereaved parents: Their relationship with grief intensity and personal growth. *Death Studies*, *39*(2), 75–83. https://doi.org/10.1080/07481187.2014.890680

Shallcross, L. (2012, June 1). A loss like no other. *Counseling Today*. https://ct.counseling.org/2012/06/a-loss-like-no-other/

Siegel, D. J. (2012). *Pocket guide to interpersonal neurobiology: An integrative handbook of the mind* (Norton Series on Interpersonal Neurobiology). W. W. Norton & Company.

Stroebe, M. S., & Schut, H. (1999). The dual process model of coping with bereavement: Rationale and description. *Death Studies*, *23*, 197–224.

Stroebe, M. S., & Schut, H. (2010). The dual process model of coping with bereavement: A decade on. *OMEGA – Journal of Death and Dying*, *61*(4), 269–271. https://doi.org/10.2190/om.61.4.a

Tervalon, M., & Murray-García, J. (1998). Cultural humility versus cultural competence: A critical distinction in defining physician training outcomes in multicultural education. *Journal of Health Care for the Poor and Underserved*, *9*(2), 117–125. https://doi.org/10.1353/hpu.2010.0233

Worden, J. W. (2018). *Grief counseling and grief therapy: A handbook for the mental health practitioner* (5th ed.). Springer Publishing Company.

Yu, W., He, L., Xu, W., Wang, J., & Prigerson, H. G. (2016). How do attachment dimensions affect bereavement adjustment? A mediation model of continuing bonds. *Psychiatry Research*, *238*, 93–99. https://doi.org/10.1016/j.psychres.2016.02.030

CHAPTER 2

Grief and Trauma: A Complex Convergence

As stated in the basic tenets of the strengths-based framework of grief and loss in Chapter 1, grief in response to the death of a loved one is a natural, expectable, and health-producing process that aids the individual in adjusting to the absence of the loved one. The term "expected" grief will be used to describe the predictable grief experience that reflects the healthy process of separation from the deceased individual. While it can take a wide variety of forms and varies according to the cultural context of the mourner, this type of grief is what we would "expect" to see with someone who has lost a loved one. Expected grief reactions have the potential to produce healthy growth.

Grief is a universal response to the loss of a loved one and while it clearly creates tumult in one's life for a period of time, it is a process that propels mourners to alter their lives and potentially grow in response to the loss. This health-producing quality of grief encourages a person to struggle with the new reality – one without their loved one – and transition to a new way of living. Regardless of the outcome, the process of grief is a human and predictable reaction to loss.

Grief reactions that correspond to what is expected given the separation from an important attachment figure include symptoms that affect mourners cognitively, emotionally, behaviorally, physically, socially, and spiritually. For many, grief is an all-encompassing experience that impacts all or most areas of their life for a period of time. For example, after the death of his wife of 26 years, Norman found that he was more forgetful and had trouble concentrating at work. He spent many hours yearning to see his wife again and would become teary when allowed to talk about her. Normally outgoing and active, in grief Norman was more withdrawn and sedentary. He reported feeling lethargic, had trouble sleeping, and often felt a tightness in his chest. He felt that many of his friends didn't understand what he was experiencing and didn't know how to support him in his loss. He clung tightly to his religious beliefs in an attempt to find comfort, but he also had moments of feeling intensely angry at God for allowing him to suffer in this way. Norman's experience is just one example of the way expected grief reactions may appear in a bereaved person's life. Expected grief reactions will be discussed more extensively in subsequent chapters.

With time and support, the intensity of expected grief lessens, though it is common for mourners to experience a resurgence of strong reactions, particularly on important

DOI: 10.4324/9780429053634-2

dates such as birthdays and the anniversary of the death. For some, grief is solely an experience of endurance and survival. Grief can, however, result in positive life changes such as greater self-awareness and self-efficacy, improved personal relationships, and renewed appreciation for life (Rubin et al., 2012).

COMPLEX GRIEF

Terminology

There are times when adapting to the absence of the deceased is extraordinarily difficult and becomes stalled and complicated. Mourners' reactions to the loss may persist and pose significant barriers to their ability to function and continue life without their beloved. In an attempt to distinguish these responses from expected grief reactions, the bereavement literature uses various terms including "complicated," "prolonged," "pathological," "unresolved," and "traumatic" grief reactions. Despite numerous efforts to classify these responses to loss, there is no clear consensus on the terminology and associated symptoms of this grief condition. Compounding this difficulty is the considerable overlap in the symptoms experienced between "normal," "complicated," and "traumatic" grief, particularly when grief is new and acute. Furthermore, in the fifth edition of the *Diagnostic and Statistical Manual of Mental Disorders* (*DSM-5*), the only mutually exclusive category for grief is "bereavement" listed under V codes. V codes are reserved for areas of mental health that are not considered mental disorders (American Psychiatric Association [APA], 2013).

While there are certain symptoms that appear to be commonly associated with "normal" versus "abnormal" grief reactions, it seems more likely that there is a continuum of bereavement reactions that could legitimately be called expected, complex, and traumatic based on the mourner's capacity to accept the loss, invest in life without the deceased, as well as the unique circumstances related to the loss and the impact of those circumstances on the individual.

BOX 2.1 AMERICAN GRIEF THROUGH THE LENS OF CAPITALISM

The prevalence of medicalized views of grief in the United States, including efforts to diagnose prolonged or complicated grief, is influenced by the greater context of capitalism, which values production, profit, and consumerism to its maximum potential (Harris, 2016). When grief has gone on for "too long" and interferes with an employee's ability to work, it is viewed as problematic. As Rosenblatt (2017) suggests, "perhaps the pathology to be examined is not in how much someone grieves but in what is expected or necessary in many workplaces" (p. 620).

Conceptualizing Complex Grief

For the purposes of this book, the term "complex" grief will be used to describe a grief process that along with separation distress is encumbered with internal or external complications that interfere with the health-producing growth process of expected grief. Complex grief persists longer than expected grief and impedes daily functioning (Shear, 2015). Complex grief responses can further be classified as traumatic or non-traumatic. Complex grief that is traumatic occurs because the circumstances surrounding the loss overwhelm the mourner's ability to process the event. Complex grief without trauma occurs when the circumstances are not traumatic but for other reasons, the grief becomes stalled, delayed, maladaptive, or prolonged.

Sufferers of complex grief experience

> frequent intense yearning, intense sorrow and emotional pain, preoccupation with the deceased and/or circumstances of the death, excessive avoidance of reminders of the loss, difficulty accepting the death, feeling alone and empty, and feeling that life has no purpose or meaning without the deceased person.
>
> (Shear et al., 2013, p. 3)

Complex mourning results in the bereaved feeling "stuck" between efforts to avoid the pain associated with life without their loved one and also holding on to the loved one and protesting the reality of the loss. The result is an inability to integrate the loss and obtain renewed fulfillment in life (Shear et al., 2013; Solomon, 2019).

How the mourning process unfolds is influenced by many variables. The presence of the following factors is believed to increase the likelihood that grief will become complex:

- Previous history of mental illness or substance abuse
- Multiple losses
- Adverse experiences in childhood
- Insufficient social support
- Significant friction with friends or family
- Substantial financial difficulties following the death
- Avoidant, anxious, or insecure attachment style
- Finding the body, if violence was involved
- Dissatisfaction with how they were told about the death
- High degree of dependency on the loved one.

(Burke & Neimeyer, 2013; Shear, 2015)

Marilyn's experience of grief following the death of her mother is indicative of complex grief. At the time that her mother died by natural causes due to her elderly age, Marilyn was 62 years old. Following her divorce 12 years prior, Marilyn had moved in with her mother. She has a tense relationship with her adult son which was often provoked when Marilyn made attempts to see her grandchildren. Because of their living arrangement, the death of Marilyn's mother left her feeling very alone and with significant financial stress.

A heavy drinker throughout her life, Marilyn's alcohol consumption increased after her mother's death. While Marilyn needed to find more affordable housing, she felt intensely disloyal to her mother for "moving on" without her. Though they were often angry with each other, Marilyn described her mother as her "best friend" and felt hopeless at the idea of a future without her. At the same time, she allowed for little expression of her grief for fear that doing so would permanently incapacitate her.

Traumatic Grief

Complex grief that is also traumatic will be the primary focus of this book. While many deaths may feel traumatic from the perspective of the mourner (Rando, 1993), there are also circumstances that are clearly and undeniably traumatic from an objective standpoint. These include deaths that:

- are unexpected
- occur out of sequence with what is considered natural, such as when children die before their parents
- involve violence or disfigurement
- are perceived as preventable
- are perceived to involve suffering
- are perceived as unjust or undeserved
- are perceived as random
- are committed by someone with the aim of causing harm
- are witnessed by the survivor
- involve multiple deaths
- involve threat to the survivor's life.

(Pearlman et al., 2014)

Circumstances that typically lead to traumatic grief include natural disasters, such as hurricanes and tsunamis, and accidental disasters such as an airplane crash or a structural collapse. Additionally, intentional acts such as arson, homicide, suicide, and terrorism result in traumatic grief for the survivors. Sudden deaths from medical emergencies such as heart attacks or strokes can also elicit traumatic grief responses as well as deaths resulting from a loved one's extended illness that includes exposure to their painful deterioration (Kosminsky & Jordan, 2016).

TRAUMA

A fundamental understanding of trauma and its impact on individuals is essential to effectively help those who are experiencing traumatic grief. While it is beyond the scope of this book to fully explore the vast field of traumatology, the following overview will provide a foundational understanding.

The term trauma has been used interchangeably to refer to both the events that are extremely difficult and overwhelming for individuals as well as the physical, mental, emotional, and spiritual responses that result from the distressing experience. The Substance Abuse and Mental Health Services Administration (SAMHSA) states that:

> Individual trauma results from an event, series of events, or set of circumstances that is experienced by an individual as physically or emotionally harmful or life threatening and that has lasting adverse effects on the individual's functioning and mental, physical, social, emotional, or spiritual well-being.
>
> (2019)

In addition, Judith Herman describes traumatic events as those that "overwhelm the ordinary systems of care that give people a sense of control, connection, and meaning. Traumatic events are extraordinary, not because they occur rarely, but rather because they overwhelm the ordinary human adaptations to life" (Herman, 1992, p. 33). Herman's definition highlights the key elements of an event that characterize it as traumatic: that is, feeling powerless, helpless, and overwhelmed in one's ability to cope and adapt. This subjective baseline explains why the same event can elicit a trauma reaction in one person but not in another. Unhealed trauma has the potential to negatively alter the health, temperament, and functioning of those who have been traumatized. It can dramatically alter the way survivors navigate their world and interact with others.

Trauma Theory

The first known conceptualization of trauma can be traced back to Freud's psychoanalytic perspective and theory of self-determination which promoted the idea that basic psychological needs may be repressed (Piers, 1996). Freud's theory maintains that the overwhelming anxiety caused by traumatic events compels the ego to push the event into "forgetfulness" (Lynch, 2012). While the content of the trauma may not be remembered, there will still be expression of the trauma in the person's affect. Frequently these expressions are somatic in nature.

Present-day theories of trauma emphasize the process of dissociation over repression. This perspective speaks to the way that traumatic memories are stored and encoded separately from other memories. The traumatic event continues to impact thoughts, behaviors, and physiological arousal though this may occur outside of conscious awareness. In addition, memories of the trauma may be triggered by relationships or by environmental cues that are associated with the traumatic event and cause the person to feel as though they are re-experiencing the trauma (Herman, 1992; Putnam, 1989; Siegel, 1995; van der Kolk & van der Hart, 1991). While the phenomena associated with trauma are consistent across all cultures (Lopez Levers, 2012), the lived experiences of traumatic events are unique to the individual and influenced by personal perspectives and interpretations (Lynch, 2012).

Types of Trauma

It's important to understand that trauma comes in a variety of forms. A single incident of trauma refers to an isolated, one-time event. In contrast, the term "complex trauma" refers to the severe psychological harm that occurs with prolonged, repeated trauma.

Complex trauma is prevalent among those who have experienced multiple traumas which may include physical and sexual abuse as children, prisoners of war, or victims of sex trafficking. Individuals with complex trauma have often experienced a variety of traumatic events throughout their lives culminating in symptoms of Post-Traumatic Stress Disorder (PTSD). In addition to the symptoms associated with PTSD, survivors of complex trauma persistently experience low self-worth and difficulty adapting to stressful events. Though the term is not yet recognized in the *DSM*, complex trauma is an increasing focus of attention in clinical and research settings.

Developmental trauma refers to the impact of repeated abuse, neglect, separation, and adverse experiences that occur between children and their caregivers. The effects of developmental trauma are long lasting and severe because of the "pervasive vulnerability of young children including their immature neurological development" (Kosminsky & Jordan, 2016, p. 44). Survivors often have difficulty managing impulses, solving problems, and using executive functioning skills. They become locked into "survival mode," rely on unhealthy coping mechanisms, and often use dissociation as the primary way to regulate their emotions (Kosminsky & Jordan, 2016).

Historical trauma refers to the cumulative emotional and psychological wounding that occurs to a group of people and is passed down and transmitted across generations. With historical trauma, a community or culture's descendants are affected, even if they did not experience the trauma directly (Boulanger, 2018). This concept came into being after researching the impact of the Holocaust on the children of survivors. Other events causing historical trauma include the enslavement of African Americans, the government creation of reservations for Native Americans in desolate regions of the country, mandatory boarding schools for Native American children, and the Japanese Internment in the 1940s. The coping mechanisms that were developed in order to survive these traumatic events are passed down through generations and lead to erosion in cultural, communal, tribal, and family systems.

Vicarious trauma, also sometimes referred to as secondary trauma or compassion fatigue, is notably present in helping professionals who work for an extended period of time with clients who are in crisis and experiencing trauma. Practitioners who develop vicarious trauma experience disruptions to their core sense of self which impacts their personal worldviews. It can compromise the practitioner's professional capacity and negatively impact their personal life (Hazen et al., 2020; Iqbal, 2015). Vicarious trauma will be discussed in greater detail in Chapter 8.

Trauma Symptoms

The impact of trauma on one's life can be devastating. Those who have survived traumatic events often experience profound and lasting changes in their physiological arousal, emotion, cognition, and memory. Defenses that at the time of the distressing event served to protect the individual from greater harm, persist even after the danger has passed. The body and mind are frozen in the experience of helplessness and terror, remain continually on alert to danger, and are unable to rest peacefully in the present moment.

Some, but not all, who experience trauma develop PTSD. This *DSM* diagnostic category is used when symptoms from one or more of the following symptom clusters remain present one month after the traumatic event and were not present before the traumatic event.

The first symptom cluster is intrusive symptoms which include recurrent and unbidden thoughts and memories about the traumatic event, recurrent and distressing dreams about the event, persistent re-experiencing of the event as with flashbacks, and physiological reactions to things that symbolize or are associated with the event. For example, Betty, whose husband was murdered by a burglar wearing a blue sweatshirt, experiences severe anxiety when she sees a man wearing a blue sweatshirt while shopping for groceries.

The second symptom cluster focuses on avoidance symptoms which include persistent efforts to avoid thoughts, feelings, people, or situations that are associated with the trauma. Using the same scenario as before, an example of an avoidance symptom would be that Betty refuses to sleep in the bedroom where her husband died.

The third symptom cluster involves thought and mood symptoms. These include an inability to remember specific components of the event, inappropriate self-blame for the event, a pervasive negative emotional state such as anger, horror, guilt, or shame, and feeling detached from others. Thought and mood symptoms may also take the shape of excessive negative beliefs about oneself or the world, such as, "I am bad" or "No one can be trusted." In addition, survivors may be unable to experience positive emotions. In Betty's case, she exhibits these symptoms when she blames her husband's death on her inability to protect him and subsequently questions her competence in other aspects of her life.

The fourth category involves symptoms of arousal. This can include irritability, aggressive behavior, self-destructive behavior, an exaggerated startle response, hypervigilance, trouble concentrating, and sleep disturbances. Betty demonstrates this symptom when she becomes panicky upon hearing noises in her home and persistently worries for her safety.

PTSD may also be accompanied with dissociative symptoms such as depersonalization and derealization. Depersonalization refers to the feeling of being outside of one's self. Betty experiences this when she observes herself from a distance. Derealization is when one feels detached from the environment and one's surroundings feel unreal, distant, or distorted as if in a dream.

Neurobiology of Trauma

Advances in medical technology have greatly enhanced the understanding of trauma, how it impacts the brain and influences the survivor's behavior in both the short and long term. A basic understanding of the neurobiology of trauma is essential when working with clients who have been traumatized. In general, the neurobiological responses to trauma are as described in the following paragraphs, though individual differences caused by genetics and life experiences also shape the brain's response. Additionally, substance use can complicate these processes. The following explanation of the brain's response to trauma is greatly simplified for ease of understanding and begins with an outline of brain structures that are critical to the process. Numerous resources exist that can provide readers with more in-depth explanations.

Brain circuitry, also known as *neural networks*, refers to the sharing of information between neurons (brain cells) and the rest of the body. The way these networks respond to trauma is intrinsic and automatic, occurring without logic or conscious thought. In addition, these reflex responses can be lasting and will arise even years after the traumatic event.

The *prefrontal cortex (PFC)* is the outer brain area located behind the forehead. It is responsible for logical thinking and planning, consolidating details of experience into narrative stories (memories), and controlling where to focus attention.

The *limbic system* is a set of structures located below the PFC. In addition to being the seat of emotions and encoding memories, the limbic system contains the defense circuitry which detects and responds to danger. This includes continually monitoring the surroundings to catch anything unpredictable and potentially dangerous. This watchful state, referred to as vigilance, occurs below conscious awareness and serves as a safeguard from danger.

A key part of the defense circuitry within the limbic system is the *amygdala* which warns the brain of danger in the environment. Another structure, the *hippocampus*, inspects aspects of the situation and compares it with the individual's knowledge of what is safe and what is dangerous. If a disturbance in the environment is associated with fear or danger, there is a moment of freezing during which the individual scans the environment to determine if there is a threat to one's safety. If a credible threat is detected, the amygdala releases a flood of the stress hormone, *cortisol*, to ready the brain and body to react to the danger. This activation of the defense circuitry occurs in a millisecond and overtakes the PFC. Thus, there is no capacity to think clearly, choose where to direct one's attention, or convert details recalled from the event into a coherent narrative. By relying on habitual and instinctive actions instead of pausing for thinking and planning, this automatic response is able to effectively provide protection (Wilson et al., 2016).

Once the defense circuitry has been triggered, an array of survival reflexes are activated. Though commonly known as "fight or flight," current research suggests that the term *defense cascade* is a more accurate description of these responses (Kozlowska et al., 2015). Frequently, the defense cascade starts with momentary freezing, during which the body prepares to take action. This evolutionary response developed so that predators, who are attracted to movement, won't see their prey. It also allows the prey to evaluate the danger and then take protective action. Depending on the circumstances, the defensive actions may be "active" or "passive."

Active defense responses include fleeing, the most common response, or fighting. Passive survival reflexes that may be activated include dissociation, tonic immobility, and collapsed immobility. Dissociation is often employed when escape is perceived as impossible. It enables coping with the situation by allowing the brain to disconnect from what's occurring in the body. Tonic immobility refers to the inability to move or talk. It may accompany dissociation or the individual may remain fully alert and cognizant of what's happening. Collapsed immobility involves being unable to speak or move, along with decreasing heart rate and blood pressure which may cause the individual to feel faint or pass out. Frequently referred to as "playing possum," this is a misnomer as it implies an intentional choice on the part of the victim. On the contrary, it is a reflexive response not under the individual's control. Both tonic immobility and collapsed immobility occur when the person experiences intense apprehension, actual bodily contact with the threatening person or animal, physical restraint, and the belief that escape is impossible (Kozlowska et al., 2015; Wilson et al., 2016). After the danger has passed, the PFC aids in taking actions that reduce risk, enables learning from the experience, and assimilates the information into the individual's understanding of safety and danger.

Once a threat has been detected, the activated defense circuitry directs attention to aspects of the situation that will enable survival or assist in coping with and enduring the threat. These targets of attention are referred to as *central details*. All other aspects of the situation are the *peripheral details* which are given less attention and thus remembered with less accuracy, if at all. Additionally, when encoding memories, the hippocampus favors information about what happened just prior to and at the beginning of the danger. This is done to help the individual foresee and evade danger in the future. This explains, in part, why memories of traumatic experiences are fragmented and contain incomplete accounts of the event (Wilson et al., 2016).

After enduring a traumatic event, the brain's vigilance increases. The amygdala is now keenly attuned to stimuli that are correlated with the trauma and, out of an abundance of caution, will react as if the danger was again present. The trigger may be a sensory cue such as a sound or smell, or a contextual cue, such as a couch resembling one on which an assault occurred. In this way, trauma undermines the brain's capacity to accurately detect danger, because it codifies many things into danger signals, even though the associations may be loose. Another outcome of trauma is an increased difficulty in utilizing the hippocampus to help distinguish safety from danger. This accounts for why some individuals struggle to regain a sense of calm after being triggered. They are unable to observe their environment and recognize that the traumatic event is not actually happening (Siegel, 2012). "This is not a sign of weakness or mental illness: It's just the brain doing what the brain does when an individual has experienced trauma but not yet recovered from that experience" (Wilson et al., 2016, pp. 36–37).

Furthermore, while animals typically return to their regular functioning after the danger has passed, the human experience is complicated by the subjective interpretations of the body's reactions and the meaning that is attached to the experience. Thus, images of past feelings and events along with imaginings about what lies ahead can also provoke the body's defense systems, though there is no external danger.

In the case of loss, trauma triggers may be related to how the bereaved was informed of the death, distressing aspects of the death scene, disturbing images of the deceased's body, associations with the person who caused the death, or other moments in which there were intense feelings of helplessness. Traumatically bereaved individuals may also become acutely distressed when they imagine what their loved one experienced in the moments leading up to the death (Solomon, 2019).

Neuroplasticity refers to the "ability of the brain to change its structure in response to experience" (Siegel, 2012, chapter 8, p. 1) and provides the pathway for recovery from traumatic stress. Thanks to modern understanding of the neurobiology of trauma, there are now numerous interventions that, when delivered in the context of safe relationships, help amend the neural patterns that have been altered by the survivor's experience of trauma. These interventions help to restore a sense of power and influence over the survivor's body and mind (Kozlowska et al., 2015; van der Kolk et al., 2014).

STRENGTHS-BASED APPROACH TO TRAUMA

As with grief, when viewed through a strengths-based approach, trauma has the potential to promote profound and positive personal growth. Tedeschi and Calhoun (1995) first noted in the literature what has been an ancient observation: that trauma can have beneficial outcomes, including "more meaningful interpersonal relationships, an increased sense of personal strength, changed priorities, and a richer existential and spiritual life" (Tedeschi & Calhoun, 2004, p. 1). Tedeschi and Calhoun used the term "posttraumatic growth" (PTG) to refer to the positive and transformative changes that can be outcomes of trauma, resulting in a return to functioning that is more advanced than previous functioning.

Drawing from the understanding of the neurobiology of trauma and PTG, the following perspectives on trauma developed by the authors provide a complement to the strengths-based framework of grief and loss. Incorporating these principles enables helping professionals to compassionately and effectively accompany survivors on their healing journey.

1. Trauma-based symptoms are a natural and expected reaction of a biopsychological system that has been overwhelmed with the threat of real or perceived danger.
2. Trauma-based symptoms emerge from an innate drive to protect the human organism from pain and danger and do not symbolize deficiency or weakness of the individual. Rather, they are reflective of resiliency, endurance, and a deep-seated resistance to surrender to pain, discomfort, and maltreatment.
3. Many symptoms of trauma represent what were once adaptive responses to the distressing event. Their continued use in the absence of danger represents an inherent instinct for self-protection and survival.
4. Trauma survivors can become empowered by learning how and why trauma symptoms develop, how they function as a mechanism of protection, and how they naturally impact functioning in various life areas.
5. In addition to reducing trauma-based symptoms, emphasizing and employing individual and environmental strengths is fundamental to restoring hope and self-agency, thereby promoting healthy recovery from trauma and enhancing resiliency.
6. The conditions of the survivor's environment and relationships play a central role in their capacity to heal from trauma, with the felt sense of safety being a critical element.
7. Healing from trauma is possible when there is a reverent respect for the biopsychosocial and neurological systems that support trauma reactions combined with care practices that facilitate the reregulation of these systems to a non-trauma state.

8. The process of healing from trauma provides fertile ground for personal growth, the development and enhancement of individual strengths, and fosters a profound appreciation for life.

As with grief, restoring the disruption caused by trauma can only occur in the context of safe and reliable relationships based on compassion, respect, and non-judgmental acceptance. When these qualities are skillfully demonstrated and used in conjunction with evidence-based interventions, the capacity for healing and growth appreciably expands (Pomeroy & Garcia, 2018).

BOX 2.2 THE FUNCTION OF MOURNING RITUALS

Though they come in a variety of forms, the actions performed around death and mourning are ceremonial rituals that are culturally decreed. While assisting mourners to realize that their loved one has died, they also reinforce connections between the bereaved and family, friends, and the community. This provides security for the mourner as they confront the intensely painful feelings of grief and loss. Rarely do the bereaved participate in mourning rituals alone, as one of the primary purposes is to prevent the mourner's isolation (Hidalgo, 2017; Markin & Zilcha-Mano, 2018).

Death rituals in mainstream Western culture are minimal compared to other cultures. Many researchers believe this came about as a result of the Black Death. The overwhelming number of deaths made it difficult to carry out the mourning rituals for all who needed them. Furthermore, practices of bathing the deceased, laying them out in the home, and visitation of family and friends were abandoned due to the mystery surrounding what had caused the deaths. People were reluctant to participate in these traditions for fear they would become contaminated. The sheer number of dead filled church cemeteries to capacity and many corpses were disposed of in ditches or mass graves (Kelly, 2006).

INTERSECTION OF TRAUMA AND GRIEF

Historically, trauma and loss have remained separate fields of study. There is a growing realization, however, that while the two phenomena are distinct, there is also considerable interrelatedness and overlap between them (Djelantik et al., 2020; Rando, 2015; Stroebe et al., 2001). Both loss and trauma are stressful life events. All trauma involves an element of loss as mourners are confronted with challenges to their worldview and their assumptions about fairness, faith, control, and other beliefs about internal and external safety (Pearlman et al., 2014; Solomon, 2019). Similarly, the loss of an important attachment figure also involves elements of trauma as mourners face the "psychological threat" of separation from the deceased. "In this sense, all losses through death may include some degree of trauma since the individual can never 'escape' the threat of separation from their loved one" (Kosminsky & Jordan, 2016, p. 92).

The experiences of bereaved persons during the acute stage of grief are similar to the symptoms experienced by survivors of trauma (Howarth, 2011; Solomon, 2019). With both loss and trauma there is a feeling of overwhelm as the individual struggles to cope with what feels like too much. Both trauma and loss give rise to cognitive, emotional, behavioral, physical, social, and spiritual disruptions. This is compounded when trauma and loss exist simultaneously.

Often the responses to trauma block the natural process of mourning. This occurs when a bereaved person avoids thoughts and memories of their loved one because they elicit traumatic memories, images, and experiences related to the death. In addition, reminders of the changes that have occurred due to the loved one's death can trigger intrusive and distressing thoughts and feelings related to the trauma (Howarth, 2011). Bereaved persons will often respond to this distress with attempts to push it away from awareness or in some manner numb themselves to the pain. These reactions may represent a deliberate attempt to avoid pain or they may occur at a subconscious level. This understandable movement away from painful reminders obstructs the natural process of grief (Howarth, 2011; Pearlman et al., 2014) and complicates the task of revising the mourner's relationship to their deceased loved one (Rubin et al., 2012). Effective intervention, therefore, addresses both the traumatic elements of the loss in tandem with facilitation of the mourning process (Pearlman et al., 2014).

CASES

CASE 2.1

Identifying Information:

Client Name: Ralph Nesbaum
Age: 38 years old
Race/Ethnicity: African American
Marital Status: Married with three children
Education Level: College degree
Occupation: Engineer

Intake Information:

Ralph Nesbaum was referred to Collinville Bereavement Center by the local police department's victims' services social worker. Ralph told the intake worker that he needed to talk to someone about a death reported in the local news and that it would help if someone would read it before he came to the center. You read the news to learn about the murder of Ralph's wife, which occurred in his home a few weeks earlier.

Initial Interview:

Ralph comes to his appointment at the scheduled time and appears very distracted but congenial. He firmly shakes your hand and follows you to your office in a very business-like manner. He sits in the chair next to your desk with his legs spread apart and elbows on his knees. You can tell he's ready to begin the session.

"When I made this appointment, I asked them to have you read the news about my situation. Were you able to do that?" Ralph begins.

"Yes, I did. You've been through a lot. How has all this publicity been for you?" you reply.

"Well, I realized a couple of days ago that the events of the last month and a half are all blurring together. I don't know up from down right now. I haven't had much sleep and I'm trying to keep it together as much as I can for the kids' sakes." Ralph sits back in the chair and wipes his forehead. "It's not only been a nightmare, but I'm actually having nightmares."

"I can only imagine how awful this must be for you," you empathize. "What would be most helpful for you right now?"

Ralph sighs, "I don't know, really. The victims' counselor really thought I should see you. I'm just trying to sort things out in my mind, I guess. I really don't know."

"It's completely okay that you don't know. Perhaps you could tell me how the last month or so has been for you?" you respond.

"Okay, well, how do I begin? Let's see.... Well, let's see. This all started about six weeks ago. I got up and went to work as usual. Around 10 o'clock in the morning, I called Becky, my wife, to find out if she'd picked up my clothes at the cleaners and she didn't answer the phone. I left a message at the house and then on her cell phone but never heard back. She's usually really good about returning my calls. I called a couple more times and still didn't hear anything and then I began to get worried. I just had a bad feeling, you know? So at about 2 p.m., I had a break and decided to go home just to check and make sure she was okay. When I got there, the side door was slightly open and then I really started to panic. We never leave that door open. I got out of the car and ran into the house through the kitchen calling her name. She didn't answer but her car was in the driveway so I thought she must be out in the backyard. I walked through the den, opened the sliding door and there she was in the corner of the deck. She was lying face down and there was blood everywhere." Ralph pauses. His breathing has become more labored and he has a distant look in his eyes. You wait patiently and then he continues, "The minute I saw her I knew she was dead but I didn't want to believe it. I rolled her over to check for a heartbeat and there was nothing. I ran to the phone to call 911 still thinking that there must be some way I could save her. Next thing I know, the house is swarming with police and they're asking me all these questions like it's my fault."

"Oh, Ralph," you say quietly.

"It was the worst day of my life," Ralph replies. "It still feels like a bad dream. I just want to wake up and find out that it never happened and that Becky's still alive."

"Of course you do," you affirm. "From what I read in the news, it sounds like they are still investigating."

"Yeah," Fred says. "They don't know who did it. Or why. I keep getting called to the police station to answer more questions. Well, it's more like an interrogation. I guess they have to rule me out as a suspect. Man, it's hell!"

"Oh, I'm sure. As if losing your wife weren't hard enough," you say. "How have you been able to manage so far?"

"Well, I can't sleep because every time I close my eyes, I see her…" he puts his head in his hands and cries, "...I see her on the deck and I imagine how she must have felt right before she died." After crying for a few seconds, Ralph takes a deep breath and continues, "When I am able to get some sleep, one of the kids crawls into bed with me and tells me they're scared. So, I'm exhausted right now. Putting one foot in front of the other is a tremendous effort."

"I bet," you say. "Okay, so you aren't getting much sleep. How about the rest of the day? How do you feel you're functioning throughout the day?"

"I'm numb. I don't feel much of anything. But, I'll tell you, every time I hear a loud noise I jump out of my skin. I react as if someone's trying to shoot me and I can't seem to stop it. I'm on edge all the time. I'm snapping at my kids over nothing and then I feel so guilty because I think about how they must feel with their mom gone. I try to help them with their homework but I'm pretty useless. Just can't seem to pull it together."

"Yes. That must be so difficult for you. I want you to know that what you are describing is typical for someone who has had a trauma like you've experienced," you suggest. "Do you have any friends or family that are being supportive?"

"Well, my mother came and stayed for the first couple of weeks, but she had to go back home last week. She helped out a lot when the police were constantly at the house and asking questions. I didn't want the younger kids exposed to all of that. And my church has been great. They've organized for someone to bring food by every night. They've been amazing, actually. I'm really grateful for the support, but, I don't know. I guess I'm just not used to all this attention…I miss our normal ordinary life."

"Yes, your world has been turned completely upside down in just about every way. What's it been like to be the focus of so much attention?"

You allow Ralph to talk more about his interactions with the police, his church group, his children's teachers. When you ask about how it is for him when he is able to get a quiet moment, he says, "I miss her...and then I think about when it happened." Ralph pauses for a while and then adds, "I probably shouldn't tell you this, but sometimes I actually see Becky out of the corner of my eye for a minute. I don't know. Maybe I'm totally losing my mind."

"Actually, that's not all that unusual. People often report experiences like that after a loved one has died."

"Hmm..." Ralph says thoughtfully. "Okay."

After giving him a moment to ponder this, you ask, "How about your job, Ralph?" you ask. "Have you started back to work yet?"

"I've started going back part-time, but it's difficult," he replies.

"Tell me about the difficulties you've had," you suggest.

"Well, first of all, I can barely get out of bed in the morning. Sometimes, I just lay there wondering why it was Becky and not me. Then when I finally get up and going, I have to get the kids taken care of and off to school. By the time I get them to school, I'm already exhausted. It's really been tough. I'm not even interested in work right now. It doesn't seem to matter that much anymore." Ralph leans back in his chair and sighs deeply.

"How is it once you are able to get to work?" you ask.

"Well, people don't really know what to do with me. You can tell they're really uncomfortable. Either they ignore me completely or they say something irritatingly stupid like 'maybe it was all in God's plan' or 'at least you've got your kids.' I want to scream at the top of my lungs, 'my wife has just been murdered and I have three kids with no mom!' Are they out of their minds? I feel like I'm living in a different dimension from the rest of the world right now."

You validate the difficulty of having people not know how to act and explain that this is a complaint you hear a lot. "Is there anyone at work that you can talk to about how you're doing?" you ask.

"I just don't want to talk about it to anyone right now. For example, the day it all hit the news I took the day off so I wouldn't have to dredge it up again. I sit inside and don't even want to go get the mail because I might run into a neighbor who wants to talk about it. Sometimes, I'll sit there for hours and don't even bother turning the lights on."

"Do you ever think about hurting yourself?" you question.

"I'd love to just disappear but I'd never do that to my kids. Even when I feel like I can't take anymore, I know in my head that my kids need me to be strong."

"It sounds like you've been through one of the most difficult things a person can face in life – having to live through the murder of your wife. I'm not surprised you're having great difficulties. There's so much to manage between the police, the kids, adjusting to life without Becky, not to mention your own grief and how your body is reacting to the trauma."

Ralph rubs his forehead and says, "Yeah, I haven't been doing so well and it seems to be getting worse instead of better. Feels like it's going to go on like this forever."

As you and Ralph continue to talk you fold in some education about traumatic grief as well as things he might do to help with sleep. You close with teaching him a skill that can help him regulate his emotions when he becomes agitated.

"Perhaps you'd like to come in again and we can continue working together to help you find ways to manage all these stresses?"

"You know, this is the first time I've really discussed how I'm feeling outside of police interrogations. I think I do need help sorting all of this out."

2.1-1. Identify the reasons you would categorize Ralph's grief as traumatic.

2.1-2. In addition to his grief, does Ralph qualify for a diagnosis of PTSD? If so, explain why.

2.1-3. Research information about how trauma affects sleep and write a summary. Include three recommendations for sleep that you could share with Ralph.

2.1-4. What information about traumatic grief would be helpful to share with Ralph? How would you present it to him?

2.1-5. What are some of Ralph's strengths?

CASE 2.2

Identifying Information:

Client Name: Fred Mathers
Age: 43 years old
Race/Ethnicity: White
Marital Status: Divorced
Education Level: Vocational school
Occupation: Construction pipefitter

Intake Information:

Fred called your office to inquire about counseling over the death of his sister five months ago. His voice was a bit shaky as he asked questions about what grief counseling usually entails. He specifically wanted to know if he would have to review his entire childhood and past. You gave some general answers to his questions, adding that it depended on each person's unique situation as well as what they wanted to explore. You assured him that he would remain in control and would be allowed to choose how he wanted to participate. You seemed to have secured his trust with your statements and he scheduled an appointment to see you.

Initial Interview:

Fred greets you cordially, although you sense immediately that he is in significant distress. After being seated, you acknowledge his sister's death and gently ask him to tell you more about his decision to seek counseling.

Fred's eyes well up in tears as he says, "My sister died about five months ago and I'm a complete mess. I'm not getting any better and I didn't know what else to do. I have been to a counselor before and it was an awful experience. I said I would never go to therapy again but I'm at the end of my rope. I can't seem to get through this."

You respond, "It's courageous of you to try counseling again after a bad experience with it. At some point, I'd like to know more about that experience so I can ensure that I will be helpful to you. Please know that I am always open to your feedback and, as I indicated on the phone, we'll go at this at a pace that feels right for you."

Fred nods, looking at you intently. "Okay," he says.

"Would you like to tell me about your sister?" you ask.

"She was in a terrible motorcycle accident. She was divorced and had one adult child who is married and lives out of the country. We grew up in an abusive family and were very close. I was her emergency contact. They put her on a ventilator and then said she wasn't going to get better. I had to make the decision to remove the ventilator..." Fred puts his head in his hands and bursts into tears.

"What was your sister's name?" you ask softly.

"Flossy. Her real name was Felicia, but we always called her Flossy," Fred quavers in a tearful voice.

"How was it for you to have to make that decision?" you ask gently.

"Oh my God! It was the hardest thing I've ever had to do. It was bad enough that this drunk driver pulled out of the side street and hit her full force. But then to see her in the hospital…" Fred devolves into heavy tears. "I feel so guilty about it. I feel like I killed my sister!"

You try to reassure Fred and reframe the experience by saying, "It's a horrible position to be put in, to have to decide to discontinue life support. I've talked with many people who had similar experiences to yours. It happens to families across the country every day. Allowing someone to die when there is no hope of surviving is an excruciating situation, but it doesn't mean you are responsible for your sister's death."

"I hear what you are saying but I have a really hard time believing that. The doctors told me that this would be the best thing for her and so I signed the papers. But now I wonder what would have happened if I had let her stay on it a few more days. Maybe she would have gotten better. I'm a total failure." Fred's tears continue.

"Were there any other family members that were involved in making that decision for your sister?" you inquire.

"No, I had to do it by myself." Fred explains, "I have two brothers but we don't get along very well. Our relationship has gotten even worse since this happened. They pretty much disappeared just like they did when we were kids. They were older than me and Flossy and took off as soon as they could. Now I think they hate me for taking her off the ventilator. Why do I have to be the one to do all the dirty work?"

You try to clarify the situation by asking, "Have your brothers told you that they are upset with you about Flossy's death?"

"No. They will hardly talk to me," Fred says.

"Do you have any other family members or friends that are supportive?" you ask.

"I have one friend who I work with," Fred says. "We're good friends, but she just found out that her husband has been cheating on her so she's got a lot going on right now. As for my family – no, I can't rely on them. I have some cousins and a couple of aunts but they… they stress me out. No, I wouldn't call them supportive."

"So you are pretty much alone with all of this, aren't you?" you ask.

"Yes, I am. And I feel like I'm dying. I can't eat and I stay awake all night reliving her last days in the hospital. I went to my doctor last week and he scolded me for losing so much weight. He says I need to let Flossy go. But I can't let her go!" Fred says fervently. "She was all I had!" He begins to cry heavily again.

"Yes, sounds like this has been a huge loss for you. Tell me more about your relationship with your sister," you suggest.

"We kind of took care of each other. I mean, we bickered some, too, but in the last year or so we got to be really close. She needed me, especially after she got divorced. I had a purpose in life. Now I have nothing. My life is meaningless. I just need to figure out how to get over this."

"It is perfectly appropriate, Fred, to have a difficult time after the death of a loved one," you say reassuringly. "For many people the hardest part of the grieving experience begins a few months after the loss. That this is a painful time for you does not mean that there is something wrong with you."

"Something must be wrong with me! I have taken leave from work because I kept making mistakes. I'm supposed to go back in a week but I'm not any better. I'm really nervous that my boss will end up firing me. I can't handle this. I just want her back! It just hurts so much!"

"I know it's hard," you say softly. You sit quietly for a moment while Fred cries. He uses a tissue to wipe his tears and blow his nose.

"I'm pathetic," he finally says.

You respond, "No, Fred, you are not pathetic. You are grieving. And unfortunately, you are having to do all of this by yourself without supportive friends or family. That makes a bad situation twice as hard." You ask Fred about his daily experiences and learn that he has trouble concentrating and often feels anxious. "Do you have a sense of what's causing the anxiety?"

"I keep seeing her in the hospital. And then when they removed life support. I just can't get those pictures out of my head," Fred squeezes his eyes shut and winces at the thought.

"Yes, those are very difficult images to have hanging out in your head," you say. "What do you usually do when those images pop up?"

"Well, I try to push them away. Try to find something else to do."

You proceed to give Fred information on both trauma and grief and the ways they interact with each other. Fred listens intently as you try to help him see that his responses make sense given the situation.

Fred looks at the floor and shakes his head. "I was just getting over my mother's death ten years ago and now Flossy!"

"It's tremendously difficult to lose a sibling. And it sounds like you two went through a lot together. To have this happen so suddenly makes it even harder." You hope to get a sense of some of Fred's strengths, so you ask him, "Can you remember what helped you get through the grief of your mother?"

"Well, I had Flossy to talk to, for one," Fred says. "I don't know. I just stayed busy, I guess. I went to the cemetery a couple of years ago and something changed. I was able to leave something there – eight years later. I felt like I had finished with the grief. Flossy's death, though, just brings it all back."

"Yes, sometimes that happens. New losses can trigger feelings from old losses. Have you had any mental or emotional struggles outside of your grief experiences?" you ask.

Fred nods and tells you about anti-depressant medication he has been taking for several years. He also told of numerous health problems for which he takes several additional medications.

Then he adds, "I was hospitalized for a nervous breakdown about 15 years ago, but I've been better since that. This has been hard, though. What am I doing wrong?"

"It doesn't mean you're doing anything wrong. Unfortunately, grieving a loved one is a lot more difficult than most people expect it to be. And it sounds like you had a lot going on in addition to Flossy's death. We can work together to help you get through this. Fortunately, the pain changes with time and attention. It won't always feel the way it does right now," you explain.

"I hope you're right. I don't know how much longer I can hold on," Fred says.

"Fred, do you ever have thoughts about hurting yourself?" you ask.

Fred takes a deep breath and says, "I've thought about it, but I'm afraid I'll go to hell if I commit suicide. I have been praying, though, that God would just take me. Sometimes I feel like he is punishing me."

You continue to assess Fred for suicidality and determine that he is not currently at risk of hurting himself, though you are concerned about his long-term ability to tolerate the emotional pain he is feeling. You give him the 24-hour crisis line and encourage him to call should he need support before you see him again. You also talk to Fred about the importance of self-care while grieving, such as eating well, getting rest, exercise, and engaging in pleasurable activities.

"Are you doing any of these things already, Fred?" you ask.

"No, I mostly just lay on the couch and surf the web," he answers. "Or drink."

You inquire more about Fred's drinking and learn that he has one to two beers each night. He also hints that sometimes he may have more than that. You talk more about how physical health influences how we deal with stress. He seems receptive and by the end of your discussion he has set a goal of going for a walk three times next week.

As you begin to arrange for a subsequent appointment, Fred says, "So you think you can help me?"

"Yes, Fred," you reply confidently. "If we work together, we'll get you through this difficult process."

"Okay. Thank you," Fred says. "Thank you so much. I feel better just knowing I've got someone to help me with this. I really appreciate it."

2.2-1. How would you categorize Fred's grief? What leads you to this conclusion?

2.2-2. What are some ways Fred's family history might play a role in his current experience?

2.2-3. How has Fred's grief impacted his coping skills?

2.2-4. Do research on how self-care strategies are important for managing stress. What would you say to Fred when explaining the importance of self-care while grieving?

2.2-5. What are some of Fred's strengths? How could these strengths be used to assist him with his grief?

CASE 2.3

Identifying Information:

Client Name: Mimi Roberts
Age: 55 years old
Race/Ethnicity: African American
Marital Status: Widowed
Education Level: Master's degree
Occupation: Chemist

Intake Information:

Mrs. Roberts requested an appointment due to multiple deaths in her family from the coronavirus. Due to concerns about virus transmission, you arrange for her to see you via telehealth.

Initial Interview:

You log on to find Mrs. Roberts waiting for you. "Hello, Mrs. Roberts," you say. "It's nice to meet you."

"Call me Mimi," she says. "Nice to meet you, too."

"Okay, Mimi. Did you have any trouble getting logged on?" She tells you it was easy. You go over a few details related to telehealth appointments, what to do if there are glitches with the technology, and confirm that you have a correct phone number for her should you lose connection completely. As you are discussing this, her dog crawls into her lap and makes himself comfortable. You use this as an opportunity to build rapport and engage with her in a conversation about her Shih Tzu dog named Prince. You move the conversation to her reason for seeking counseling.

"How can I be helpful to you, Mimi?" you ask.

"Well, I'm not even sure where to start. I'm really struggling with everything that's happened over the last six months." She goes on to explain that her husband of 30 years died after a three-month battle with the coronavirus, in addition to an elderly aunt, and a younger brother.

"Oh, Mimi," you say empathetically. "That is a lot of loss."

"It is. It's a lot. It's pretty overwhelming to be honest," she says.

"I would think so!" you say. "Were all of these deaths related to the coronavirus?"

"Yes," they were. With some prompting from you, she goes on to explain that her husband got it first and was hospitalized for two months before he died. While he was in the hospital, her aunt died. "I didn't even get to see her except for once over the phone. She had been in a nursing home and we weren't allowed to visit due to concerns about contamination." She continues explaining that her brother got sick shortly after her husband's death. She said he recovered and left the hospital but died a couple of weeks later due to complications from the virus.

"How have you been holding up, Mimi?" you ask.

"Not so great, really. I'm just…" she begins tearing up, "...so sad."

"Yes," you say softly. Her tears are now flowing freely. You attentively sit with her as she experiences these emotions. After a few moments, you say "This might be a hard question to answer, Mimi, but do you know what part about this has been the hardest?"

"That is kind of hard to answer," she replies. Through tears she continues, "I really miss my husband…. And I still can't believe this happened! One minute we were packing for our vacation and the next minute the whole country was shut down. And then... he's gone!"

"That is a lot to get your head around, much less your heart," you say.

Mimi nods in agreement. "I'm just in constant fear now. I won't leave my house. I have panic attacks when I watch the news. But I feel like I have to stay informed. I see people wearing masks and it just tears me up inside."

"Can you tell me more about that?" you ask.

"I see Marcus in the hospital, hooked up to all these tubes, on the ventilator…" Mimi starts breathing heavily, her face becomes flush, her eyes are wide, and she starts shifting in her chair.

"Mimi, come back to this moment. Right here. Tell me about the room you are in. What do you see?" You continue to guide Mimi to reconnect with the present moment, noticing what she sees, hears, and encouraging her to focus on the sensation of touch. After doing this for a while, she appears calmer and you ask, "How are you doing right now?"

"I'm better," she says with a deep breath. "What was that? What's happening to me?"

"I know it feels disconcerting, Mimi. I think you were having a trauma reaction to your experience with Marcus. Is that similar to what happens when you watch the news?"

"Yes," she says. "Though I usually can't keep it on for long, so I just turn it off. Am I going to be okay? This is terrifying. I feel like I'm going crazy." It appears she is becoming agitated again.

"Mimi, let's take some deep breaths together and I'll explain to you what's happening." You do some deep breathing in tandem with her and encourage her to pet her dog to help soothe herself. You then explain trauma responses and the physiological and emotional reactions they can cause. She seems able to take in your explanation and expresses some relief.

"Do you think about Marcus often?" you ask.

"I guess he's always there in the back of my mind, but it's just so hard. I'm trying to focus on getting through the day, taking care of the house, taking care of Prince," she explains.

"For some people, when a death has been traumatic it can be hard to deal with the loss or even think about their loved one because it brings up disturbing memories which we naturally want to push away. Does that resonate with what you experience?" you ask. Mimi considers this and then answers, "I think so. When I think about Marcus, I think about how I didn't get to spend his last days with him. That was so hard. Then I think about the video calls we had, how I could barely see his face. Then I wonder if he really got the care he needed, and if I'm going to get sick. It's just too much. The thoughts I have, the fear I feel, it just gets too scary so I try to just focus on being okay."

You normalize this experience for Mimi, again placing it in the context of traumatic loss. You spend the remainder of your time together, discussing the things that trigger traumatic reactions for Mimi and do some problem solving on how she can minimize exposure to those triggers and manage them when they do happen.

As the session comes to a close, Mimi says, "Thank you so much. I'm so glad I called you. It helps just understanding what's going on. I'll try these things you suggested. Can we meet again?"

"Absolutely," you say. "I feel very hopeful that we can get you through this. I know that may be hard for you to see right now. In the meantime, you can borrow my hope, okay?"

"Okay," Mimi says with a small smile. "Thank you."

2.3-1. Why would Mimi's losses be considered traumatic?
2.3-2. What is the value of educating Mimi about trauma reactions? What would you say to help her understand her experience?
2.3-3. What are some of the triggers Mimi identified? Given the circumstances of the loss, what other things might trigger grief and trauma reactions?
2.3-4. How do you interpret Mimi's statement, "so I try to just focus on being okay"?
2.3-5. Research three methods for managing flashbacks, panic attacks, or emotional flooding. Write how you would explain these techniques to Mimi.
2.3-6. What are Mimi's strengths?

REFERENCES

American Psychiatric Association [APA]. (2013). *Diagnostic and statistical manual of mental disorders* (5th ed.). https://doi.org/10.1176/appi.books.9780890425596

Boulanger, G. (2018). When is vicarious trauma a necessary therapeutic tool? *Psychoanalytic Psychology*, *35*(1), 60–69. https://doi.org/10.1037/pap0000089

Burke, L. A., & Neimeyer, R. A. (2013). Prospective risk factors for complicated grief: A review of the empirical literature. In M. Stroebe, H. Schut, & J. V. Bout (Eds.), *Complicated grief: Scientific foundations for health care professionals* (pp. 145–161). Routledge.

Djelantik, A., Robinaugh, D. J., Kleber, R. J., Smid, G. E., & Boelen, P. A. (2020). Symptomatology following loss and trauma: Latent class and network analyses of prolonged grief disorder, posttraumatic stress disorder, and depression in a treatment-seeking trauma-exposed sample. *Depression and Anxiety*, *37*(1), 26–34. https://doi.org/10.1002/da.22880

Harris, D. L. (2016). Social expectations of the bereaved. In D. L. Harris & T. C. Bordere (Eds.), *Handbook of social justice in loss and grief: Exploring diversity, equity, and inclusion* (pp. 165–175). Routledge.

Hazen, K. P., Carlson, M. W., Hatton-Bowers, H., Fessinger, M. B., Cole-Mossman, J., Bahm, J., Hauptman, K., Brank, E. M., & Gilkerson, L. (2020). Evaluating the facilitating attuned interactions (FAN) approach: Vicarious trauma, professional burnout, and reflective practice. *Children and Youth Services Review*, *112*. https://doi.org/10.1016/j.childyouth.2020.104925

Herman, J. L. (1992). *Trauma and recovery*. Basic Books.

Hidalgo, I. M. (2017). The effects of children's spiritual coping after parent, grandparent or sibling death on children's grief, personal growth, and mental health (Doctoral dissertation). https://digitalcommons.fiu.edu/etd/3467

Howarth, R. (2011). Concepts and controversies in grief and loss. *Journal of Mental Health Counseling*, *33*(1), 4–10. https://doi.org/10.17744/mehc.33.1.900m56162888u737

Iqbal, A. (2015). The ethical considerations of counselling psychologists working with trauma: Is there a risk of vicarious traumatisation? *Counselling Psychology Review*, *30*(1), 44–51.

Kelly, J. (2006). *The great mortality: An intimate history of the Black Death, the most devastating plague of all time*. HarperCollins.

Kosminsky, P. S., & Jordan, J. R. (2016). *Attachment-informed grief therapy: The clinician's guide to foundations and applications*. Routledge.

Kozlowska, K., Walker, P., McLean, L., & Carrive, P. (2015). Fear and the defense cascade. *Harvard Review of Psychiatry*, *23*(4), 263–287. https://doi.org/10.1097/hrp.0000000000000065

Lopez Levers, L. (2012). An introduction to counseling survivors of trauma: Beginning to understand the context of trauma. In L. Lopez Levers (Ed.), *Trauma counseling: Theories and inventions* (pp. 1–22). Springer Publishing Company.

Lynch, M. F. (2012). Theoretical contexts of trauma counseling. In L. Lopez Levers (Ed.), *Trauma counseling: Theories and inventions* (pp. 45–58). Springer Publishing Company.

Markin, R. D., & Zilcha-Mano, S. (2018). Cultural processes in psychotherapy for perinatal loss: Breaking the cultural taboo against perinatal grief. *Psychotherapy*, *55*(1), 20–26. https://doi.org/10.1037/pst0000122

Pearlman, L. A., Wortman, C. B., Feuer, C. A., Farber, C. H., & Rando, T. A. (2014). *Treating traumatic bereavement: A practitioner's guide*. Guilford Publications.

Piers, C. (1996). A return to the source: Reading Freud in the midst of contemporary trauma theory. *Psychotherapy*, *33*(4), 539–548. https://doi.org/10.1037/0033-3204.33.4.539

Pomeroy, E. C., & Garcia, R. B. (2018). *Direct practice skills for evidence-based social work: A strengths-based text and workbook*. Springer Publishing Company.

Putnam, F. W. (1989). *Diagnosis and treatment of multiple personality disorder*. Guilford Press.

Rando, T. A. (1993). *Treatment of complicated mourning*. Research Press.

Rando, T. A. (2015). When trauma and loss collide: The evolution of intervention for traumatic bereavement. In J. M. Stillion & T. Attig (Eds.), *Death, dying, and bereavement: Contemporary perspectives, institutions, and practices* (pp. 321–334). Springer Publishing Company.

Rosenblatt, P. C. (2017). Researching grief: Cultural, relational, and individual possibilities. *Journal of Loss and Trauma*, *22*(8), 617–630. https://doi.org/10.1080/15325024.2017.1388347

Rubin, S. S., Malkinson, R., & Witztum, E. (2012). *Working with the bereaved: Multiple lenses on loss and mourning*. Taylor & Francis.

Shear, M. K. (2015). Complicated grief. *New England Journal of Medicine*, *372*(2), 153–160. https://doi.org/10.1056/nejmcp1315618

Shear, M. K., Ghesquiere, A., & Glickman, K. (2013). Bereavement and complicated grief. *Current Psychiatry Reports*, *15*(11). https://doi.org/10.1007/s11920-013-0406-z

Siegel, D. J. (1995). Memory, trauma, and psychotherapy: A cognitive science view. *Journal of Psychotherapy Practice and Research*, *4*(2), 93–122.

Siegel, D. J. (2012). *Pocket guide to interpersonal neurobiology: An integrative handbook of the mind* (Norton Series on Interpersonal Neurobiology). W. W. Norton & Company.

Solomon, R. (2019, April). *The utilization of EMDR therapy with grief and mourning* [Presentation]. Compassion Works, Dallas, Texas, United States.

Stroebe, M. S., Hansson, R. O., Stroebe, W., & Schut, H. (2001). Introduction: Concepts and issues in contemporary research on bereavement. In M. S. Stroebe, R. O. Hansson, W. Stroebe, & H. Schut (Eds.), *Handbook of bereavement research: Consequences, coping, and care* (pp. 3–45). American Psychological Association.

Substance Abuse and Mental Health Services Administration [SAMHSA]. (2019). *Trauma and violence*. www.samhsa.gov/trauma-violence

Tedeschi, R. G., & Calhoun, L. G. (1995). *Trauma & transformation: Growing in the aftermath of suffering*. Sage Publications.

Tedeschi, R. G., & Calhoun, L. G. (2004). Target article: "Posttraumatic growth: Conceptual foundations and empirical evidence." *Psychological Inquiry*, *15*, 1–18. https://doi.org/10.1207/s15327965pli1501_01

van der Kolk, B. A., Stone, L., West, J., Rhodes, A., Emerson, D., Suvak, M., & Spinazzola, J. (2014). Yoga as an adjunctive treatment for posttraumatic stress disorder. *The Journal of Clinical Psychiatry*, *75*(06), e559–e565. https://doi.org/10.4088/jcp.13m08561

van der Kolk, B. A., & van der Hart, O. (1991). The intrusive past: The flexibility of memory and the engraving of trauma. *American Imago*, *48*(2), 425–454.

Wilson, C., Lonsway, K. A., & Archambault, J. (2016). *Understanding the neurobiology of trauma and implications for interviewing victims*. End Violence Against Women International. www.evawintl.org/Library/DocumentLibraryHandler.ashx?id=842

CHAPTER 3

Expected and Traumatic Grief Interviewing and Assessment: Using the Strengths-Based Framework of Grief and Loss

As a helping professional, there is a natural tendency to focus on the problems and challenges that are causing clients distress. That is, after all, why people seek support, to get relief from the problematic aspects of their lives. While it is necessary to attend to these difficulties, practitioners should also listen attentively for aspects of the client and the situation that represent strengths, resources, and opportunities. Awareness of these assets provides direction for appropriate interventions and can be positively leveraged to support the client's healing process. Actively highlighting client strengths has the additional effect of instilling hope and helping clients feel empowered with the notion that the process of grief is not insurmountable.

When assessing with the strengths-based approach, there is no implied assumption of a disorder or pathology that needs to be fixed. On the contrary, the client's grief reactions are viewed as an expected reaction to their loss. In addition, it is assumed that the client has both individual and environmental resources to aid them throughout the grief process, though they may need assistance in discovering and utilizing these assets.

ESTABLISHING RAPPORT

The primary goal when first meeting clients is to establish rapport and create an atmosphere of trust and safety. This is done by using an affirming and respectful demeanor and allowing the client to choose what they will share with the practitioner (Pomeroy & Garcia, 2018). This is especially relevant for clients who have experienced trauma. Their heightened state of vigilance often results in a wariness of new situations, fears and apprehensions about not being in control, and increased difficulty trusting others. Practitioners must play an active role to ensure that the therapeutic environment,

DOI: 10.4324/9780429053634-3

which includes the relationship with the practitioner, feels physically, socially, and emotionally safe so as to not re-traumatize the individual (Menschner & Maul, 2016). Providing predictability (e.g. explaining what will happen in the session), choice (e.g. allowing the client to decide where to start), and pacing (e.g. not encouraging detailed traumatic material to be disclosed before the client is ready) are some ways that practitioners can establish safety in the therapeutic setting and communicate to clients that their right to self-determination will be honored.

Rapport is also established when practitioners are attentively present to clients, communicate authentic empathy, and demonstrate tolerance for hearing the client's story without themselves becoming emotionally dysregulated. When clients become emotionally dysregulated the therapist assists them in stabilizing, or reregulating, their emotions. Not only does this encourage richer participation on the part of the client, it also "serves as a reregulating function that is in many respects similar to the reregulation that an attuned caregiver provides to a distressed child" (Kosminsky & Jordan, 2016, p. 123). As one client described her therapist, "She heard all of the grisly details of my story and never flinched. She stayed with me in all parts of this tragedy. She was my rock." The gathering of assessment information is most effective when it flows naturally from the rapport-building process.

BOX 3.1 TRAUMA-INFORMED CARE

In recent years, there has been a push to provide care in ways that are sensitive to how trauma survivors could be re-traumatized by the way in which services are delivered. Referred to as Trauma-Informed Care (TIC), this strengths-based approach "emphasizes physical, psychological, and emotional safety for both providers and survivors, and creates opportunities for survivors to rebuild a sense of control and empowerment" (Hopper et al., 2010, p. 82). TIC is anchored in a comprehensive understanding of trauma and is deliberately infused into all aspects of service delivery. TIC includes the following elements:

- **Safety:** ensuring that all aspects of the service setting promote feelings of physical and emotional safety for survivors.
- **Trust:** Practicing appropriate, consistent, and clear boundaries with clients and being forthright and specific regarding what services involve, how they will be delivered, and by whom.
- **Collaboration:** Acknowledging that survivors are the experts of their experience and encouraging them to be active in decisions about their care.
- **Choice:** Providing thorough information about intervention options so that survivors can make well informed decisions about their care.
- **Empowerment:** Recognizing that the sense of powerlessness endemic to many trauma survivors may be reversed by emphasizing choice and collaboration, and by providing opportunities to develop trust in others and the self.

(Knight, 2018)

STRENGTHS-BASED QUESTIONS

Using strengths-based questions in the initial interview can illuminate rich information about the client. The intentional wording of these questions facilitates the discovery of client strengths and resources. The following are some examples of interview questions that can be utilized with a person experiencing expected or traumatic grief:

- "How have you managed to survive (or thrive) thus far, given all the challenges you have had to contend with?"
- "What people have given you special understanding, support and guidance?"
- "Who are the special people on whom you can depend?"
- "What parts of your world and your being would you like to recapture, reinvent, or relive?"
- "What are your hopes, visions, and aspirations?"
- "How can I help you achieve your goals or recover those special abilities and times that you have had in the past?"
- "What is it about your life, yourself, and your accomplishments that give you real pride?"
- "What are your ideas or theories about your current situation?"
- "What are your ideas about how things – thoughts, feelings, behaviors, relationships, etc. – might change?"

(Saleebey, 2006, pp. 86–87)

In addition to Saleebey's questions, we would add:

- Are there moments when you feel at peace? Safe?
- What has helped you in the past?
- How are you currently adapting to this change?
- What would be a sign that you are managing this situation better?
- What do you imagine you would be doing if you weren't avoiding thoughts connected to the deceased or the traumatic event?
- What would be different in your life, if your grief felt manageable?

ASSESSING WITH SYSTEMS THEORY AND THE PERSON-IN-ENVIRONMENT (P-I-E) PERSPECTIVE

While listening for assessment information, practitioners must remember that mourners do not experience their grief in silos untouched by the environment around them. When clients talk about their grief, it is often based on the social construction of loss. They are governed by emotions and cognitions that are culturally grounded as well as social rules of politeness and other societal beliefs. Many people are multicultural and have a variety of societal rules that influence their behavior (Rosenblatt, 2016).

For this reason, ecological systems theory and the P-I-E (Person-In-Environment) perspective are particularly useful for understanding a client's grief experience. Ecological systems theory holds that all development is contextual and an outcome of human relationships within the social environment (Bronfenbrenner, 1979). This framework reveals how conditions in different levels of the environment play a role in the client's grief experience. At the microsystem level, the focus is on individuals, small groups, and families. The mesosystem considers the context of communities and organizations, e.g. churches, schools, neighborhoods, and social clubs. The macrosystem includes influences from the larger environment such as national, international, political and legal systems, societal values, and mass media. These subsystems are critical to understanding the dynamics and interrelationships that impact personal behaviors, including responses to loss. Ecological perspectives are useful for improving the client's functioning by shifting the focus of interventions from the individual (e.g. client's behavior/deficits) to the client's system or interrelationships (e.g. family, school, and community) in an effort to capitalize on the client's strengths and resources in their environment (Bronfenbrenner, 2005).

The following variables can be influenced by all levels of the environment and are particularly relevant to the grief experience: physical health, mental health, attachment style, social support, individual strengths, environmental strengths, culture, race and ethnicity, social status (e.g. privileged/marginalized), spirituality, relationship to the deceased, circumstances surrounding the loss, and secondary losses. Depending on the

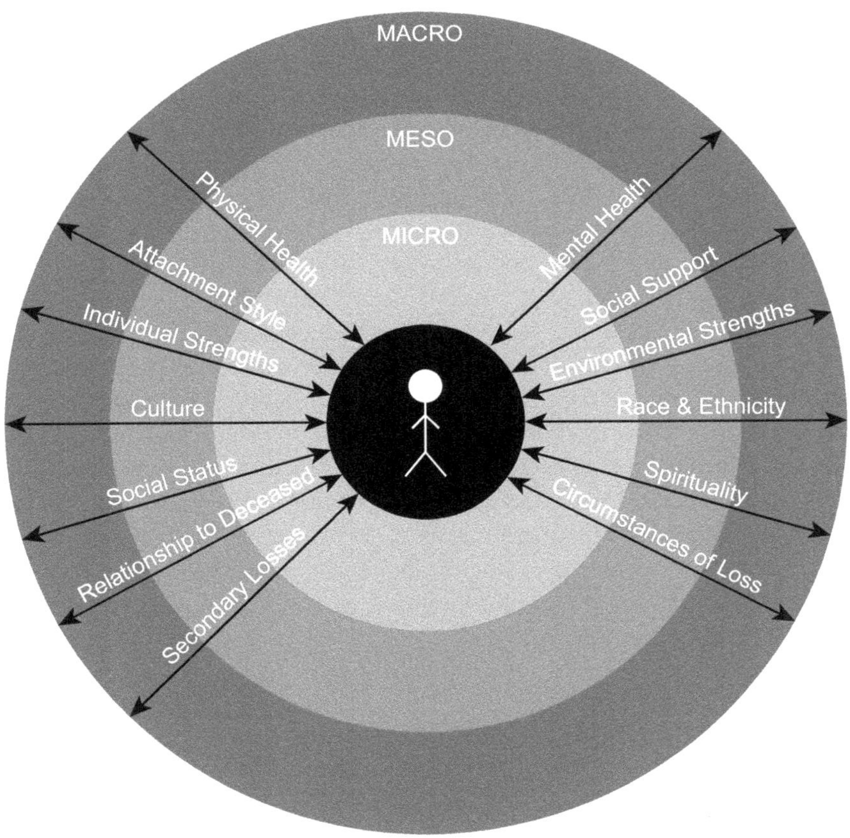

FIGURE 3.1 P-I-E Perspective of the Grief Experience

unique circumstances of the mourner and the loss event, the expression of some variables may either facilitate or impede healthy grieving. For example, a mother mourning the death of her black son who died at the hands of a police officer will have a very different grief experience from a mourner who lost her elderly mother due to natural causes. Grief assessments that use the P-I-E view to consider the client's experiences as they relate to all levels of the environment can more fully elucidate the unique grief experience of the mourner. By paying particular attention to when these variables interfere with the mourner's ability to adapt to their loved one's death, practitioners can have a clearer understanding of how they can most effectively intervene.

FACILITATING THE CLIENT'S STORY

Often, the assessment begins with clients telling the story of their loss. The "death narrative" or "event story" (Neimeyer, 2012) serves as a springboard for gathering information, developing the therapeutic relationship, and guiding the choice of intervention. The recounting of these events in and of itself can also provide therapeutic value to the client as they endeavor to grasp the reality that their loved one is deceased. Practitioners should pay particular attention to salient features of the story, including when the death occurred, how the bereaved was informed of the death, if the death was expected or a surprise, support that the bereaved received, and any aspects of the story that are difficult for the client to discuss or evoke emotional responses. As practitioners learn about the client's relationship to the deceased, how the client's functioning has been affected by the loss, and the primary focus of the client's attention, they begin to gather clues as to the client's orientation to the loss (recall the DPM model of loss orientation versus restoration orientation) and the mourner's attachment style as discussed in Chapter 1. Practitioners will also want to listen for the client's perceptions of causality and preventability, feelings of guilt, how the loss has affected their assumptive worldview, and any additional aspects of the situation that may have been experienced as traumatic. Information and comments that hint to the client's personal value system are also important to note.

It is critical that practitioners listen with an open mind, being careful not to make assumptions about the intensity of the experience for the client or what aspects of the situation are causing the client the most distress. For example, when working with a father who accidentally ran over his daughter with a motor vehicle, the therapist presumed that the parent felt enormous guilt. However, as the assessment interview unfolded it became evident that guilt was not the dominant emotion. Furthermore, choosing which aspects of the grief experience to focus on during the session must occur in collaboration with the client.

PRIOR LEVEL OF FUNCTIONING

When working with grieving clients, it can be particularly helpful to obtain information about the chronology of events and the onset of symptoms related to the loss. This provides information about the client's functioning prior to the death and thus helps determine what symptoms may be directly related to the loss experience. Learning about the client's previous experiences with grief, loss, and trauma is also useful. As these details are discussed, the practitioner can begin to get a sense for where the client is in regard to accepting the loss and what obstacles may stand in the way of effectively adjusting to it. This information also helps reveal client strengths which may not be readily apparent when the client is in distress.

Whenever possible, multiple sources of information are preferred over relying solely on the client's perspective. Additional sources of assessment data include information from other professionals (e.g. medical, psychological, social, educational, spiritual, legal, etc.), relevant family members, and other persons who provide social support.

THE CONTEXT OF CULTURE IN THE ASSESSMENT PROCESS

Culture can be defined as "the integrated pattern of human behavior that includes thoughts, communications, actions, customs, beliefs, values, and institutions of a racial, ethnic, religious, or social group" (Gilbert et al., 2007, as cited in National Association of Social Workers [NASW], 2015). Cultural context may greatly influence a client's reactions to grief, loss, and trauma, and the assessment activities and demeanor while interviewing should reflect this understanding. As Rosenblatt (2016) explains, "I try not to create more social justice issues by interviewing in a closed-minded, controlling, not-hearing way. Instead I try to interview with openness to what people have to offer" (p. 69).

Practitioners must be cautious about interpreting assessment data through the lens of their own cultural experience which can lead to mislabeling or erroneously pathologizing what is expected and adaptive behavior within the client's cultural milieu. Likewise, practitioners should not assume that all persons from a particular culture will grieve in a prescribed manner. While each culture has its expectations for how mourning should be expressed, private expressions of grief can vary with individuals and families (Rosenblatt, 2016).

Therefore, learning about the client's familial grief culture can be very informative. Family grief culture refers to those unique customs, values, beliefs, rituals, communications, and behaviors that frame acceptable norms around death, loss, and bereavement within a specific family. For example, in one family the norm may be that the deceased is rarely, if ever, mentioned. In another family, the deceased can be discussed but only positive feelings may be expressed. In a third family, it may be acceptable to joke, laugh, and tell stories about the deceased one's foibles. All of these behaviors represent acceptable norms within these specific families but may be considered unusual or even irreverent behaviors outside of the family. The following questions can elicit information about the client's familial grief culture:

- What was your first experience with death within your family?
- What are some of your family's rituals around the loss?
- What messages did you receive directly or indirectly about the expression of grief?
- How does your family's spiritual traditions influence their response to loss?
- How are children treated in relation to a death?

- What are some of the family roles related to the death?
- What are some of the family values related to death?
- What were some of the spoken and unspoken rules about behaviors related to the bereavement period and the person who died?

BOX 3.2 MOURNING RITUALS: AFRICAN AMERICANS

Many African American mourning rituals have their origins in African funeral traditions. Community support for the mourners begins with a wake, during which supporters, often with food in hand, visit the bereaved and share memories of the deceased. Generally, the casket is open during funeral services and participants may touch, kiss, or lay hands on the body. In the United States open casket funerals may also represent a testimony to the injustices experienced by African Americans. This was the case when Mamie Till, the mother of Emmett Till, who was lynched to death in 1955, demanded an open casket so others could witness the violence that killed her child. The congregation numbered in the thousands to mourn his tragic death. Today, once again, thousands of people congregated at the funeral of George Floyd, who also died as a result of racial injustice.

As was the custom in West African cultures, funeral services involve significant community wide participation and may be extravagant and long lasting events. Often, there is fervent weeping. Church leaders stand ready with tissues and fans to assist mourners.

The jazz funerals in New Orleans continue the traditions of their Kongolese ancestors. After intense expressions of sorrow through weeping and wailing, the dead are accompanied to the graveyard with jubilant dancing, singing, and music played by brass bands as they dance the soul to its heavenly destination (Hidalgo, 2017).

GRIEF IN THE CONTEXT OF A MENTAL HEALTH ASSESSMENT

Conducting an assessment with a grieving client includes an evaluation of the total mental health of the individual. In doing so, it is important to decipher the symptomatology of mental disorders as well as that of grief and trauma. While an extended grief reaction may be expected for some clients, it could also indicate the coexistence of trauma or mental health challenges that were present prior to the loss.

Assessment of Bereavement according to the *Diagnostic and Statistical Manual of Mental Disorders*, Fifth Edition (*DSM-5*)

Historically, bereavement has received minimal attention from the American Psychiatric Association (APA) and was included in the *DSM-5* and *DSM-4-TR* as a V code (other conditions that may be a focus of clinical attention). The definition of bereavement included a two-month time period, which was considered a major limitation by the field of experts in grief and loss. Moreover, a diagnosis of Major Depressive Disorder prevented the practitioner from diagnosing bereavement.

Although the *Diagnostic and Statistical Manual of Mental Disorders*, fifth edition (*DSM-5*) recognizes the differences between uncomplicated bereavement, which is still defined as a V code, and Major Depressive Disorder, it also allows for a person experiencing a severe grief reaction and depression to be diagnosed with a Major Depressive Disorder. Although the major symptoms of grief involve feelings of emptiness and loss that come and go in waves, the symptoms of major depression include hopelessness and persistent depression that pervasively influence the person's mood (American Psychiatric Association [APA], 2013). In addition, persons with Major Depressive Disorder will have low self-esteem while those with a grief reaction may keep their self-esteem intact. However, the authors of the *DSM-5* recognize that there can be significant overlap in symptoms and a bereaved individual can become clinically depressed.

Bereavement is also noted in the *DSM-5* in the Trauma- and Stressor-Related Disorders category under Other Specified Trauma- and Stressor-Related Disorder. An individual who experiences the death of a close relation (friend or family member), and who continues to long for the deceased, has significant emotional pain, and who is preoccupied with the deceased may have a complicated grief condition that would be classified as a Persistent Complex Bereavement Disorder (APA, 2013). In addition, the individual experiences symptoms similar to a trauma reaction, such as emotional numbing, anger, excessive avoidance of situations that remind one of the death, a desire to die in order to be with the deceased, loneliness, role confusion, and lack of interest in pleasurable activities. A specifier of "with traumatic bereavement" can be included if the death was of a traumatic nature such as homicide or suicide. Persistent Complex Bereavement Disorder is also being considered as a unique diagnosis; however, presently it is in the Appendix under "Conditions for Further Study." Therefore, to diagnose a client who is experiencing these symptoms, a practitioner would have to use the "Other Trauma- and Stressor-Related Disorder" classification (APA, 2013).

Finally, Uncomplicated Bereavement remains in the *DSM-5* under "Other Conditions That May Be a Focus of Clinical Attention" as a V code. Uncomplicated Bereavement is considered a normal expression of grief over the loss of a loved one and not a mental disorder (APA, 2013). The duration of a normal grief reaction is not specified in the *DSM-5*, with an acknowledgment that culture may play a significant role in the length of the grief process.

Bereavement can also be found in the *DSM-5* (APA, 2013) under Adjustment Disorders. In the case of the death of a loved one, the grief reaction must surpass what is customary in that person's environment and culture. In addition, the developmental level of the person must be taken into consideration (APA, 2013). For example, a young child who develops behavioral problems after the death of a distant relative might be given a diagnosis of Adjustment Disorder with the specifier, "with mixed disturbance of emotions and conduct."

Assessment of Grief and Depression

Understanding the distinction between clinical depression and bereavement-related depression and how they may coexist informs the assessment process and guides practitioners to providing clients with the most effective interventions. Many of the symptoms that are characteristic of major depression, such as sadness, tearfulness, sleeplessness, and reduced appetite, are also considered to be common, and in fact, expected for someone who is in the initial stages of grief (Friedman, 2012). While depressive symptomatology includes feelings of self-hate, self-blame, and despair as well as somatic fatigue and lack of energy (Lichtenthal et al., 2004; Ogrodniczuk et al., 2003), expected grief reactions may or may not involve these depressive emotions.

A critical distinction between a major depressive episode and a grief reaction is that in depression the symptoms are continuous and chronic, dominating the daily life of the individual and pervading multiple areas of the individual's life. With grief, however, there can be an ebb and flow of both positive and negative emotions and the negative symptoms of grief may be intermittent and vary in intensity. In addition, self-recrimination and utter despair tend to be focal points for the depressed individual, whereas sadness interspersed with periods of normalcy characterize the person who is experiencing an expected grief reaction (Solomon, 2019). Frequently, the depressed person feels little hope that life will improve while the person with expected grief can usually recognize that grief is a temporary state that will eventually feel less dispiriting.

The distinction between depression and grief is further blurred when considering complex grief. Depressive symptoms exclusively related to the loss often have the deceased or the absence of the deceased as their focus (Shear et al., 2013). For example, a bereaved woman who is very critical of herself for the way she spoke to her brother just prior to his unexpected death but does not berate herself in other areas of her life suggests that she is suffering from bereavement, as opposed to clinical depression. When grief and depression coexist, interventions must be tailored to address both issues and include a referral for a medical evaluation.

As stated earlier, knowledge about a client's functioning prior to the loss, including any history of depression, is important. As with many life stressors, loss can precipitate a recurrence of depressive episodes. In addition, if a client is experiencing suicidal thoughts, a thorough suicide risk assessment is warranted followed by the appropriate interventions. There are many assessment tools available to help practitioners identify and assess suicidal clients, including John Klott's book, *Suicide & Psychological Pain* (2012). Additional information about suicide can be obtained from the American Foundation for Suicide Prevention (afsp.org) and the Suicide Prevention Resource Center (sprc.org).

Assessment of Grief and Trauma

Careful listening and respectful inquiry will assist practitioners in assessing the presence or absence of trauma. If it appears that the client was traumatized by the death, practitioners should inquire about symptoms related to PTSD and their impact on the client's daily functioning. This information will be folded into determining the best approach to interventions. As with depression, knowledge of previous traumatic experiences can be useful in identifying risks and strengths.

While specific details about the traumatic aspects of the loss such as sensory memories of the death or imaginings about how the loved one suffered may be an important focus of attention, practitioners should not pressure clients to reveal such vivid details before sufficient safety and trust have been established and it has been determined that the client is ready to do so (Kosminsky & Jordan, 2016). Preferably, direct focus on these details occurs as one piece of a thoughtfully designed intervention plan.

Knowledge of the kinds of triggers that activate a client's trauma response is important for crafting interventions. It also helps practitioners ensure that the therapeutic interaction does not inadvertently evoke trauma-related symptoms. Again, strengths-based questions that yield information about how clients have tried to adapt to their trauma-induced symptoms provide useful information while also communicating belief in the client's ability to heal. The authors' grief assessment instrument provided at the end of this chapter includes elements that address traumatic loss and trauma symptoms.

ASSESSMENT INSTRUMENTS

Some of the common assessment instruments used to evaluate grief, depression, and PTSD are listed here. These scales can provide a baseline for the client's functioning and lead to consistent interpretation of symptoms by all practitioners involved with the client.

Depression:

- Beck Depression Inventory II (BDI-II; Beck et al., 1996)
- Center for Epidemiologic Studies Depression Scale (CES-D; Radloff, 1977)
- Hamilton Rating Scale for Depression (Hamilton, 1967)

Grief:

- The Inventory of Complicated Grief (Prigerson et al., 1995)
- Brief Grief Questionnaire (Shear et al., 2006)
- Texas Revised Inventory of Grief (Faschingbauer, 1981)

Stress and Trauma:

- Traumatic Grief Inventory Self-Report version (TGI-SR) (Boelen et al., 2019)
- Acute Stress Disorder Scale (ASDS) (Bryant et al., 2000)
- Trauma Symptom Checklist-33 (TSC-33) (Briere & Runtz, 1989)
- Mississippi Scale for Combat-Related Posttraumatic Stress (Keane et al., 1988)
- Impact of Event Scale (IES) (Horowitz et al., 1979)
- Centrality of Event Scale (CES) (Berntsen & Rubin, 2006)
- Adverse Childhood Experiences Scale (Felitti et al., 1998)
- The Harvard Trauma Questionnaire PTS subscale (HTQ) (Mollica et al., 1992).

These instruments are some of the most commonly used and well-researched assessment tools in the field of grief, loss, and trauma. Other instruments are being developed and researched. Standardized instruments require field testing with a wide number of diverse populations to prove reliability and validity. As with pharmaceutical drugs, it can take many years to develop a standardized assessment instrument.

ASSESSMENT INTERVIEWING

Assessment information is commonly gathered in a semi-structured interview. The psychosocial assessment outlined in the next section delineates the range of data that would yield a thorough assessment of expected and traumatic grief, though some information may be more or less relevant depending on the client's situation. Practitioners can use this outline as a guide for the kinds of information to listen for and inquire about as the client discloses information over time. By gathering information in a manner that is in keeping with the natural flow of conversation, rather than a rigid and linear manner, clients will feel more at ease disclosing information and clarifying their responses (Pomeroy & Garcia, 2018).

It is also important to note that gathering this information typically occurs over several meetings and within the context of developing a safe and trusting environment for the client. As Kosminsky and Jordan (2016) explain, "excessive focus on assessment with a newly bereaved and traumatized client, to the exclusion of building safety and the feeling of being understood in the therapeutic relationship, runs the risk of empathic failure with clients" (p. 157). In addition, the ongoing nature of assessment is especially relevant with grief and loss as there are expected changes over time in the grief experience.

PSYCHOSOCIAL ASSESSMENT OF GRIEF, LOSS, AND MOURNING

In addition to the information typically covered by a psychosocial assessment (e.g. identifying information, mental status exam, medical history, developmental history [for children and adolescents]), the following outline delineates the types of information most relevant to assessing expected grief and traumatic grief reactions in bereaved individuals:

I. General Information about the Loss

- A. Date of death, manner of death
- B. Role the deceased played in client's life (e.g. spouse, parent, child, friend)
- C. Nature of the relationship with the deceased (e.g. close, amicable, conflictual, detached)
- D. Secondary losses (e.g. financial status, family role, home, school)

II. The Death Experience

- A. The story of the death and the circumstances surrounding the loss
    1. How did the client learn about the death?
    2. Does the client have any regrets about what happened when the loved one died?
- B. Trauma in Relation to the Loss
    1. Which of the following can be said about the loss?

        ____ Unexpected
        ____ Out of sequence with what is considered natural (i.e. child dying before parents)
        ____ Violent or gruesome in nature

____ Perceived as preventable
____ Perceived to involve suffering
____ Perceived as unjust or undeserved
____ Perceived as random
____ Committed by someone with the aim of causing harm
____ Witnessed by the survivor
____ Involved multiple deaths
____ Involved threat to the survivor's life

III. Impact of the Loss as Compared with Pre-Death Functioning

A. Cognitive Functioning (e.g. concentration, forgetfulness, preoccupation, confusion)
B. Emotional Functioning (e.g. sadness, anger, loneliness, disbelief, anxiety)
C. Behavioral Functioning (e.g. withdrawal, high risk-taking behaviors, compulsive behaviors, substance use)
D. Physical functioning (e.g. sleep, appetite, aches and pains, fatigue)
E. Spirituality

1. What is the client's basic philosophy or belief system?
2. What gives the client meaning and purpose?
3. Does the client's spiritual belief system provide comfort or create distress?
4. Have the client's perspectives on life or the world been altered as a result of the loss?

F. Overall Impact and Adjustment to the Loss

1. How are the changes noted in the previous areas impacting the client's ability to function in daily life?

    1. In family roles and obligations?
    2. At work or school?
    3. In personal relationships?

2. What is the client's demeanor while discussing the loss? (e.g. emotional, detached, dissociative)
3. Does the client present as being overly focused on the loss, reluctant to confront the loss, or alternating between both of these?
4. What life-enhancing versus life-depleting grief reactions does the client exhibit?
5. How has the client attempted to cope with the loss?

    1. Are these coping mechanisms life-enhancing or life-depleting?

6. What aspects of the loss event are the most distressing to the client?

IV. Symptoms Related to the Traumatic Nature of the Loss

A. Intrusive symptoms (e.g. involuntary and intrusive memories, distressing dreams, flashbacks related to the loss)

B. Avoidance thoughts and behaviors (e.g. attempts to avoid thoughts, feelings, or reminders associated with the loss)

    1. Thought and mood disturbances (e.g. distorted thinking about self or the circumstances that caused the loss, persistent difficulty experiencing positive emotions)
    2. Symptoms of arousal (e.g. increased irritability, exaggerated startle response, hypervigilance, sleep disturbance, difficulty concentrating)
    3. For how long have these symptoms continued following the loss event?

V. Social Support and Relationship Functioning

A. Does the client have close family or friends?

    1. What is the quality of these relationships? Do they feel supportive to the client?
    2. How has the client's support system responded to the loss? To the client's grief reactions?

B. Is the client able to ask for help from friends and family when needed?

C. What needs is the client's support system able to address? Unable to address?

VI. Attachment Style

A. What was the client's attachment to the deceased prior to the death? (e.g. secure, anxious, avoidant)

B. Does the client experience continuing bonds with the deceased? (e.g. recalling memories of deceased, talking to deceased, engaging in memorialization activities)

    1. Does the client feel a connection with the deceased?
    2. Do these connections provide comfort or distress?
    3. Do these connections aid the client in accepting and adjusting to the loss? Or do they provoke avoidance?

VII. Psychosocial History

A. Significant childhood experiences

B. Previous losses
Who was lost? How? When did this occur? How did it impact the client's life?

C. Previous traumas (e.g. abuse, natural disasters, accidents, major life changes)

D. Mental health challenges (e.g. depression, anxiety, PTSD, severe mental disorders)

    1. Diagnoses given
    2. Current and past treatment received
    3. Past suicide attempts
    4. Current suicide ideation

VIII. Familial Context of Loss

A. What is the client's familial grief culture?
How is the client's expression of grief similar to or different from their family?

B. Are there specific family values that impact the client's grief experience?
C. What role/roles does the client hold in the family system?

1. How are the family roles impacted by the loss?
2. Are family relationships functional and supportive or dysfunctional and harmful?

IX. Cultural Context of Loss

A. What are the client's cultural rituals around loss?

1. What are some of the spoken and unspoken rules regarding behaviors related to grief and mourning within the client's culture?
2. How is the client's expression of grief similar to or different from their culture?

B. What is the impact of cultural traditions on the client's grief reactions?
C. What is the impact of spiritual traditions on the client's grief reactions?

X. Spirituality and Meaning Construction

A. What is the client's narrative about the life of the deceased and the role the loved one played in their life?
B. How is the client trying to make sense of the loss?
C. Since the death, which of the following has the client experienced?

____ Changes in assumptive worldview (e.g. safety, fairness, benevolence, control, trust)
____ Values (e.g. morals, priorities)
____ Religious/spiritual views

D. Does the client indicate motivation to search for new meanings?

XI. Strengths and Resources

A. Individual strengths

1. Does the client appear to have purpose/meaning in their life?
2. What strengths are evident in the client's worldview?
3. Does the client demonstrate evidence of any of the following?

___ openness to receiving help
___ willingness to engage with the practitioner
___ readiness to experience relief from distress
___ spiritual resources (i.e. belief system, community)
___ resiliency
___ self-efficacy
___ history of using effective coping skills
___ other individual strengths: ____________________________________

B. Environmental strengths

1. Are there indications of any of the following?

___ basic needs of food, shelter, healthcare, etc. are being met

___ sufficient means for acquiring professional assistance
___ sufficient access to informal support systems
___ sufficient access to culturally relevant resources
___ sufficient information and ability to utilize resources
___ other environmental strengths: ______________________________

CASES

CASE 3.1

Identifying Information:

Name: Linh Nguyen
Age: 26 years old
Race/Ethnicity: Vietnamese American
Marital Status: Married
Education Level: Vocational school
Occupation: Licensed massage therapist at a local spa

Intake Information:

Linh called your office and asked for counseling regarding the death of her sister. In visiting with her briefly on the phone, she tells you that her sister was five years older than she and that she died in a car accident.

Initial Interview:

Linh arrives for her appointment at the scheduled time. She is fashionably dressed and greets you amicably. You begin the session by gently prompting, "So, I understand you are here because you lost your sister."

"Yes", she says. "It happened about nine months ago. She had a car wreck. It was raining. She took her eyes off the road for just a moment and looked up to see something dart into the road. She started skidding out of control and crashed into a tree. My brother-in-law was in the car with her when it happened. They rushed her to the hospital, but she died about four hours later." Linh's eyes begin to well up with tears.

"I see that her death is hard for you. I believe you told me that she lived in a different city, is that right?" you ask.

"Yes, she lived about three hours away. I was in a massage session when the call came in. By the time I got the message, cancelled my appointments, and got on the road she had already died." Tears are now rolling down Linh's face. You quietly move a box of tissues beside her on the couch and wait for her to continue. "I just don't know how I'm going to get through this!" Linh says amidst her tears.

"Tell me more about that," you prompt.

"It's just so hard! I miss her so much! I feel like I'm falling apart! I thought I was doing okay but lately it seems to be getting worse," Linh says, still crying.

"You know, a lot of people who have lost a loved one really struggle around six to nine months after the death. In what way is it getting worse for you?" you ask.

Linh explains, "I want to cry all the time. I'm irritable. I'm unmotivated. It takes everything I have to get myself to work. I always feel so tired."

"Have you been able to sleep?" you ask.

"I have been sleeping a lot," Linh admits. "It's all I want to do."

"How is your appetite?" you inquire.

"I haven't been eating much. Nothing really sounds good. I have about one meal a day with a few snacks," she says.

"I know that it's dreadfully uncomfortable, Linh, but you should know that it is expected that you would be having a hard time, even after nine months. And all the symptoms you are describing – low motivation, fatigue, changes in your sleep and appetite, irritability – these are all normal for someone who has lost a loved one."

"Oh, well that's good to know, I guess," she responds. "I keep thinking I should be farther along by now."

"Tell me more about how this is going for you. Have you been able to get yourself to work?"

"Yes, I have. I've only had to call in once since this happened and that was because I had come down with a cold or something. It's hard to pull myself out of bed, but I am able to do it. Once I get there I can usually manage okay, although my boss has really been making me angry lately. So far, I've been able to hold my tongue, though. Thankfully, I'm usually in session with someone so I don't have to deal with her too much.... I used to love what I do. I was getting ready to start my own practice and go into business for myself. I was so excited about it, but now...I just can't get myself to take any action on it." Linh begins to cry again. "I just want my sister back!"

"Of course, you do," you reply softly. "Tell me about her. What was your relationship with her like?"

"Mai was my best friend," Linh explains. "We talked at least two or three times a week on the phone. We talked about everything – the big important stuff like fights with our husbands and stupid stuff like the latest shoe sales. Any decision I had to make, I called her to get her thoughts and advice and she did the same with me. She was always there for me. She was my biggest cheerleader and was really encouraging me to start my own business. She was totally convinced I could do it even when I wasn't so sure. I just feel so lost without her!"

"I would imagine so!" you affirm. "Her death has left a huge hole in your life!"

"Yes," Linh nods as she cries. "It really has. And my husband doesn't really get it. Whenever I try to talk about her, he changes the subject. If I get sad he starts making jokes. I guess he is trying to cheer me up, but it doesn't work. I feel like lately, he's just getting sick of it. Sometimes, if I get sad, he just leaves the room without saying anything."

"How is that for you?" you ask.

"It really hurts," Linh says. "I try to be happy, especially when he's around. I don't want to bring him down with me. But it's hard...."

"As much as you may wish you could be happy all the time, I don't see that as being realistic right now. You are in the throes of grief over your sister and best friend.

That is a significant loss! It can be even more difficult when you feel misunderstood or unsupported. Do you have other people in your life that give you support with this?" you question.

"I talk to my mom some. I know she's having a real hard time with this, so I try to be strong for her. I have one friend that I've talked to a little bit, but I can only lean on her so much. I have several friends that I have hardly seen since this happened. They seem to feel uncomfortable around me. The thing is…the person who I would have been talking to about this, who would be helping me through it, is Mai!" Linh becomes teary again. "And she's not here!"

"This must feel very lonely for you," you venture. Linh nods and you continue. "Unfortunately, I hear stories like this quite often. It seems that a lot of people are very uncomfortable around the subject of death. They don't know what to do or how to help someone who is grieving. It leaves people in your situation feeling very alone at a time when they are most in need of support."

"Yes," Linh agrees. "If I could just get through this, maybe things would get back to normal again, but I don't know how."

"What have you tried so far?" you ask.

"I've tried to get my mind off of it and to stay busy. But I have no energy to do anything so that has been kind of hard. Like I said, I just can't seem to get excited about anything. I've told myself to be grateful that I had such an awesome sister and to appreciate the time we had, but…." Linh shakes her head and reaches for a tissue.

"I'm guessing that that hasn't gotten you very far," you say. Linh shakes her head in agreement. You continue, "You can be grateful for what you had and also want more time with her. For such an awesome person to suddenly disappear from your life is devastating. It's very hard to see the positive side of this right now. Do you ever allow yourself to cry about Mai? To really let go with the tears or do you try to quickly stuff them and pull it together?"

"It depends on who is around. Sometimes if I am by myself I will just let loose. I usually feel a little better afterwards, but it also feels so lonely. If my husband is around, which is most of the time, I try to keep it together," Linh responds.

"I'm glad to hear that you allow yourself to lean into it a little bit. When you honor those emotions and let yourself express them, they will gradually begin to dissipate. Also, many times people who are grieving have to educate other people about what they need. It may feel kind of like a chore to have to do that when you are already so spent, but it can be worth it in the long run. Do you have a sense of how you wish your husband would respond?" you ask.

Linh dries some of her tears and says, "I just want him to hold me and let me cry without trying to make it okay. It's not okay and nothing will ever make it okay!"

"All right," you say. "Is there anything else that you need from him?"

"I need him to understand that I can't get over this in nine months. It's too painful. I need him to be patient with me and give me some time with this," she pleads.

"Have you expressed these needs to him?" you ask.

"No," Linh says. "No, I haven't and I guess I should. He's never lost anyone before, so he can't relate to this at all. I don't know if I can get him to understand how hard it is."

"It is very difficult for people who have not experienced the death of someone they love to understand how overwhelmingly painful and powerful grief can be. Though you probably won't be able to make him fully understand, you can teach him about what you need from him as you go through this. Also, I can send you back with some information that talks about grief. That might give him some added insight into what it's like for you," you offer.

"Okay. That sounds good." Linh pauses then looks directly at you. "So, what is going to happen? When will this ever get better?" she asks.

"I know that it's hard to imagine a time when this will be easier, but grief doesn't last forever if you give it some attention, just as you are doing now and as you do when you allow yourself to have your emotions. Eventually, you will start having a few good days, and gradually the good days will outnumber the bad days. There will always be a hole in your heart for Mai. Nothing will ever be able to fill that hole. But with time you will become more accustomed to that empty space and the pain won't be as intense as it is for you now," you explain.

"I hope so. How long does it take?" Linh asks.

"That's a common question and there's no formula for calculating a time frame for grief. You may hear people say that the first year is the hardest. Others will tell you that the second year feels just as hard. But it's a gradual process. Sometimes it feels like you are taking two steps forward and one step back," you pause to gauge her reaction. She nods silently and seems to be taking this in. After a moment you continue, "I'm very glad you chose to come in and get some support with this, Linh. People tend to do better when they can be with others who understand what they are experiencing."

"It feels good to talk to someone who gets it. And to not have to feel like I have to censor myself," she says.

"I'm glad to hear that. It sounds like it would be helpful for you to continue coming here so that you can have a safe space to have your grief in whatever form it takes. You might also want to consider attending one of the local support groups," you add.

"I don't know about a group. I don't think I could open up in front of a bunch of people," Linh says.

"Group is not for everyone, but many people find it to be extremely helpful. There is something quite powerful about being with others who are in the same situation. Most people feel relieved to learn that other people are having similar experiences with their loss," you explain.

"Okay. I'll think about that. In the meantime, I think I want to continue with individual counseling," Linh says.

"That sounds great," you assure her. "Let's schedule a time when you can come in again."

3.1-1. Based on this initial assessment, would you categorize Linh's grief as expected, complex, or traumatic?

3.1-2. What are some strengths-based assessment questions you could ask Linh?

3.1-3. Write three questions to ask Linh that would help you understand the cultural context of her grief.

3.1-4. What additional assessment information would you like to get in future sessions?
3.1-5. How has Linh's grief experience affected her relationships with others?
3.1-6. What are some of Linh's strengths?
3.1-7. Find an article on sibling loss. Identify at least three reasons that sibling loss is difficult.

CASE 3.2

Identifying Information:

Client Name: Naomi Witherspoon
Age: 46 years old
Race/Ethnicity: White
Marital Status: Single
Education Level: College degree
Occupation: High school math teacher

Intake Information:

Naomi called your office and asked detailed questions about the counseling sessions that your agency provides. She said her best friend had died five months ago and she wanted to know if people often came in for grief counseling, if they found it helpful, how many sessions you thought she might need and if it was appropriate for her to seek help for the loss of a friend, rather than a spouse or parent. At the end of the call she agreed to make an appointment to see you.

Initial Interview:

Naomi arrives for her appointment, breathless from rushing to get there on time. You slowly lead her to your office and offer her some water hoping that this will help her catch her breath and relax. She explains that she was detained at her school by a call from the parent of one of her students.

After settling into your office, she begins to talk about her loss by saying, "So, as I told you on the phone, I lost my best friend." She swallows and looks at the floor.

"What was her name?" you ask softly.

"Melanie," Naomi says as tears fill her eyes.

"How did Melanie die?" you inquire.

"She had cancer," Naomi reports. "She was diagnosed in September and she died three weeks later."

"Three weeks?" you voice sympathetically. "She declined very quickly!"

"Yes, she did," Naomi agrees. "It all happened so fast. When she first got diagnosed I admit I feared the worst, but I never thought it would be just three weeks. I assumed we'd have some time – several rounds of treatment, that sort of thing."

"So this was pretty sudden and unexpected," you say.

"Oh yes," Naomi says emphatically. "And it has really rattled me. Sometimes I think I'll be okay but it seems like most of the time I'm just limping along. I feel like I'm barely able to keep my head above water."

"Tell me more about that," you prompt.

Naomi explains, "Work has been especially difficult. Some days I just have to grit my teeth to keep from completely losing my temper with my students. They are just being normal teenagers but it really sets me off. I am just so low on patience with them. I used to never be like that. I find myself counting the minutes until the bell rings so I can get a little break."

"Are your co-workers aware of the trouble you are having?" you ask, hoping to get a sense of the kind of social support Naomi has.

"I don't really think so. Many of them knew Melanie because she was an assistant principal at the other high school in town. When I've tried to explain it to a few people they are nice, but I don't think they really get it. It seems that since she was just a friend, they don't see why I should be having such a hard time. I think that if I had lost a spouse or someone more significant, they would be more understanding." Naomi holds her temple in her hand. "I feel like I'm blowing this all out of proportion."

"But she was significant to you, wasn't she?" you ask.

"Yes, she was," Naomi says softly. She covers her eyes and begins to cry.

"Tell me more about your relationship with her," you say.

"She was my best friend. I could talk to her about anything. We got together every Friday after work. We'd usually go out to eat and to a movie. Or go shopping or something. We talked about work a lot – you know, compare notes, complain, share ideas. And we'd talk about our families and…well, everything. We could talk about anything and everything." Naomi begins to cry again. "She knew me better than anyone else."

"It's no wonder you are having a hard time with this, Naomi," you empathize. "A friend like that is truly a treasure. I would expect you to be having a great deal of difficulty after such a loss."

Naomi nods while she continues to cry silently.

"I'm glad you are letting yourself have these feelings, Naomi. I know it's hard." After a few moments, you encourage her to continue by saying, "What does it feel like to have Melanie gone?"

"It's awful!" Naomi says. "The pain is just unbearable sometimes. And I feel so lonely. I really need a friend right now but my friend can't be here for me! I don't know what to do with myself. I just want it to go away. I keep trying to talk myself into being happy, but it's not working. I need to know how to get through this."

"Well, positive thinking can help sometimes, but there is no escaping the pain of grief. What are some of the other ways you have tried to deal with this?" you inquire.

Naomi thinks for a moment then says, "Well, I usually feel better after I exercise and I have been trying to get to the gym more. It's been hard to make myself go, however. I'd much rather lie on the couch and watch TV. I do visit the cemetery every so often and take her some flowers. Somehow that seems to help a little."

"Those are some very good things to do. Consciously taking good care of your body is very important while grieving. And as with exercise, try to eat well and get plenty of rest. And sometimes you have to force yourself into action, rather than wait until you feel like doing something that would help you." You add, "That can be hard to do. I'm impressed that you've been able to get yourself to the gym."

"That makes sense that I need to take care of my body. I could probably get myself to exercise more if I took my workout clothes to school with me. I've also thought about joining an aerobics class. I want to make some new friends…but it's hard." Naomi sighs. "I spend all day pretending that I'm happy and okay. It's exhausting. And who wants to be friends with someone who is depressed?"

"I think the aerobics class sounds like a good idea," you affirm. "Even if you don't make any friends there, you will be getting some exercise. I know it can be hard to make friends when you feel sad and needy. I'm glad, however, that you have the desire to do so. It will come with time."

Naomi nods in understanding and after a moment says, "I guess you can't just make it go away, huh?"

"I wish I could but, unfortunately, no," you say empathically. "The pain won't always feel this intense, though. In the meantime, you have to focus on caring for yourself as you find a way to get used to Melanie's absence."

Naomi sighs deeply. "Just taking it day by day?"

"Day by day is generally a good strategy," you agree. "You may find that on some days you have to take it five minutes at a time."

"Oh, yes! I have many days like that," Naomi says.

"On those days you might find it helpful to really focus on the present moment, whatever that entails. If you are folding clothes, for example, direct your attention to how the cloth feels in your hands, to the way the cloth moves as you fold it, the smell of the clean clothes. Focus on experiencing the world around you through your senses," you explain. "But just as important as getting through the day is letting yourself experience the grief. After such a loss, I would expect you to be very tearful and irritable and low on motivation. It's okay to honor those feelings – to give yourself permission to have them."

"So if I want to cry just let myself cry?" Naomi asks. You nod in agreement. "What about all this anger? This desire to strangle my students?"

"Well, deep breathing while you are in the moment can help," you offer. "Physical activity, as we mentioned earlier, is also a great release for tension and anger. You might need to run up and down the stairs a few times or go for a walk around the track during your lunch break or go to your car and sing an angry song or have a good cry. Also, recognizing that your reserves are low right now and that you need to get plenty of rest may help you be more patient with yourself and with your students. Remember Naomi, that now is a time when you really want to be gentle with yourself. It's not the time to aim for the Teacher of the Year award." You pause while Naomi takes in the information you have given her. You add, "And of course, talking about it can help, which is how I can be useful."

"Yes," Naomi agrees. After a moment of silence she says, "There is something else that I want to ask you about."

"Go ahead," you encourage.

"I have always been very active in my church and I've relied on my faith to help me get through some tough times, but since this happened…." Naomi's voice trails off and her eyebrows furrow. You wait patiently and attentively. She continues, "Since this happened, I don't want to have anything to do with God or church. Whenever I go to worship, I sit there seething with anger the whole time. I don't understand how God could let this happen! Melanie was such a good person. All she wanted was to help kids and show kindness to others! What kind of God would do this?" Naomi's tone suggests feelings of anger and desperation.

You try to put feelings to what Naomi has expressed and say, "You feel angry with God? You feel that God has let you down?"

"Yes, I do! It doesn't make sense to me." Naomi pauses. "And it really scares me to be having these thoughts. I have never questioned my faith before."

You inquire into Naomi's faith tradition and she tells you that her church is oriented in fundamental Christianity. She explains that she has subscribed to this belief system since childhood. You direct the conversation back to her feelings about her current experience of spirituality.

"You have relied on these beliefs and shaped your life around them and now they don't seem to fit," you venture. "That can be very disconcerting. It might even feel like another loss."

"Yes!" Naomi agrees. "My anger at God is so strong and I feel really guilty about it!"

"Actually, I hear this quite a bit," you reassure Naomi. "Many people begin to question their previously held perspectives or spiritual beliefs after losing a loved one. Often people will feel angry with God or begin to doubt everything they once believed. This even happens to people who have been very strong in their faith. This is a common component of the grief process for some. As with the pain of grief, though, it doesn't have to be permanent."

"What do I do about it? Just endure it?" Naomi asks.

You respond, "Sometimes just expressing your feelings toward or about God can be helpful, just as you would with a friend or family member. I have heard many pastors tell people in your situation that God is strong enough to handle the anger. But it would probably also be helpful for you to discuss this more with a church leader who can speak with you in the language of your faith. Would you be open to doing that? Do you know of someone you could talk to about this?"

Naomi thinks for a moment. "There is a woman named Nancy, who is married to one of the deacons. I think I might feel comfortable talking to her. It's not something I want everyone in my church to know about but I'm sure she would keep it confidential."

"Sounds like she could be a helpful resource for you. Just explain to her how important your confidentiality is to you."

"Yes, it would probably be good for me to talk to her." Naomi sighs heavily, then continues, "This is so hard. I had no idea it would be this hard."

"Yes," you affirm. "It's excruciating. I hope you won't feel that you need to minimize this. It's a time when you want to take extra good care of yourself – pamper yourself a little. The grief over a best friend is an extremely stressful experience."

"I feel better just hearing you say that to me," Naomi says. "I have been trying to pretend it's not such a big deal. But it is."

"You have made a good start in caring for yourself by coming to see me. What would you like to do about coming in again?"

"I think I'd like to come again in about two weeks," Naomi responds. "What you have told me today helps a lot. Next week I'm going to try to talk to Nancy – the woman at church. Then I can tell you how that went."

"That sounds like a good plan," you say.

3.2-1. Using the ecological systems and P-I-E perspective, discuss Naomi's grief experience.
3.2-2. What are some secondary losses that Naomi is experiencing?
3.2-3. What additional information would be useful to have as you work with Naomi?
3.2-4. What are some of Naomi's strengths?
3.2-5. What are some strengths-based questions you could ask Naomi?

CASE 3.3

Identifying Information:

Client Name: Janice Richards
Age: 26 years old
Race/Ethnicity: White
Marital Status: Single
Education Level: Some college
Occupation: Clerk in shipping and receiving

Intake Information:

Janice Richards was referred to the Capitol Mental Health Center by a crisis hotline worker. She had called the crisis hotline the night before concerning the recent death of her boyfriend of six months. She told the hotline worker that she felt like "killing herself" although the worker determined that she was not suicidal. Janice contacted the mental health center the following day and said she desperately needed to talk to someone.

Initial Interview:

Janice arrives for her appointment 15 minutes early and is pacing in the waiting room when you go out to greet her. She is dressed in sweatpants and T-shirt with her hair pulled back in a ponytail. She is wearing no make-up and has a very disheveled appearance. You introduce yourself and Janice begins talking on the way to your office.

"I'm just a wreck – a walking wreck today. I got up this morning and just knew I couldn't go to work. I don't think I've slept in a week."

"Maybe you'd like to sit down and tell me what's been going on," you suggest as you close your office door.

Janice plops down on the couch and begins to cry uncontrollably. You hand her some tissue and lean forward attentively. "I just don't know where to begin," she coughs out. "It's been a nightmare. I just can't believe this is happening to me. We were going to get married someday and then he's just gone."

"It sounds like you really cared about him," you reflect.

Janice looks at you with a hopeless expression and bursts into tears again. She buries her face in her hands and blurts out, "He's dead!"

"Okay, Janice," you gently encourage, "would you like to tell me the story of what happened from the beginning?" You're trying to understand what Janice is telling you.

Janice sighs deeply and sits back in the chair. She seems to be trying to pull herself together. "Yes, I'd really like to tell someone the whole story."

"Great, where would you like to start?" you suggest.

"Well, I'll start from the beginning. I've been dating this guy named Jack for a little over six months. We'd had our fights like all couples do, but we really loved each other." Janice sighs deeply.

"Were you living together?" you ask.

"It was kind of on and off. Living together I mean," Janice replies.

"Okay, so sometimes you were living together. At your home or Jack's?" you question.

"My home – most of the time. What I mean is our relationship kind of had its ups and downs. Most of the time it was great but sometimes it just seemed like he got tired of being with me and would go off with his own friends and didn't even seem to be thinking about me."

"Okay, so sometimes Jack needed some space. How did it make you feel when he would go off with his friends?" you query.

"Well, it was devastating; like he didn't really care about me. We'd argue about it all the time and sometimes he would just tell me he needed a breather from the relationship. I would just go ballistic and tell him that if we were in a committed relationship, he couldn't just go off and leave me alone." Janice sits up. It's apparent that she is angry.

"And how did he respond to you when you told him he couldn't leave you alone?" you question.

"He'd just walk away from me and wouldn't discuss it. Then eventually he'd come back and say he really wanted to be with me. I'd be so angry at him but when he apologized, I just melted. I was so glad he was back, I didn't care about anything else." She pauses and stares out the window. "Now he's gone forever. I'm so alone."

"Okay, I think I understand that Jack was a very important person in your life. Would you like to tell me how he died?"

"We were having one of our fights because Jack insisted on going to a lake party with his guy friends and I wasn't invited. I couldn't believe he was doing this to me because we had just had a big discussion about how much I needed him to be with me. I told him if he walked out that door, just never come back. Those were my exact words." Janice begins sobbing again and then adds, "And he never did."

"What happened after he went to the party?" you ask.

"Well, I was so frustrated, I didn't know what to do. I tried to watch some shows but it was hard to focus so I decided to call him. I wanted to tell him that I was sorry I got so angry and that I wasn't mad anymore. I called several times over about a two-hour period but he never answered. Finally, I just fell asleep on the couch. Next thing I know the phone is ringing; it's 3 a.m. and they want to know if Jack is at my house. I told them no and some police guy tells me Jack is missing. He was last seen swimming in Target Lake. They wanted to know when the last time I saw him was. I thought I was having a dream. I didn't really put all of the pieces together. I just figured he'd come home. Twenty-four hours later, they find him at the bottom of the lake. I just can't believe it."

"This has really been a major blow to you," you respond.

"It has! I feel so empty without him! I feel like I'm nothing without Jack. Sometimes I just think I'd be better off dead. I can't imagine ever being able to fill all this emptiness inside me. I just feel so unlovable." Janice curls her knees up to her chest and whispers, "How could this be happening again?"

You say, "This has happened before, Janice?"

"Well, not exactly. But people are always leaving me."

"You mean other boyfriends or family?" you query.

"Every guy I've ever dated, ends up leaving me. I don't understand it. What's wrong with me?"

"It sounds like you have felt a lot of abandonment in your life. Can you tell me a little more about that?" you ask.

"Yea, well, all my relationships – they start out okay, but then something happens and they always leave. I don't get it. I'm scared to death of being alone. I desperately want someone to take care of me. Why does everyone leave me?" she looks at you imploringly.

"You know, some of what you're feeling may be related to this recent loss you've experienced and some of how you're feeling right now may be touching other losses you've had. Can you tell me more about yourself? Your family?"

Janice describes a childhood lived in the suburbs punctuated by three moves for her father's job. She has a younger sister that she speaks to occasionally and describes a tense relationship with her mother.

"Do you have any friends that are supportive?"

"I have a couple of people from work that I hang out with sometimes," she replies. "I've tried to talk to some of Jack's friends but they don't really like me. I just want to get information about the funeral and stuff. God, that's going to be hell. His friends hate me. I don't know how I'm going to get through that."

"That would be hard under any circumstance," you say.

Janice proceeds to tell you about some of Jack's friends and how they have treated her rudely in the past. You validate the pain and frustration this has caused her.

"It sounds like you've had a lot of loss, Janice, so it's no wonder you're feeling so distraught about Jack. Grief can trigger many of the feelings you are describing and working through it is a process that will take some time. I know how difficult it is to manage these feelings and that's why I'd like to continue seeing you. I think it would be helpful to talk more about your losses and how they have affected you," you offer.

"Yeah, but isn't there something you could do right now to make me feel better?" she pleads. "I just can't stand this empty feeling! It's like a deep, dark hole I can't fill up. It makes me feel worthless and ugly."

"I know you're experiencing a lot of intense emotions right now. Would it help to go over some things you could do when these feelings become overwhelming?"

"Yes," Janice says.

In addition to suggesting journaling and exercise, you also teach Janice how to regulate her breathing and explain how that can be helpful. Janice seems agreeable to try these. After a thorough suicide assessment, you determine that Janice is okay to dismiss without additional intervention other than a subsequent appointment.

"I'm really glad you reached out for help, Janice. I'm looking forward to working with you."

3.3-1. How would you characterize the grief Janice is experiencing?
3.3-2. List three strengths-based questions that you could ask Janice.
3.3-3. What are some of Janice's strengths?
3.3-4. What else might be going on for Janice, in addition to her grief?
3.3-5. What additional information would you like to obtain in future sessions?
3.3-6. List four possible goals for your work with Janice.
3.3-7. What additional resources might be useful for Janice?

REFERENCES

American Psychiatric Association [APA]. (2013). *Diagnostic and statistical manual of mental disorders* (5th ed.). https://doi.org/10.1176/appi.books.9780890425596

Beck, A. T., Steer, R. A., & Brown, G. K. (1996). *Manual for the Beck Depression Inventory* (2nd ed.). Psychological Corporation.

Berntsen, D., & Rubin, D. C. (2006). The centrality of event scale: A measure of integrating a trauma into one's identity and its relation to post-traumatic stress disorder symptoms. *Behaviour Research and Therapy*, *44*(2), 219–231. https://doi.org/10.1016/j.brat.2005.01.009

Boelen, P. A., Djelantik, A. A. A. M. J., de Keijser, J., Lenferink, L. I. M., & Smid, G. E. (2019). Further validation of the Traumatic Grief Inventory-Self Report (TGI-SR): A measure of persistent complex bereavement disorder and prolonged grief disorder. *Death Studies*, *43*(6), 351–364, DOI: 10.1080/07481187.2018.1480546

Briere, J., & Runtz, M. (1989). The Trauma Symptom Checklist (TSC-33): Early data on a new scale. *Journal of Interpersonal Violence*, *4*, 151–163.

Bronfenbrenner, U. (1979). Contexts of child rearing: Problems and prospects. *American Psychologist*, *34*(10), 844–850.

Bronfenbrenner, U. (2005). *Making human beings human: Bioecological perspectives on human development.* Sage.

Bryant, R. A., Moulds, M. L., & Guthrie, R. M. (2000). Acute stress disorder scale: A self-report measure of acute stress disorder. *Psychological Assessment*, *12*, 61–68.

Faschingbauer, T. (1981). *The Texas Inventory of Grief—Revised.* Honeycomb Publishing.

Felitti, V. J., Anda, R. F., Nordenberg, D., Williamson, D. F., Spitz, A. M., Edwards, V., & Marks, J. S. (1998). Relationship of childhood abuse and household dysfunction to many of the leading causes of death in adults: The Adverse Childhood Experiences (ACE) Study. *American Journal of Preventive Medicine*, *14*(4), 245–258.

Friedman, R. A. (2012). Grief, depression, and the DSM-5. *New England Journal of Medicine*, *366*(20), 1855–1857. https://doi.org/10.1056/nejmp1201794

Gilbert, J., Goode, T. D., & Dunne, C. (2007). *Curricula enhancement model: Cultural awareness.* Washington, DC: National Center for Cultural Competence, Georgetown University Center for Child and Human Development.

Hamilton, M. (1967). Development of a rating scale for primary depressive illness. *British Journal of Social and Clinical Psychology*, *6*, 278–296.

Hidalgo, I. M. (2017). The effects of children's spiritual coping after parent, grandparent or sibling death on children's grief, personal growth, and mental health (Doctoral dissertation). https://digitalcommons.fiu.edu/etd/3467

Hopper, E. K., Bassuk, E. L., & Olivet, J. (2010). Shelter from the storm: Trauma-informed care in homelessness services settings. *The Open Health Services and Policy Journal*, *3*(1), 80–100.

Horowitz, A., Wilner, N., & Alvarez, W. (1979). Impact of event scale 4: A measure of subjective stress. *Psychological Medicine*, *41*, 209–218.

Keane, T. M., Caddell, J. M., & Taylor, K. L. (1988). Mississippi Scale for combat related post traumatic stress disorder: Three studies in reliability and validity. *Journal of Consulting and Clinical Psychology*, *56*, 85–90.

Klott, J. (2012). *Suicide & psychological pain: Prevention that works*. PESI Publishing & Media.

Knight, C. (2018). Trauma-informed supervision: Historical antecedents, current practice, and future directions. *The Clinical Supervisor*, *37*(1), 7–37. https://doi.org/10.1080/07325223.2017.1413607

Kosminsky, P. S., & Jordan, J. R. (2016). *Attachment-informed grief therapy: The clinician's guide to foundations and applications*. Routledge.

Lichtenthal, W. G., Cruess, D. G., & Prigerson, H. G. (2004). A case for establishing complicated grief as a distinct mental disorder in DSM-V. *Clinical Psychology Review*, *24*, 637–662.

Menschner, C., & Maul, A. (2016). Key ingredients for successful trauma-informed care implementation [PDF file]. Center for Health Care Strategies. www.chcs.org/media/ATC_whitepaper_040616.pdf

Mollica, R. F., Caspi-Yavin, Y., Bollini, P., Truong, T., Tor, S., & Lavelle, J. (1992). The Harvard Trauma Questionnaire: Validating a cross-cultural instrument for measuring torture, trauma, and posttraumatic stress disorder in Indochinese refugees. *Journal of Nervous and Mental Disease*, *180*(2), 111–116. https://doi.org/10.1097/00005053-199202000-00008

National Association of Social Workers [NASW]. (2015). *Standards and indicators for cultural competence in social work practice*. National Association of Social Workers.

Neimeyer, R. A. (2012). Retelling the narrative of the death. In R. A. Neimeyer (Ed.), *Techniques of grief therapy: Creative practices for counseling the bereaved* (pp. 86–90). Routledge.

Ogrodniczuk, J. S., Piper, W. E., Joyce, A. S., Weideman, R., McCallum, M., Azim, H. F., & Rosie, J. A. (2003). Differentiating symptoms of complicated grief and depression among psychiatric outpatients. *Canadian Journal of Psychiatry*, *48*, 87–93.

Pomeroy, E. C., & Garcia, R. B. (2018). *Direct practice skills for evidence-based social work: A strengths-based text and workbook*. Springer Publishing Company.

Prigerson, H. G., Maciejewski, P. K., Reynolds, C. F., Bierhals, A. J., Newsom, J. T., Fasiczka, A., Frank, E., Doman, J., & Miller, M. (1995). Inventory of complicated grief: A scale to measure maladaptive symptoms of loss. *Psychiatry Research*, *59*(1–2), 65–79. https://doi.org/10.1016/0165-1781(95)02757-2

Radloff, L. S. (1977). The CES-D scale: A new self-report depression scale for research in the general population. *Applied Psychological Measurement*, *1*, 385–401.

Rosenblatt, P. (2016). Cultural competence and humility. In D. L. Harris & T. C. Bordere (Eds.), *Handbook of social justice in loss and grief: Exploring diversity, equity, and inclusion* (pp. 67–74). Routledge.

Saleebey, D. (2006). *The strengths perspective in social work practice* (4th ed.). Pearson Education.

Shear, M. K., Ghesquiere, A., & Glickman, K. (2013). Bereavement and complicated grief. *Current Psychiatry Reports*, *15*(11). https://doi.org/10.1007/s11920-013-0406-z

Shear, K. M., Jackson, C. T., Essock, S. M., Donahue, S. A., & Felton, C. J. (2006). Brief grief questionnaire. PsycTESTS Dataset. https://doi.org/10.1037/t62516-000

Solomon, R. (2019, April). *The utilization of EMDR therapy with grief and mourning* [Presentation]. Compassion Works, Dallas, Texas, United States.

CHAPTER 4

Expected and Traumatic Grief in Adults

The symptoms, emotions, and behaviors associated with expected grief reactions represent a process of healthy adaptation and are not inherently pathological. Grief in response to the death of a significant loved one is, however, intense, disruptive, and painful. Mourners frequently express fears that they are "going crazy" or "losing my mind" and often feel relief upon learning that their responses are not abnormal. Thus, an important role for the practitioner is to educate clients about the nature of expected grief and assist them to cope with the fluctuations in emotions that the loss introduces into their lives. While focusing on ways to cope with grief is important, the goal is not to fix grief or make it go away. Rather it is to assist the client in experiencing the grief reactions in a way that helps them transition to living without the deceased while also allowing them to function adequately with the here and now issues in their lives. Much like a midwife assists a laboring woman during childbirth, counselors help mourners safely navigate through the changing and turbulent journey of loss.

RESPONSES TO GRIEF

As with other stresses, grief has a way of awakening fears and sensitivities from childhood (Hart et al., 2006; Smid et al., 2015). Past experiences and unprocessed wounds may resurface and be re-experienced. Although difficult, this brings with it the possibility for new understanding, insight, and growth (Kosminsky & Jordan, 2016).

The manner in which bereaved persons respond to the loss of a significant loved one is believed to be largely influenced by the attachment style they developed in childhood (see discussion on Bowlby in Chapter 1) and the attachment they had with the lost loved one (Burke & Neimeyer, 2013; Parkes & Prigerson, 2013; Zech & Arnold, 2011). When mourning becomes stalled, it may be related to the bereaved person's expectations about the capacity to trust and rely on others (Kosminsky & Jordan, 2016).

Similar to a child's response to prolonged separation from an important caregiver, adults respond to the death of a loved one with strategies designed to obtain safety and emotional regulation. Hyperactivation, the strategy typically employed by anxiously

DOI: 10.4324/9780429053634-4

attached individuals, is characterized by escalated attempts to restore proximity to the attachment figure. Mourners who use this strategy are likely to display dependence on others while fearing that support will not be available. They are highly focused on the loss, the painful feelings it brings, and are consumed with worries about their ability to cope without their loved one. Their open expression of emotion represents their attempt to seek support from others (Kosminsky & Jordan, 2016).

Deactivation is the strategy often employed by avoidantly attached individuals. This response is designed to protect the individual from the unavailability of the attachment figure by suppressing the need for comfort and reassurance. When confronted with grief these individuals avoid reminders of the loss, are reluctant to be vulnerable with others, and often minimize the difficulty of their experience and their need for assistance. They have difficulty accessing the emotions that accompany loss and may have successfully trained themselves not to feel, a phenomena Bowlby called "defensive exclusion" (Bowlby, 1982). Deactivation may lead to a variety of somatic symptoms or maladaptive behaviors, including drug abuse or dysfunction in relationships (Kosminsky & Jordan, 2016).

Bereaved clients with a disorganized attachment style employ elements of both hyperactivation and deactivation in their attempt to obtain comfort after a loss. This is understandable in light of their history of early childhood trauma and unpredictable caregivers. These clients tend to have the most difficulty trusting others, including the practitioner. They are likely to dismiss positive remarks made about their strengths or abilities and struggle to stay engaged in the healing process (Kosminsky & Jordan, 2016).

Securely attached individuals will also experience significant emotional distress upon the death of a loved one. However, their ability to trust in others and seek support enables them to more easily oscillate between hyperactivation strategies and deactivation strategies which facilitates healthy adaptation to the loss (Mikulincer & Shaver, 2008).

While there are differences in the degree of severity, the length of recovery, and the manner of expression, the universal experience of grief has an all-encompassing impact on mourners, affecting their capacity to function cognitively, emotionally, behaviorally, physically, socially, and spiritually. The following discussion summarizes the responses that characterize both expected and traumatic grief. Considering these two types of grief in comparison can be helpful to understanding the broad continuum of grief reactions that bereaved persons may exhibit.

BOX 4.1 MOURNING RITUALS: NATIVE AMERICANS

There is vast diversity among the Native American population. The customs of each tribe are shaped by acculturation, relocation, and education in boarding schools. In addition, Native Americans observe a variety of Christian religions.

For Navajo Americans death is viewed as another stage in a person's life, and the customs surrounding burial and mourning facilitate their journey beyond the earthly realm. If rituals are not carried out as specified by tradition, both the deceased's spirit and the remaining family members will be negatively impacted. Within four days of the death, the body is cleansed, adorned, and blessed to ensure a safe journey. The belongings of the deceased are buried with the body, given to others, or burned. On the fourth day, the family will cleanse themselves which then allows the loved one's spirit to begin traveling to the next life. Following this ritual, any conversation about the deceased, even years after the death, is believed to risk physical and mental harm to the loved one's surviving family and descendants (Hidalgo, 2017).

COGNITIVE FUNCTIONING

Cognitive Functioning with Expected Grief

Grieving clients commonly report significant disruption in their cognitive functioning at the onset of grief. Cognitive disruptions may present as forgetfulness, disorientation, difficulty concentrating, distractibility, preoccupation, impaired judgment, and distortions in reality testing (Stroebe et al., 2001). When grief is acute, there are typically periods of disbelief and the mourner may temporarily forget that the loved one is dead or have difficulty grasping the reality of the loss. This may serve a protective function to give the bereaved time to gather supportive resources as well as to gradually adjust to the permanence of their loved one's absence. Many clients state feeling as if they are "in a fog" or "just going through the motions." They also report problems with thinking clearly and making decisions. These symptoms often result in frustration because they impair the client's ability to work, read, and accomplish tasks. For example, one female client described great difficulty finding her counselor's office despite the fact that she was familiar with the location. Another client who was an avid reader prior to his loss, stated that it took great effort for him to finish reading just one page.

Clients may report visual or auditory perceptions of the deceased or dreams in which the person has communication with the deceased. This does not necessarily indicate unresolved loss nor does it always represent a continuing bond relationship with the deceased, particularly when it occurs soon after the death (Field et al., 2013). While these changes in cognition can be alarming to clients, with expected grief, they eventually abate over time (Stroebe et al., 2001).

Cognitive Functioning with Traumatic Grief

Along with the expected grief reactions outlined in the previous paragraphs, additional, enduring, and more disruptive cognitive difficulties are experienced when grief is traumatic. Intrusive thoughts and images of the deceased or the mode of death can permeate mourners' daily activities. The bereaved may obsessively ruminate about aspects of the loss such as if the loved one suffered, ways the death could have been prevented, or ways to get justice for the loss (Pearlman et al., 2014). Additionally, it is common for traumatically bereaved individuals to experience confusion, distractibility, impaired judgment, memory problems, and a general lack of concentration that lingers over time.

Neurological research on trauma supports a connection between PTSD, including traumatic grief, and problems with memory, attention, planning, and problem solving (Hayes et al., 2012; Shear, 2015). It is believed that many of the cognitive resources that would be used for processing information are, in sufferers of PTSD, instead focused on identifying threats. They often perceive harmless stimuli as dangerous and maintain heightened focus on potential danger at the expense of other cognitive and executive functions (Hayes et al., 2012). When thinking of the loss provokes intense distress, the bereaved may avoid such thoughts or become so emotionally dysregulated that it stalls the grieving process and impedes successful adaptation to the loss (Wortman & Pearlman, 2016).

EMOTIONAL FUNCTIONING

Emotional Functioning with Expected Grief

Society tends to focus primarily on the emotional impact of loss felt by grieving individuals. Although adults anticipate emotional difficulties following the death of a loved one, they are often surprised by the depth and intensity of their feelings. These feelings may fluctuate throughout the day or week depending on the client's attachment with the deceased, circumstances surrounding the death, and current life situation. The very nature of grief involves oscillation of the mourner's emotions with varying degrees of strength and force (Stroebe et al., 2016). Although the continual and unpredictable change in emotional state can be unsettling, it is one of the life-enhancing aspects of expected grief. It allows the mourner the capacity to move between confronting the emotional pain of the loss, orienting oneself to life without the deceased, and taking needed respites from the exhausting work of grief (Stroebe & Schut, 2010).

Some of the feelings associated with expected grief include sadness, loneliness, anger, guilt, irritability, periods of numbness, disbelief, relief, regret, anxiety, emptiness, and restlessness. Because of the unbidden and ever-shifting emotional state of the mourner, individuals often report feeling as if they can't control their emotions. For example, a woman who recently lost her mother reported having to leave work early due to a sudden and irrepressible surge of tears that drew the attention of her co-workers. She not only felt embarrassed but worried that it would happen again and that she wouldn't be able to maintain control of her feelings.

Individuals may also be highly sensitive while grieving and experience intense anger, irritability, and frustration. They may explode in anger or crumble in despair over mild irritations. While their response may be out of proportion to the actual circumstances it is not unusual during acute grieving and speaks to the tremendous toll that grief extracts, leaving little in reserve for buffering stress. Such emotional upsurges are characteristic of expected grief reactions and represent the body's attempts to process the stresses evoked by the loss (Nagoski & Nagoski, 2019). Unfortunately, they may also cause damaging social and occupational consequences.

Emotional Functioning with Traumatic Grief

Emotional impairment is perhaps the most noticeable component of complex grief. With traumatic loss, mourners may also suffer from PTSD or associated symptoms such as hypervigilance, numbness, dissociation, hypersensitivity, emotional lability, terror, irritability, guilt, and rage (American Psychiatric Association [APA], 2013). Some individuals experiencing traumatic bereavement may become severely depressed, experience frequent panic attacks, or emotional flooding. These reactions can make mourners feel out of control, adding to their fears. In contrast, some traumatically bereaved individuals may suppress their emotions in an attempt to maintain self-control and thereby further exacerbate the inner turmoil they experience.

From an emotional standpoint, the survivor of trauma is attempting to process not only the loss of a loved one but the traumatic circumstances surrounding the loss. There is often a strong tendency to avoid thoughts and feelings about the deceased because they bring up disturbing images and sensations. These emotional states interweave and influence each other, and may cause the mourner to become stuck and unable to continue through the natural grief process (Howarth, 2011). With traumatic grief, suicidal ideation is of particular concern and should be continually assessed and monitored by a trained practitioner (Shear, 2015). Consultation or supervision is highly recommended if suicidality is suspected or present in any form regardless of the practitioner's expertise.

BEHAVIORAL FUNCTIONING

Behavioral Functioning with Expected Grief

While in mourning, people engage in a wide variety of behaviors as they try to adjust to the absence of their loved one (Stroebe et al., 2001; Worden, 2018). Because feelings and behaviors are inextricably tied together, when a person's feelings are in turmoil, their behavior can also be erratic and unstable. For example, when experiencing overwhelming sadness and loneliness, one may become more withdrawn and isolated as socializing with others becomes more difficult. Similarly, decreased feelings of motivation can make it very difficult to accomplish simple daily tasks.

A person's behavior reflects their attempt to cope with the grief experience. These behaviors exist on a continuum from life-enhancing to life-depleting that can either help or hinder the adaptation process. Life-enhancing behaviors are those activities that nourish and promote healing within the mourner. These behaviors have health-promoting benefits and cause no harm to self or others. Life-depleting behaviors, on the other hand, may have damaging consequences to the mourner or others. These behaviors stifle the grief process by directing energy into unhealthy and unproductive activities. Table 4.1 provides some examples of life-enhancing and life-depleting behaviors.

TABLE 4.1 Examples of Common Behaviors Associated with Grief

Life-Enhancing Behaviors	Life-Depleting Behaviors
• Crying • Talking about the loss • Reaching out for support • Accepting assistance • Getting rest/sleep • Exercising • Taking care of oneself • Seeking symbolic connection with the deceased • Forming and maintaining new attachments	• Substance abuse • High risk-taking behaviors • Compulsive/excessive behaviors (e.g. eating, shopping, working, gambling) • Withdrawal and isolation • Agitated, aggressive, and demanding behaviors • Anxiety-driven behaviors • Suicidal gestures or attempts

At any given time during the grief process, some of these behaviors may be life-enhancing at one point and life-depleting at another time. For example, while crying can provide a healthy release of emotions, endless and excessive crying may exhaust the mourner to the extent that they are unable to carry out daily and necessary tasks. In this case, the bereaved individual can benefit from learning strategies for regulating emotions in order to manage the sadness they experience. This doesn't mean clients are advised to suppress their tears or made to feel that crying is inappropriate. Rather, the practitioner recognizes that the inability to regulate emotions drains the mourner of needed energy for daily living and building a life without the deceased. Therefore, an understanding of the subtle complexities of grief and its behavioral expression is an important component of counseling bereaved individuals.

Behavioral Functioning with Traumatic Grief

The behaviors of mourners experiencing traumatic grief often have a more complicated motivation behind them as compared with expected grief: fear and avoidance. They may be more inclined to engage in activities that distract them from thoughts about the loved one or the death event. In addition, the traumatic aspects of the loss may prompt actions that have the goal of managing their felt sense of danger, such as withdrawal, isolation, and hypervigilance.

According to neuroscientists, many behavioral responses can be attributed to the seeking circuitry of the brain. Also referred to as the reward circuitry, this grouping of interconnected neurons provides motivation to put effort into a behavior. Often this is done as a means to try and avoid unpleasant experiences. When distress is especially high, the seeking circuitry may become intensely concentrated on quick fixes to provide an instantaneous escape from the discomfort (Hopper, 2015). Compulsive behaviors, such as substance abuse, overeating, gambling, excessive working, shopping, watching television, or being on social media may be attempts to push away the distress brought on by the loss.

BOX 4.2 ATTACHMENT ORIENTATION AND BEHAVIORS IN COUNSELING

A mourner's attachment orientation may also explain their behavior in relationship with counselors (Mikulincer & Shaver, 2014; Shaver & Mikulincer, 2011). Because they doubt their ability to deal with life stresses, anxiously attached individuals are more likely to openly express their emotions and seek help from others. They may bond easily with the counselor, prolong therapy sessions, and seek contact with the practitioner between sessions due to their desperate need to attach to someone who can provide the strength and insight they do not have. They may be open to suggestions that will help them but lack follow-through. These behaviors reflect their learning that hanging on to their pain and declaring it to others improves the probability that their needs for connection and security will be met (Kosminsky & Jordan, 2016).

Avoidantly attached individuals tend to minimize their feelings and often reject the suggestion that they need assistance in managing the loss. They find themselves in counseling at the insistence of others or when their strategy of suppressing their feelings stops working. They may give the impression that they are not in touch with their feelings about the loss or speak about it on an intellectual level and not an emotional one. They gravitate toward concrete advice and tools that can help them "move on with their lives" (Kosminsky & Jordan, 2016). Avoidantly attached individuals may be more likely to engage in life-depleting behaviors in an effort to avoid or minimize their distress.

PHYSICAL FUNCTIONING

Physical Functioning with Expected Grief

Many people experience physical changes or ailments after the death of their loved one. It is as if bereaved persons are "hard-wired" to grieve, with the repercussions of the loss manifesting in their physical being. These symptoms vary widely among individuals and different cultural groups and often include fatigue, tightness in the chest, headaches, stomachaches, insomnia or hypersomnia, increase or decrease in appetite, and a wide variety of aches and pains. There is evidence linking acute grief to increases in heart rate, blood pressure, cortisol levels, as well as disruptions in the sleep cycle and immune system functioning (Shear, 2015). In addition, medical conditions that were present prior to the loss may become more severe during the grieving process. The discomfort of physical or medical problems has a synergistic effect on a person's cognitive, emotional, and social functioning as they struggle to cope with the loss.

An additional influence on physical functioning relates to the role that individuals who share an attachment bond have on each other. There is considerable research suggesting that co-regulation occurs in close relationships between individuals and assists in maintaining emotional and physiological homeostasis (Butler & Randall, 2012). Sbarra and Hazan (2008) suggest that losing a loved one that had provided that regulation accounts for the physical symptoms experienced during bereavement. Though taxing and unpleasant, these changes assist the bereaved to recalibrate in the absence of their co-regulator, the deceased.

Individuals who present with physical complaints should be referred to a medical professional for a thorough assessment and treatment. Following a medical examination, practitioners can often help individuals with physical symptoms that appear to be stress related, rather than medical in nature. With consent of the client, practitioners can collaborate closely with physicians to provide a holistic intervention.

Physical Functioning with Traumatic Grief

When grief is traumatic, the tie between emotional and physiological responses is often intensified and persists in duration. The ongoing state of arousal and hypervigilance experienced by sufferers of trauma is a function of the body's continual secretion of cortisol, the essential hormone activated when responding to a threat. When the danger, or *perception* of danger, does not relent, physical symptoms associated with stress may become severe and lead to long-term health problems.

Research has firmly established that trauma causes health problems. In 1998 doctors Robert Anda and Vincent Felitti, in collaboration with the Centers for Disease Control and Prevention (CDC) and Kaiser Permanente, published an extensive study on the childhood experiences and medical histories of over 17,000 patients. The revelations were startling in their enormity and scope. With regards to physical health alone, those who experienced trauma in their family as children were significantly more likely to develop one of the leading causes of death in the United States, including chronic obstructive pulmonary disease (COPD), ischemic heart disease, and liver disease, as well cancer, emphysema, and substance dependence (Felitti et al., 1998). Dependence on alcohol or other drugs may also develop as mourners attempt to numb their pain or avoid distressing thoughts involving the loss (Dyregrov, Cimitan, et al., 2014).

SOCIAL FUNCTIONING

Social Functioning with Expected Grief

While grieving, an individual's social environment (friends, family, co-workers, and neighbors) can be very influential in how well the mourner is able to cope with the loss and the events that follow (Mancini & Bonanno, 2009; Mikulincer & Shaver, 2009; Rubin et al., 2012; Scheidt et al., 2012). A strong, active, and sensitive social support system can greatly ameliorate the painful feelings associated with grief (Dyregrov, De Leo, et al., 2014). Any support, both tangible and intangible, that reduces the stress and strain that comes with losing a loved one can contribute significantly to the life-enhancing aspects of the grief process. For example, a neighbor might volunteer to mow the yard of a newly widowed man. A close friend may give a grieving spouse a needed break by keeping her children for an evening. Organizations, churches, or work colleagues may coordinate the delivery of meals to a family who has lost a loved one. A trusted friend can listen patiently as the bereaved talks about the deceased and the new challenges that come with the loss. Mourners who are able to accept such offers of support are often able to adjust and adapt more easily than individuals who isolate themselves from support with their grief.

Grief, however, can also present multiple challenges for mourners in their relationships with others. The taxing effects of grief on the bereaved often leave little energy for socializing, which over time may create distance in social relationships. Furthermore, with their renewed perspective on what is important and the loss of the person with whom they could have intimate and meaningful interactions, mourners may crave a deeper level of intimacy from their relationships. They often report a diminished tolerance for superficial conversations which can feel trifling and tiring (Dyregrov & Dyregrov, 2008). Some friendships will be up for this task while others will fall by the wayside.

Some members of a mourner's support system may attempt to be helpful in ways that are insensitive and inappropriate. For example, mourners often report feeling angry and discounted upon hearing clichés about grief such as "He's in a better place now" or "At least he's no longer in pain." Such statements and actions reflect little understanding of grief and are often felt as unsupportive by the mourner despite the good intentions with which they were offered. Even close friends of the mourner may feel awkward and ill-equipped to provide support or assistance. Instead, they may avoid the person or avoid discussions about the loss due to their own discomfort. When mourners perceive that their support system does not understand their grief, it can be experienced as a secondary loss, heightening feelings of loneliness, abandonment, and despair.

Additionally, the attachment orientation of the bereaved person may also play a role in how mourners function socially. While securely attached individuals will have an easier time utilizing existing social connections and making new ones, anxiously attached and avoidantly attached individuals will face greater difficulty. Their support system is typically fewer in number, and they often report feeling disappointed with the support they are given (Collins & Feeney, 2004; Dykas & Cassidy, 2011).

Social Functioning with Traumatic Grief

Individuals experiencing traumatic grief often face intensified challenges in their social environment. While the initial response to survivors of traumatic loss may be extremely supportive, assistance and understanding over the long term often wanes dramatically. This may be in part due to the horror associated with traumatic deaths, such as homicide and suicide. For example, while the death of an aging parent may be expected and ordinary, the death of a loved one to murder or suicide is unexpected and unnerving.

As a consequence, traumatically bereaved persons often feel out of place and uncertain about how to interact with others. As Dyregrov and Dyregrov (2008) explain,

> Interaction with others is characterized by a number of questions. Who can we speak with? How should we behave? Can we say what we really feel? Shall we explain what happened? Do we have the energy to explain? What do I reply when they ask how it's going? What will they think of us? What if I meet someone who does not know what has happened? When is it appropriate to start going out again, to laugh and live a normal life, etc.?
>
> (p. 47)

Mourners must also contend with the reactions of others when the loss is brought up during social interactions. Bereaved survivors of suicide, for example, often report that conversation about the deceased can quickly become awkward when the cause of death is disclosed. One mourner explains, "When the death of my husband's uncle came up everyone expressed lots of caring and sympathy. But when the conversation turned to my friend and that she died by suicide, everyone got very quiet and changed the subject."

Mourners who become stalled in their grief may find that connecting with others is difficult and unfulfilling as they remain focused on their loss. This can result in estrangement from their support system. Additionally, trauma survivors who face a minefield of potential triggers when they leave the safety of their home may be more inclined to isolate from others. Furthermore, distance in relationships may increase when others try to be of assistance but their attempts are not helpful. Over time this becomes frustrating to family and friends who then further withdraw from contact with the mourner (Shear, 2015).

SPIRITUAL FUNCTIONING

Spiritual Functioning with Expected Grief

The death of a loved one often has profound effects on the spiritual well-being of the survivors who are mourning the loss. Because there is a vast diversity of spiritual beliefs and expressions among individuals that may or may not overlap with religious ideology and institutions, a broad interpretation of spirituality is helpful for understanding how this fundamental human quality intertwines with the grief experience. Hence, spirituality can be explained as "the aspect of humanity that refers to the way individuals seek and express meaning and purpose and the way they experience their connectedness to the moment, to self, to others, to nature, and to the significant or sacred" (Puchalski et al., 2009, p. 886).

Witnessing or being closely tied to the dying process is for many people a life-altering experience that provokes existential questions of why we exist and what is the meaning of life. This spiritual examination by the bereaved "provides both a place to stand and a potential point of leverage that can alter and reorganize the meaning of life, the relationship with the deceased, the deceased's life, and the meaning of the loss" (Rubin et al., 2012, p. 217). For some mourners, their faith is an internal strength that provides an anchor of comfort, hope, and security during a turbulent time. Their relationship with God serves as a symbolic attachment figure that is looked to for comfort during times of duress (Granqvist & Kirkpatrick, 2013). While research confirms that observance of religious beliefs and practices generally lessens distress (Burke & Neimeyer, 2014), it is common for believers to also experience transitory moments of disappointment, blame, and anger with God (Exline & Martin, 2005).

When facing the death of a loved one, some individuals will find themselves on a quest to ascertain the meaning of their experience and more generally the meaning of life. Beliefs, goals, and values may be questioned and re-considered in light of the loss. Some mourners search for a larger meaning in the loss as a way to mitigate the pain and regain a sense of safety and control. With time, many bereaved emerge from this experience with a renewed and clearer perspective on what is important and subsequently make alterations in their lives to reflect these priorities.

Spiritual Functioning with Traumatic Grief

Grief that is traumatic has considerable potential to unravel the very essence of a mourner's spiritual constitution (Sangster & Lee, 2017). Survivors of traumatic grief are more likely to experience severe and extensive doubt and disillusionment about their entire faith system (Pearlman et al., 2014). Questions such as "What kind of God would let this happen?" or "Is there really a God?" may become prominent as they try to process their grief. They may feel disappointed, angry, and betrayed when their faith is insufficient in alleviating their pain. While momentary anger with God is an expected component of the grief process, traumatically bereaved persons may experience this for a prolonged time which can contribute to poor adjustment (Exline & Rose, 2005). Some report feeling that they are being punished by God or that, if only they could believe more fervently in their faith, the pain from their loss would be tolerable. Insensitive responses from church representatives can also cause mourners to feel alienated and abandoned from their faith or faith community. Often the result is that mourners vigorously question or reject their existing beliefs and find themselves in a spiritual crisis (Burke & Neimeyer, 2014). In all of these situations, the disconnection from one's faith is often experienced as a secondary loss.

Similarly, traumatic grief often catalyzes mourners to question their assumptions and beliefs about how the world works (Wortman & Pearlman, 2016). Subconscious beliefs about the world and the self supply fundamental feelings of safety and security. Presumptions that the world is fair and predictable, that the self is invincible, and that others are altruistic provide the feeling of being in control and protected from danger. These assumptive worldviews distract us from our mortality and enable us to go about our lives with a felt sense of security and minimal anxiety (Smith et al., 2015). When a trauma occurs, such as with traumatic loss, these assumptive worldviews rupture. Without the protection of these beliefs, mourners may experience prolonged and chronic distress (Smith et al., 2015).

Additionally, survivors of traumatic grief are more likely to experience pervasive feelings of guilt related to the loss and find ways to blame themselves for the death (Kosminsky & Jordan, 2016). This may be an unconscious attempt to fit the loss into the mourner's existing worldviews. For example, it may be less distressing to believe that the death could have been prevented than to believe that random, horrible things happen which ruptures illusions of control.

ASSESSING GRIEF IN ADULTS USING STANDARDIZED INSTRUMENTS

Though standardized instruments for issues for grief and loss can be useful in counseling at times, they are primarily used in research. For issues related to trauma, however, standardized instruments are more often used. Many times, clients whose presenting problem is grief also have a co-occurring condition such as depression, anxiety, or other mental health issue. Useful assessment instruments for adults with expected and traumatic grief are listed in Chapter 3.

BOX 4.3 MOURNING RITUALS: BUDDHISM

Buddhist rituals are designed to assist with the transition from death to rebirth. Buddhists believe that the person's state of mind at the time of their death influences their process of rebirth. For this reason, chants of the Buddha's teachings are performed to calm the dying individual. After death, the corpse is positioned on its right side and covered except for the crown of the head. The body is kept in the home or temple with depictions of Buddhas and burning incense placed nearby. Outside of where the body rests, family members make offerings, such as flowers or fruit, to sway the deceased's soul to leave the body. Additionally, a priest provides guidance to the corpse to assist in the transition between life forms (Hidalgo, 2017). Generally, the corpse is cremated as this is believed to help the soul vacate its physical form. Among Buddhists in the United States there is great diversity in mourning rituals depending on location and cultural origins. Some families blend Christian beliefs into their funeral rituals, while others exclusively follow Buddhist practices (Buddhist Funerals Guide, n.d.).

THE INFLUENCE OF CULTURE ON GRIEF REACTIONS

As discussed in Chapter 1, practitioners must exercise cultural humility when working with bereaved persons and consider the client's needs within the context of their cultural environment, including their family grief culture. Outside of the fundamental, internal experience of loss, the primary measure of how one is managing their grief is often shaped by the broader context in which they must function. Many who grieve do not require intervention. For those that seek help, it is often because they are being told by family and friends that they are not grieving correctly or have in some way absorbed the message that their experience is at odds with their community's expectation of them. Even in cultures that provide ample permission and space for mourners to experience their grief, if bereaved persons do not want or need to grieve in that way, they may experience difficulty (Rosenblatt, 2017).

When a person's grief experience – including their way of expressing (or not expressing) their grief, their level of functioning, and how they adapt to the loss – is at odds with the paradigm of their community or the broader culture, this may cause distress. In working with persons of different cultures, practitioners must set aside their own preconceived notions about what constitutes healthy versus unhealthy grief responses. Only when considered within the context of the client's own cultural environment can the counselor know how to be helpful. For example, while it is commonly presumed that talking about the loss can be helpful, some cultures believe this invites misfortune. This was the experience of Hsu et al. (2004) in studying the experience of Taiwanese women who had a stillbirth. They faced enormous difficulty persuading women to talk to them due to the prevailing belief among the women that discussing the loss would bring bad luck and incur disfavor from their families.

Practitioners will want to make note of grief reactions that are blocking the client's ability to receive social support, maintain basic functioning, and, with time, adapt to the loss. Practitioners must be acutely aware when making determinations that a client's grief is lasting too long, not long enough, is too emotional, or not emotional enough. Such appraisals must be checked, with the inquiry of "according to whom?" (Rosenblatt, 2016). What may seem strange or intolerable to the practitioner may be customary and helpful for the client. Mourners must be allowed the dignity and respect to respond to their loss in ways that are authentic and best fit their needs.

In addition to the clients' socio-cultural context, practitioners must be mindful of the role that socio-economic and broader social justice issues play in how clients experience their grief. This includes how their grief is regarded by others, the kind of grieving that is deemed acceptable, and the availability of culturally relevant support and assistance. In addition, it must be noted that the loss experience of marginalized and oppressed populations has historical origins and cumulative implications for members of these groups (Bordere, 2019; Lipscomb & Ashley, 2018).

INTERVENTIONS

Interventions grounded in the strengths-based framework of grief and loss place particular emphasis on honoring the value and dignity of clients, incorporating the client's strengths, and cultivating hope for a fulfilling future. Any impediments to progress are viewed as opportunities to employ different strategies and help the client develop new strengths (Pomeroy & Garcia, 2018). Strengths-based interventions reinforce life-enhancing coping skills and call attention to healthy adaptations mourners make as they navigate the path toward adjustment. This may include validating and encouraging the release of intense emotions, giving permission for the bereaved to have a break from their grief and enjoy aspects of life, and recognizing and supporting positive growth that has come about due to the loss.

The primary goals of grief counseling are to help the mourner find life-enhancing ways to honor and cope with the emotions of grief, while also creating a fulfilling life without the physical presence of the deceased. Professional intervention may be needed when the natural process of accommodation to the loss is obstructed (Shear & Bloom, 2017). This involves helping clients learn to manage the difficult cognitive, emotional, physical, social, and spiritual disruptions brought on by grief, identify alternative ways of moving through life without the deceased, and assimilate the changes caused by their shaken worldview (Cole, 2021).

As mourners fluctuate between feeling the loss and creating a new life without their loved one, the practitioner must be attuned to periods when the client is stuck and needs assistance moving forward. At times, individuals may need more guidance in learning to regulate their emotions and invest in rebuilding a life without the deceased. This may be particularly relevant for anxiously attached individuals. At other times, mourners may need the practitioner's assistance in allowing and managing the emotional aspects of the loss. This may be the predominant approach used with avoidantly attached individuals (Kosminsky & Jordan, 2016). The practitioner's ability to start where the client is and skillfully nudge them in the appropriate direction is the art of grief counseling.

The specific ways that practitioners help bereaved clients depends on the unique circumstances of the loss and the challenges the mourner is facing at any given point in time. In general, grief counseling involves three components that operate together: strength building, trauma processing, and mourning the loss (Wortman & Pearlman, 2016).

STRENGTH BUILDING

Consistent with the strengths-based framework of grief and loss, the employment and development of the mourner's individual and environmental strengths is a central element of helping mourners adapt to their loss. By activating the bereaved person's competencies, confidence, aspirations, and opportunities, mourners become better equipped to persevere through the journey of loss and adaptation. Counselors assist clients with strength building in a variety of ways, that include establishing the therapeutic relationship, providing psychoeducation, teaching emotional regulation, promoting self-care, managing and mobilizing social support, problem solving, and clarifying values.

Establishing the Therapeutic Relationship

Central to the effectiveness of counseling and a component of strength building is the relationship that is developed between the counselor and the client. Counseling is a healing endeavor only when clients feel trusting of the practitioner, and this is especially true with the vulnerable experience of expected and traumatic grief. Practitioners earn their clients' trust through the use of rapport-building skills, empathic listening, unconditional positive regard, ethical and appropriate boundaries, and respect for the mourner's values and cultural influences (Pomeroy & Garcia, 2018).

Grief counselors must also demonstrate that they are capable of tolerating the client's intense emotions in a calm and non-judgmental manner. The security that mourners derive from the relationship with the practitioner creates a steady anchor for confronting the pain and fear that are endemic to the grief and loss experience. It also serves as a safeguard for exploring the uncharted territory of life without their loved one. In many ways, grief counselors serve as transitional attachment figures for bereaved persons. Just as parents help children regulate their responses to distress, connection between practitioner and client helps the client stay emotionally regulated during counseling sessions, thereby enabling them to achieve a more productive experience of the counseling endeavor (Kosminsky & Jordan, 2016). For individuals with an insecure attachment style, this function is of supreme importance and can lead to opportunities for the client to learn and experience healthy relationships.

Psychoeducation

Practitioners can use psychoeducation with great effectiveness to help clients understand their situation and know what is realistic to expect from themselves while they are grieving. Accurate information about grief and trauma attenuates the cognitive, emotional, physical, social, and spiritual changes the client experiences and mitigates negative self-judgments about how they are coping. Information can help clients adopt realistic expectations regarding the "two steps forward, one step back" nature of the grief process. It also empowers them to make more informed and reasonable decisions about their lives. The use of psychoeducation is immensely valuable in helping mourners accept and accommodate the stressful aspects of their grief process as well as empowering them to manage the larger context within which they have their experience.

Emotional Regulation

Healing from grief requires that the bereaved be capable of synthesizing new information, trying on new perspectives, and learning new skills. This is especially challenging when one is also experiencing the raw pain that naturally accompanies loss. An understanding of Polyvagal Theory, as discussed in the following paragraph, is helpful for guiding clients to learn to regulate their emotional experience.

According to Polyvagal Theory, when clients become hyper-aroused their sympathetic nervous system is activated and initiates the defense cascade. In this state, clients may experience emotional flooding, intrusive images, and racing or ruminative thoughts. They may perceive themselves to be unsafe and thus are on guard against danger. Conversely, when a client's parasympathetic nervous system is engaged, they become hypo-aroused as a last ditch way to survive what feels like an impossible situation. Just as animals will "play dead" when attempting to survive a more powerful predator, when this freeze state is activated clients shut down, display little or no emotion, feel numb and disconnected, and are incapable of clear thoughts or actions. The optimal balance exists in between hyper-arousal and hypo-arousal. It occurs in the ventral vagal system and is aptly referred to as the "window of tolerance." When in their window of tolerance, clients can access both their emotions and thoughts. This allows for social interaction, new learning, and adaptive responses (Porges & Dana, 2018).

Practitioners play a key role in helping clients access and expand their window of tolerance while coming to grips with the loss of their loved one. Therapeutic skills that can assist with this include grounding, relaxation, breath training, visualization, mindfulness, and meditation (Levine, 2012; van der Kolk, 2014). Some clients may have difficulty using these techniques without the support of psychotropic medication. In such cases, practitioners will want to collaborate closely with the client's physician.

Self-Care

Due to the physiological disruptions caused by expected and traumatic grief, it is important for practitioners to coach clients on self-care practices and encourage their use. Because mourners typically feel unmoored, overwhelmed, and uncertain in the wake of their loss, they can benefit from reminders to attend to their basic needs, e.g. rest, nutrition, and hydration. Attention to sleep is particularly important and may include education on sleep hygiene or a referral to a medical professional. In some instances, it may be useful for the practitioner to collaborate with clients' physicians. Some mourners need "permission" to simplify their life, lower their work and social commitments, and engage in activities that are soothing. With this support, mourners can more easily allow themselves to enjoy pleasant moments when they arise and get needed respites from the grief experience.

Managing and Mobilizing Social Support

Practitioners can also help mourners manage the social implications of being bereaved and coach them on developing and using social support. This may include helping them mobilize existing support and discern who among their social network can be helpful and in what manner. Practitioners can also help mourners reframe feelings of guilt they may have about requesting and accepting help. Ideally, the bereaved become empowered to educate their support system about their particular needs, both practical and psychological. Because connecting with others who are also grieving can be enormously helpful, practitioners can also provide referrals to support groups and grief retreats.

Problem Solving

Practitioners can facilitate productive problem solving as clients navigate the numerous practical challenges that emerge after the death of a loved one. They may help clients find workable solutions for dilemmas related to work, school, or family, such as finding adequate childcare, adjusting household expenses, or navigating social situations. When the death was caused by criminal activity, the bereaved may need assistance in navigating the legal system and coping with the stresses brought on by the judicial process. Practitioners can be especially helpful with challenges on how to approach holidays without the deceased, cope with the deceased's birthday and death anniversary, decisions regarding the deceased's possessions, or how the loved one will be memorialized.

Clarifying Values

Because of the fundamental way that loss can alter a person's sense of purpose and how they understand and interface with the world, mourners can benefit from reconnecting to, and in some cases redefining, their values. Shear and Bloom (2017) suggest that bereaved persons can be prompted to engage in the work of re-inventing their lives by asking "What would you want for yourself if your grief was at a manageable level?" (p. 11). The answer to this question can be used as a launching point for setting goals and subsequently outlining small steps that enable the bereaved individual to achieve these aspirations. These newly formed intentions may reflect thoughts and feelings that honor the loved one (e.g. raise money for cancer research) or new perspectives and insights that were obtained from the experience of grief (e.g. take better care of their health, spend more time with family). Additionally, Acceptance and Commitment Therapy (ACT) provides some helpful techniques in assisting clients to clarify what is important to them and then engage in actions to demonstrate that in their lives (Harris, 2009; Speedlin et al., 2016).

TRAUMA PROCESSING

Helping traumatically bereaved persons requires advanced clinical skills and a strategic approach that addresses both the trauma and the grief concurrently (Pearlman et al., 2014). Because trauma symptoms can interfere with the grief process, healing involves removing the barriers that prevent the natural process of grief from unfolding (Shear & Bloom, 2017; Wetherell, 2012). These barriers may take the form of flashbacks, intrusive and disturbing thoughts, distressing memories, disrupted sleep, avoidance of feelings, and life-depleting behaviors (Wortman & Pearlman, 2016). Interventions used for processing trauma require sufficient training and clinical expertise on the part of practitioners. Commonly used approaches include cognitive methods, exposure techniques, Eye Movement Desensitization and Reprocessing (EMDR), and body-based approaches.

Cognitive Approaches

Cognitive approaches to processing trauma involve identifying and then challenging the automatic thoughts that cause distress. The cognitions may pertain to negative thoughts that the bereaved might hold about themselves, e.g. "I'm a bad person," others, e.g. "No one can be trusted," or humankind, e.g. "The world is not safe."

Practitioners help mourners by challenging these irrational thoughts and replacing them with more helpful and adaptive thoughts (Wortman & Pearlman, 2016). Studies have shown that there are limitations to this approach because, while it addresses clients' intellectual interpretations of the trauma, it has little impact on the physiological changes that have resulted from the traumatic experience (van der Kolk, 2014).

Exposure Techniques

Exposure techniques have been used to help clients manage the emotional aspects of trauma with the goal of gradually desensitizing their responses to the loss and the traumatic aspects of the loss. In summary, this approach involves having clients repeatedly focus on distressing aspects of the loss until they no longer produce an emotional response. While there is research to support this method, it requires strong commitment and great fortitude on the part of the client to sustain the difficult emotions that are required to participate in this intervention. Clients often approach these sessions with dread, if they attend at all, and show an increase in maladaptive symptoms (Corrigan & Hull, 2015; van der Kolk, 2014).

Eye Movement Desensitization and Reprocessing (EMDR)

EMDR is a technique for treating trauma that is backed by substantial research, including studies that examine fMRI imaging of the brain. Through the use of bilateral stimulation of the right and left sides of the brain, EMDR allows survivors to revisit the trauma without being overwhelmed by it. Because they remain within their window of tolerance, survivors are able to view the event from an expanded perspective, learn from it, and integrate it. It becomes a "coherent event in the past, instead of experiencing sensations and images divorced from any context" (van der Kolk, 2014, p. 255). The administration of EMDR follows specific and precise protocols which must be followed so that clients are not further harmed while engaged with the traumatic material. Therefore, EMDR can be provided only by practitioners that receive this specialized training. For the treatment of complex PTSD, advanced certification in EMDR is strongly recommended. More can be learned about EMDR by visiting the EMDR International Association at EMDRIA.org.

Body-Based Approaches

Because of the physiological changes that occur as a result of trauma exposure, interventions that focus on the body can provide transformative results for survivors. One such intervention is Somatic Experiencing (SE) which uses knowledge of the nervous system to alleviate the lingering effects of traumatic experiences. Peter Levine developed the technique based on his observations of animals in the wild and comparing how they recover from danger to how humans respond to threats, both physical and emotional (Levine & Frederick, 1997). SE focuses on physical sensations which are believed to represent unfinished, biologically based defensive responses that were activated in an attempt to secure safety from the threat. By titrating mindful attention to those sensations, the body is allowed to gently complete the defensive action thereby releasing its need to hold on to the threat. For example, during a session of SE therapy, a trauma survivor who was held down during an assault may find his legs moving as if he were running away from the attacker. By releasing the stuck energy that he was unable to use during the attack, the biological response to the threat is complete and the trauma is healed. This resolution is able to occur without the client having to recount the trauma in extensive detail (Levine, 2012).

Other body-based techniques, such as yoga, have been used to process feelings of grief. Yoga provides relief from the somatic symptoms of grief (Stang, 2016) and lends itself to increased focus on the present moment. In addition, by involving postures that are uncomfortable, yoga teaches that discomfort is bearable (Stirling, 2016). Yoga is also beneficial as an adjunct intervention for trauma and has proven useful in helping traumatized individuals regulate their emotions through conscious attention to breath and by promoting greater awareness of the body (van der Kolk et al., 2014). When used for this purpose, the yoga environment and behavior of instructors is modified to respect the sensitivities of trauma survivors (Nguyen-Feng et al., 2019). More information about the Trauma Sensitive Yoga curriculum, developed by Dave Emerson, can be found at traumasensitiveyoga.com.

MOURNING THE LOSS

Practitioners can facilitate the client's process of confronting and adapting to the reality that their loved one is deceased in several ways. These include telling the story of the loss, remembering the deceased, mourning secondary losses, acknowledging continuing bonds with the deceased, finding meaning in the loss, and identifying and working toward new life goals.

Telling the Story of the Loss

While also important for gathering assessment information, most clients will benefit from telling the story of the loss and reflecting on how it has impacted their life. This seems to be one way the bereaved gradually puncture the numbness and sense of unreality that is typical of the days and weeks immediately following the death. As the therapeutic relationship strengthens, they may revisit the story multiple times with a focus on different pieces of the story. As this occurs, practitioners allow clients to emote freely and, if necessary, provide assistance with trauma processing while also helping them remain within their window of tolerance. Practitioners will want to listen for and encourage the gradual resolution of guilt feelings, decrease fixation on needing answers to unanswerable questions, and promote signs of acceptance which will naturally wax and wane. Life-enhancing coping skills and feelings of hope for the future are also noted and encouraged.

Remembering the Deceased

Many bereaved persons also find a measure of comfort and relief in activities that allow them to remember and reminisce about the deceased. This may take the form of simply talking to others about their loved one to more tangible projects that memorialize the deceased. There are an endless number of ways mourners try to stay connected to the memory of their beloved ranging from keeping pictures and memorabilia of the person who died nearby, making a quilt from the shirts of the deceased, planting a tree in the person's honor, or raising money for a cause that was relevant to the loved one's life. Practitioners will want to support the culturally specific ways that the bereaved remember family or friends. For example, Dia de los Muertos, or Day of the Dead, is celebrated by many Mexican families. The festivities include decorating the loved one's gravesite and building altars that contain memorabilia, pictures, and the deceased's favorite foods and drinks. These actions are believed to attract the loved one's spirit in order to receive the offerings and know they are remembered by the living.

Mourning Secondary Losses

As time goes on, mourners begin to experience the secondary losses that result from their loved one's death. Practitioners can be helpful by naming these losses and assisting mourners on recognizing how these have altered the meaning they ascribe to their lives. For example, the loss of a spouse may mean the loss of companionship, sexual intimacy, and hopes and plans for a future together. The disruption of assumptive worldviews caused by the death can also represent secondary losses that mourners must learn to accommodate.

Acknowledging Continuing Bonds with the Deceased

In addition to remembering the deceased, some mourners will naturally seek a connection with their loved ones. In a sense, they are attempting to find a symbolic place for the deceased in their lives. This follows with the Continuing Bonds theory which acknowledges the benefits that an ongoing relationship with the deceased can have for the bereaved (see Chapter 1 for more discussion on Continuing Bonds). If it has been determined that it would be helpful, practitioners can encourage mourners to develop this relationship, share with mourners the various forms that continuing bonds can take, and help them discern what types of symbolic connections will be meaningful, healthy, and adaptive (Currier et al., 2015; Field et al., 2013). There are various ways continuing bonds can be expressed, including talking to the lost loved one, writing letters to them, or participating in an activity they enjoyed.

When the relationship with the deceased was conflictual, mourners may require additional assistance from practitioners. Letter writing and the Gestalt empty chair technique can be used to repair any unresolved conflict by allowing mourners to symbolically communicate thoughts and feelings that could not be expressed when the deceased was alive. This safe expression allows for increased awareness and new insights regarding their feelings toward the deceased. These activities can help the bereaved come to a sense of resolution in their relationship with the deceased and create a new reference point from which to begin moving forward with their life.

When mourners are overwhelmed by feelings of guilt, practitioners can employ cognitive methods to methodically re-examine their experiences and understand their actions and reasoning at the time (De Leo et al., 2014). For paralyzing guilt that is not amenable to these methods, performing activities that symbolize penance for perceived or actual wrongs that were done to the deceased may be helpful. For example, a man bereaved by the suicide of his wife participated in efforts to educate others about mental illness and the warning signs of suicide. By giving others the information he wished he'd had, he was eventually able to stop berating himself for not recognizing that his wife was struggling. EMDR has also been shown to be helpful in relieving disturbing aspects of the grief process, such as guilt and anger with the loved one (Solomon & Rando, 2007).

Finding Meaning in the Loss

Many, though not all, bereaved persons are naturally inclined to ascribe meaning to the death of their loved one. Some will do this by trying to "make sense" of the death in the context of their existing worldviews of safety, justice, control, order, and predictability. When the loss does not easily align with these appraisals, they may be compelled to alter their worldviews as a way to integrate the loss. Some may approach this by identifying benefits ("silver linings") that come as a result of the death ("I've learned to appreciate life more"), or by allowing it to change how they identify themselves ("sadder but wiser") (Hibberd, 2013, p. 678). Others manage this need by seeking and clarifying their purpose in life and their reason to continue living despite hardship. An additional way that some will make meaning of their loved one's death is by finding significance in life. This approach emphasizes values that supersede the self and are worth living for, for their own sake. Approaching meaning making from this angle may be especially helpful when the death was a result of violence (Hibberd, 2013). Examples of finding life significance against the backdrop of loss can be found in the following statements made by bereaved individuals:

- "I now see every day as a gift. I spend my time appreciating all the beauty around me."
- "I realize that I, too, will die someday. I want to spend my remaining time on earth doing something that will make things better for those that come after me."
- "I no longer take for granted the time I have with the people I love. Those moments of connection are everything."

Practitioners can help with the process of making meaning from the loss by asking questions that encourage reflection and discernment.

Identifying New Life Goals

A key aspect of healing from loss involves re-engaging with life and the world that has been changed by the loved one's absence. Practitioners may facilitate this process by assisting mourners in building connections with others, clarifying their values, evaluating their current life activities, identifying new goals and, for some, finding meaning in the loss (Smid et al., 2015). They walk with mourners as they attempt to answer the questions, "what now?" and "what matters?" (Hibberd, 2013, p. 681).

Some bereaved persons will intentionally or unintentionally fight against this task, preferring to cling to their pain because it makes them feel connected to their loved one. Pearlman et al. (2014) describe how some mourners experience this:

> The active accommodation of the loss in mourning can feel like resignation, accepting precisely that which one wishes to resist. It can feel tantamount to acknowledging that it is "OK" that the loved one is gone. Such acceptance can seem intolerable. Losing a significant other can leave anyone feeling powerless. Resisting acceptance – whether by remaining within grief or by not moving through mourning more fully – can give the illusion of control, even as it ultimately robs the survivor of true empowerment.
>
> (p. 22)

EMDR has also been shown to be helpful for loved ones who cling to their pain as a way to feel connected to their loved one. Following EMDR therapy, bereaved persons commonly report feeling a stronger sense of connection with the deceased, while also experiencing a lightening of the distress that accompanies the loss (Solomon, 2019). Acceptance and Commitment Therapy (ACT) can also help bereaved persons clarify their values and identify actions that are congruent with these priorities.

COMPLICATED GRIEF TREATMENT (CGT)

Complicated Grief Treatment (CGT) is a treatment protocol that has been extensively tested and proven to be highly effective in treating people who experience complicated grief (Shear et al., 2005, 2014, 2016). Developed by Dr. Katherine Shear, CGT is a 16-session intervention that aims to help mourners adapt to their loss and remove obstacles that inhibit adaptation. Through structured sessions that employ specific methods and processes, CGT helps clients understand their experience with grief, manage difficult emotions, think about the future, strengthen relationships with others, recount the story of the death, and cope with memories of the deceased. The intervention includes techniques that focus on both the loss and on creating a life without the deceased. More information about CGT including access to training, manuals, assessment instruments, and handouts can be found at the Center for Complicated Grief at complicatedgrief.columbia.edu.

STRENGTHS-BASED GROUP INTERVENTIONS FOR ADULTS

In addition to individual counseling, group counseling has been used as a primary vehicle for working with the bereaved (Worden, 2018). Psychoeducational group interventions have been shown to improve well-being and grief resolution, increase social support, and decrease the risk of psychopathology related to unresolved grief issues (Pomeroy & Holleran, 2002). The power of group support and shared, mutual concerns can ameliorate the loneliness and isolation associated with loss. The potential benefit of being with others who share a common experience with grief is far-reaching (Brown, 2018).

The authors have found bereavement groups that combine the strengths-based framework of grief and loss with a psychoeducational format can greatly enhance mourners' feelings of competency in relation to managing grief. The provision of both information and emotional support serves to alleviate some of the painful symptoms associated with loss and allows participants to understand the process of grief in a context that includes not only themselves but others. This approach helps dispel some of the myths and unrealistic expectations associated with the grieving process. Additionally, the mutual sharing of common experiences creates a community from which participants can draw strength. These dynamics assist mourners in developing the individual and environmental strengths that are necessary for the healing process to progress. Not only are psychoeducational groups effective, they are also economically feasible for clients who cannot afford individual counseling as well as for agencies with limited resources (Pomeroy et al., 2015). Internet-based self-help bereavement groups have also been found to be very useful in providing information and support (Brodbeck et al., 2019). The following paragraphs outline a psychoeducational group design that uses the strengths-based framework of grief and loss.

THE STRENGTHS-BASED PSYCHOEDUCATIONAL GROUP DESIGN

Group Goals

The goals for this group are to provide individuals with a safe and structured environment to facilitate healthy adjustment to the absence of the loved one. This is accomplished by building an understanding of the life-enhancing aspects of grief, processing the mourner's adaptation to the loss, promoting awareness about life-depleting grief reactions, and enhancing the mourner's coping skills and resources to engage in a life separate from the loved one. These goals underlie the content of the group sessions (Pomeroy et al., 2015).

Time-limited psychoeducational groups based on the strengths-based framework of grief and loss have been found to be practical and productive because of the structured discussion topics, the life-enhancing coping strategies that are encouraged between group sessions, and the trusting relationships that develop among members. Although the first two sessions focus on the participants' losses, subsequent sessions guide the participants in strengths-based coping skills. The group is six to eight weeks in length and is compatible with agencies that specialize in end of life care, such as hospice or community outpatient clinics. The facilitator of this type of group also serves as a conduit between participants and community resources (Pomeroy et al., 2015).

Group Content

The content of a grief group will be somewhat dependent on the composition of the group members. For example, in a group composed of parents who have lost a child, discussions may focus on the need for communication between the surviving parents.

However, regardless of the specific issues that the members bring to the group, there is certain content that is covered in all groups using the strengths-based psychoeducational approach. These topics include expected grief reactions, adjustment to the loss, navigating transitions, family concerns, using community resources, and engaging in outside activities (Pomeroy et al., 2015).

A Strengths-Based Traumatic Grief Group Intervention

Group intervention can also be effective for mourners experiencing traumatic grief reactions, particularly when membership includes others whose loved ones died in a similar manner. Interventions used in these types of groups are highly specific to the population of survivors. These groups can also provide a buffer from isolation and stigmatized loss (e.g. suicide, drug use, HIV/AIDS, COVID-19).

The authors have found that traumatic grief reactions can be more effectively addressed in a group setting after the mourner has had some individual counseling or has had time to process the trauma associated with the death. While members can benefit from hearing the struggles of others in their situation, processing detailed traumatic material in individual sessions increases the risk of trauma exposure to other group members. Thus, an individual assessment prior to entering a traumatic grief group that considers the degree of trauma and level of crisis, as well as the person's overall mental health status, is recommended (Pomeroy et al., 2015).

CASES

CASE 4.1

Identifying Information:

Client Name: Peggy Mockingbird
Age: 49 years old
Race/Ethnicity: White and Native American, Cherokee tribe
Marital Status: Married
Education Level: College degree
Occupation: Legislative aide

Intake Information:

Mrs. Mockingbird called the Center for Family Survival and stated that she needed to talk to someone due to problems she was having with her job. She believes that these problems may stem from the loss of her mother approximately five months ago. She indicated that she had a very close relationship with her mother who lived in her home prior to her death.

Initial Interview:

Upon greeting Peggy, she responds in a warm and professional manner, shaking your hand firmly. As the two of you walk back to your office, she tells you that she has needed to talk to someone for quite some time. She appears affable and eager to start the session.

You begin by saying, "Tell me why you decided to come in today."

"Like I said, I have been needing to talk to someone for a while but just couldn't find the time to make an appointment. Ever since my mother died, I just don't feel like myself. I feel like I'm going crazy. It has really made things difficult at my job and I've got to get myself together. I've got a stressful job as it is and this is pushing me over the edge."

"Tell me more about work and not feeling like yourself," you say.

Peggy sighs and says, "Well, ever since my mom passed away, I've had a really hard time concentrating and find myself thinking about her a lot. Sometimes I just begin crying for no reason at all. Last week my boss noticed that I had forgotten some details in a report that he needed. He was upset and it put him in a bad position, but I think he was also surprised. That's just not like me. I couldn't tell him that I was still upset about my mother. After all, it's been almost five months. I should be over it by now."

"Actually, most people are still having a hard time after five months. That is not unusual. The grief process takes time. Are there other things you've noticed that have been difficult?"

Peggy slumps in her chair and stares out the window. "I'm just tired all the time. And I don't really care about anything. It is so hard to get myself to work in the morning and I used to love my job. It just all seems meaningless now. I wish I could stay in bed all day. And no matter what I do, I can't seem to feel better."

"Your mother's death has really shaken things up for you, hasn't it?" you ask. "Maybe you could tell me a little bit about what it was like for you when she died."

"Well," Peggy begins, "she was 82 years old when she died, but she had been having health problems for the last few years. She moved in with me and my family about five years ago. When she was diagnosed with congestive heart failure, I couldn't believe it. She seemed too young and active to be that sick. She seemed okay, so I didn't really consider it to be that serious."

"What kind of relationship did you have with your mother?" you inquire.

"We were very close. I mean, we had our occasional spats like mothers and daughters do, but over the years we became good friends and I really liked having her around." Peggy's eyes begin to tear up as she reaches for a tissue. "She was always there for me even though I was taking care of her in the end. I just really miss her!"

"So there's a big empty space in your life now," you respond. Peggy nods. "That is very difficult. Can you tell me about the rest of your family?"

"Well, it's just me and my husband at the house. I have two children but they are both away at college right now. My husband is a very kind man and he is supportive but sometimes I think he doesn't understand why I'm still upset. I also have five brothers and sisters but they don't live here and weren't around much while Mother was dying."

"So you were your mother's primary caregiver throughout her illness?"

"Yes, I had a brother who would come some weekends to see her but it was mostly up to me. I feel so bad. I just keep thinking I should have done more...." Peggy's voice trails off as she turns again to the window.

"It sounds like you were doing a lot. What else do you think you should have done?" you ask gently.

"I don't know. I guess I keep thinking about the day she died. My brother had come for the weekend and I needed to go run some errands. Every time I had to leave her I always hurried so that I could get back to her quickly. But I was so tired and since my brother was there I told myself I could take my time and take care of myself for once. Like, I stopped at the nail salon on the spur of the moment to see if I could get a manicure and they happened to have an opening. I called my brother and told him I was going to be late in getting back. He told me it was no problem and that Mom was sleeping. So, I took the appointment and got my nails done. It was about five o'clock when I started back home. I guess I was about three miles from the house when my brother called and told me to get home fast. He knew I was driving and so he wouldn't tell me what was going on, just that I needed to come home. By the time I got there, she had passed away," Peggy says tearfully. "I couldn't believe it. I've never felt so horrible in my life. I should have been there! I wanted to be there with her." Peggy looks at you with tears streaming down her face.

"So it really bothered you that you weren't there when she died?" you suggest.

Peggy nods, still crying. "I can't get it out of my mind. In our culture, it's important not to die alone and even though my brother was there I feel like I should have been there, too."

"I'm sure you wish you could have been with your mother. I'm wondering if you are blaming yourself for taking a break," you respond.

"I do blame myself in a way. I know in my head that it's not my fault. I know I didn't choose to be gone at her moment of death, but why did I have to get my nails done at *that* time?" Peggy says with a tone of frustration.

"It is normal for people to have regrets when a loved one dies," you explain. "Sometimes we feel bad about things that we can control, but also there are regrets about things that are beyond our control. It seems like you had no way of knowing that your mother was going to die on that particular day."

"You're right," Peggy acknowledges. "I didn't have the slightest idea. I wouldn't have gone out if I had known."

You allow her to digest this information for a few moments as you sit quietly with her. Peggy seems calmer, although a bit subdued.

"Do you have any good memories of your mother?" you ask.

"Oh yes," she says. "A lot. We used to cook together." Peggy continues to talk about good, everyday moments with her mom as well as difficult family transitions they experienced together, such as when Peggy's maternal grandmother died. As you listen to her, it becomes clear how devoted Peggy was to her mom's well-being and how close they were.

"I can see why not being there at your mother's moment of death is hard, Peggy. You shared so much of your life with each other."

Peggy nods in agreement, "We did. That's true."

"It might be helpful to remember some of those moments when you get really focused on not being there when she died. It would be unfair to let that one moment overshadow the truth that you were a big presence in your mom's life."

Peggy considers this and then says, "You're right. Yes, I think that would help me a lot."

"Some might even suggest that it was easier for her to go when you weren't there. That the separation with you present would have been too hard."

"Hmm," Peggy says as she reflects on what you have said. "Actually, that makes a lot of sense. I can totally see that being the case for my mom because we were just so close."

"It seems like you've begun to process some of the harder parts of the grief process," you say. "I think I can be helpful by letting you talk about the issues that are coming up for you and help you find strategies for managing some of the overwhelming feelings you are having in relation to your mother's death. Having an outlet here might also prevent this from leaking out at work so frequently."

"That would be good," Peggy says. "I actually feel a little better already. It's a relief to be able to talk to someone about all this. I feel like it's been bottled up for months."

"Great," you say. "Let's find a time to schedule our next appointment."

4.1-1. How would you characterize Peggy's grief reactions? What are your concerns for her? What are her strengths?

4.1-2. How has the grief affected various areas of Peggy's life?

4.1-3. How are Peggy's feelings of guilt impacting her grief process?

4.1-4. How might you help Peggy address the discord she is feeling at work? With her husband?

4.1-5. Based on what you currently know about Peggy, what types of interventions might be helpful to her?

4.1-6. What other resources could be helpful to Peggy?

CASE 4.2

Identifying Information:

Client Name: Grant Thomas
Age: 51 years old
Race/Ethnicity: Jamaican
Marital Status: Married with two living children, one deceased
Education Level: Associate's degree
Occupation: Civil engineering tech

Intake Information:

When setting up the appointment, Grant explained that he was referred to you by a friend who had been a client of yours in the past. "He said he trusts you completely, and I trust him so I thought I would give it a try." He explained that he is seeking help to deal with the death of his 18-year-old son who was shot by a police officer. "You may have heard about it," he mentions. "It was in the news." You clarify his son's name and the date of death so that you can read up on the story prior to meeting with Grant.

In researching the incident, you find two news stories that summarize the situation as follows: three months ago Devon Thomas, age 18, was fatally shot by a police officer after what seems to have been a case of mistaken identity. Law enforcement had been looking for a man who was accused of murder. Police received a call from a convenience store clerk at 1:30 a.m. reporting that someone resembling the suspect had entered the store. When Devon left the store in his car, police followed him and pulled him over. As Devon reached for his ID, police shot him in the chest and he died on the scene. No weapon of any kind was found on Devon or in his car. The officers have been put on administrative leave, pending investigation.

Initial Interview:

You greet Grant in the waiting room. He is cordial, though subdued and you can see what looks like weariness in his eyes. You let him choose where he will sit and offer him water which he declines.

"Grant, I wanted to let you know that I read some of the news reports about what happened to Devon. I'm really glad you reached out for help. What a tragedy! How can I be helpful to you?"

"How can you help me? Honestly, I don't know. I don't know if anyone can help me." He looks out the window and his eyes well up with tears. He pauses for a while and seems to be trying to not burst into tears.

You want to let him know you see his pain but don't want to push so you softly say, "I can see this is so hard."

Still looking out the window, he nods and finally says, "So hard." He looks at you and shakes his head, "I don't even know where to begin."

"Well, maybe let's start with how things have been in the last week or so." You ask him about sleeping, eating, and if he is able to work. He tells you that he gets about four hours of sleep a night if he's lucky, he makes himself eat, though he doesn't have much of an appetite, and it has been difficult to concentrate at work. "My job is very tedious. You have to be meticulous because there are a lot of important details that you have to get right. One little mistake can mess up the whole project. I've been messing up a lot lately. I think that's why my buddy suggested I see you. He can tell I'm having a hard time. And he's a good guy, a good friend."

"I'm glad you have him. Do you have other supportive people in your life?" you ask.

"My mom lives on the other side of town. She comes over a lot. She's trying to get us to eat. And we have lots of friends who are supportive. My wife is devastated, of course, but she's really digging into the legal part of all of this. She's the one that follows up with our attorney, talks to the community activists, talks to the press, all of that. I don't know how she does it. I try to be active in all of it and participate in those conversations but half the time, I just zone out. My wife has to explain to me what happened even though I was at the meeting with her! I don't know. I just can't get my head around it. Just not smart enough for all that legal stuff, I guess."

"I would hesitate about assuming that it's related to how smart you are, Grant. The legal field is a whole different world. Unless you've been trained in it, it's like trying to understand a foreign language – and that's true for non-emotional issues. When it relates to the tragic death of your son, that's a whole different deal. I suspect that the traumatic nature of Devon's death is what is making it hard for you to stay focused."

"You think so?" Grant asks.

"Yes, I do," you say.

"I've had nightmares, too," he continues. "And I can't drive by the Quikmart where he was." As he looks at the floor, he shakes his head, "I just can't do it. I can't even drive by a *different* Quikmart."

"What happens when you do?" you ask.

"I get really freaked out. It feels like my heart goes to my stomach. One time I had to pull over. I think I might have been hyperventilating or having a panic attack or something."

"That must be very unsettling. It's completely understandable, however. I'm not surprised you're having those kinds of reactions," you explain.

"It is?" Grant asks.

"Yes," you affirm. "Very typical for what you've experienced."

"Hmm. Okay." Grant says, then adds, "I just feel pretty useless. We had a meeting with our attorney the other day and I got lost getting there. I've been there before. It's not hard to find. I feel like I'm letting my wife down. And if I can't get it together to work, that won't be good. We can't afford for me to lose my job. I guess my wife is just stronger than me. The power of a mother's love, maybe?"

"Well," you begin, "it may also be that this is your wife's way of coping. Maybe staying focused on the legal proceedings is a way to distract her from the pain or of trying to have some feeling of control or power. I, of course, don't know her and can't say that for certain. I do know that different people deal with grief in different ways. And it may change over time. This is still a very new loss for you."

"Hmm," he responds. "I just know I've got to get better. I can't keep messing up at work. I want to be able to be there for my family and do right by my son." After pausing, he sighs and adds, "I just want to wake up and have it all be a dream."

"I'm sure you do. The loss of a child is an extremely difficult loss and the circumstances surrounding Devon's death make it especially hard." Grant nods in agreement. You go on to explain to Grant how loss and trauma affect the brain and the body.

"I guess that makes sense," he responds as he digests what you've said. "I want justice for Devon. How in the hell does an innocent kid get killed and the murderers are walking free?" Grant's voice gets louder. "My son did nothing wrong. He was a good kid. He was going to school to be a nurse! To help people! The only thing he did wrong was go to the convenience store and be black. That's the only thing!"

You nod in agreement. "I hear you, Grant. It's not right." You listen attentively as Grant continues to express frustration and anger about the circumstances of Devon's death and the injustice that has been done to his family. "I want to be hopeful. I want to believe we will get justice for Devon, but sometimes that seems like a fairy tale. It's not like this doesn't happen all the time and the cop walks free." Grant is clenching his fists. "If I really let myself think about it, I get so angry. So angry!"

"Of course you do!" you affirm. After a pause, you ask, "Do you think about Devon often?"

Instantly, Grant's eyes become wet again. "I want to, but…" he sighs and reaches for a tissue. "It's hard. I had to go identify his body. That's what I keep seeing in my head. And I keep wondering what he thought about when he was dying. Was he in pain? Was he scared? I wasn't there but I can imagine it, you know?"

"Yes," you respond. "Those are some very uncomfortable things to carry around in your head."

"They are," he agrees. "I just don't know what to do."

"There are several ways I believe I can be helpful, Grant." You give a general outline of some of the possible interventions you think might benefit him.

"Okay. Well, I'm open. I need help."

You let Grant ask any questions he has about the counseling process and discuss when he'd like to meet again.

"Since we have a few minutes left, I'd like to show you an exercise that many of my clients have found helpful for managing distressing moments. Would you be open to that?"

"Sure," Grant responds.

You conclude the session by teaching Grant a simple mindfulness exercise.

4.2-1. What aspects of Grant's situation lead the counselor to conclude he is experiencing trauma in addition to loss?

4.2-2. Using the P-I-E perspective, how do you understand Grant's grief experience?

4.2-3. In this session, the therapist spends some time explaining the effects of grief and trauma to Grant. If you were the therapist, how would you explain this to him in a way that is informative and easy to understand?

4.2-4. What are some interventions that might be helpful for Grant? How would you summarize these to him in this first session?

4.2-5. What is a simple mindfulness exercise you could show Grant? What words would you use as you teach this to him?

4.2-6. What are Grant's individual and environmental strengths? How might these be helpful to your work with him?

CASE 4.3

Identifying Information:

Client Name: Jared Nichols
Age: 23 years old
Race/Ethnicity: White
Marital Status: Single
Education Level: Some college
Occupation: Sales associate at an electronics store

Intake Information:

A victims' advocate referred Jared to you from the local police department. She had been urging him to get counseling since his girlfriend died by suicide three weeks ago.

Initial Interview:

Jared arrives for his appointment on time. He seems a bit self-conscious, though friendly when you greet him.

He sits on the couch in your office and you begin the session by saying, "Jared, I understand you are here about your girlfriend."

"Yes," he says.

"Can you help me understand what happened?" you suggest.

He takes a deep breath and rests his head in his hand as he says, "She killed herself."

"Oh, I see. That can be very traumatizing," you respond empathetically and wait for Jared to continue.

"It's kind of a long story. Do you want me to tell you everything?" he asks.

"You can go into as much detail as you like," you say gently.

"Well, I had been dating Adrianna for about a year and a half. She was...God, she was just beautiful...and crazy and fun. I loved her so much and we were talking about moving in together. But she was also kind of clingy and always worried that I was going to leave her. One weekend I went camping with my buddies. We were celebrating my friend Tim's birthday. When I got back in cell phone range, I saw that she had called me about 12 times. When I called her, she was real angry with me and was kind of freaking out. I got mad at her and we wound up in a big fight. We stayed apart for a couple of days but then we made up and got back together and I thought everything was fine." Jared starts to cry. "But then," he continues through his tears, "Then on Thursday I got off work early and went over to her place. I was going to surprise her, take her out to eat and maybe get a movie. But I knocked on the door and no one answered. I called her cell phone but just got her voicemail. I waited a while, thinking she would call me back and then I called her work to see if maybe she had had to go in unexpectedly. They told me she wasn't there. I started to get this really strange feeling. I could just feel that something wasn't right. I called her brother but he hadn't heard from her either. I tried to get in the house but it was locked. I got frantic. I tried all the windows and the back door but I couldn't find a way in the house. At this point I'm really freaking out." You notice that Jared is breathing heavily and quickly. He looks at the floor as he continues. "I called her brother again. I was hoping he would have a spare key to her place but he didn't. He rushed over and we decided to call the cops. They opened the house and I ran through it, screaming for her. I opened the door to her bedroom and...." Jared stops talking and breaks down in tears.

You remain respectfully silent for a while and then gently ask, "Do you want to continue, Jared?"

"Yeah. Yeah, I'm okay. Sorry," he answers.

"There is no need to apologize, Jared," you reassure him. "It must be difficult for you to relive this story. Take your time and continue when you are ready."

Jared catches his breath for a moment and then tearfully tells you, "She was there – she had hung herself." He stops and cries silently.

"What a horrible thing for you to find! This must really be tearing you up, Jared!" You pause and allow him to continue crying.

"The cops found her at about the same time I did," Jared continues, still very tearful. "They got her down and tried to revive her but it was too late. I completely lost it. I went totally nuts. They had to hold me down."

"Of course you lost it!" you validate.

"Yeah," Jared says. He takes a deep breath. "So that's what happened, and I'm just a huge mess."

"I would imagine so. Can you tell me what makes you feel like you're a mess?"

"I feel like I'm losing my mind. I just can't seem to get it together. I finally decided I was going to have to take some time off work but I can't afford to take off too much. I feel like I've got this cloud hanging over me. And sometimes I just want to break down and cry and scream, but I don't want to freak out my friends. I need to know how to handle this." Jared looks at you and asks you desperately, "Am I beyond repair? Am I going to be a broken, insane person for the rest of my life?"

You try to reassure Jared with some information by saying, "I know it's scary and it feels horrible, but everything you have described is typical for someone who has had a traumatic loss such as you have had. I would expect you to be feeling in a fog, feeling out of control emotionally, uncomfortable around your friends, trouble concentrating, feeling off balance – these are things that I, as a grief counselor, hear all the time. It is an awful experience, but it is an expected response to this kind of loss. And no, you are not destined to be like this for the rest of your life. Many people have lost a loved one to suicide and they learn how to get through it and be okay."

Jared lets out a big sigh. "So I'm not totally crazy? That's a relief!"

"No it's not unusual," you emphasize. "I would not expect that you would be able to 'keep it together' after such a loss. And I can help you learn some ways to get through this. Tell me first, however, how you have dealt with this so far?"

"I've been partying some, to be honest with you. I know you are probably going to tell me that that's not good, right? I'm not drunk all the time or anything like that, but

I've been hanging out with my friends a lot – I don't want to be alone – and we end up drinking and smoking weed," Jared admits.

"I can understand not wanting to be alone," you respond, "and I'm glad you have friends that can be with you. You're right, drinking or smoking is not the best way to deal with this, but it's good that you understand that. As we work together, we can talk about some other ways to handle this that would be healthier for you."

"That sounds good," Jared says. "I hate thinking about it, but at the same time I can't stop. I keep trying to figure it out. She didn't leave a note or anything."

"It's natural that you are trying to put the puzzle pieces together. How do you understand Adrianna's suicide?" you ask.

"I don't know. Her family is kind of strange. I don't know the whole story – she NEVER talked about it – but her parents are divorced, and her dad is an alcoholic. After the memorial, her brother told me that she had attempted suicide several years ago and at one time she was taking some kind of medication for her moods. I had no idea! No one ever told me any of that!" Jared's tone suggests that he feels angry about this. "And then I think about our fight and I feel so bad. Maybe if I had handled it differently…maybe that was what put her over the edge." Jared becomes tearful again. "She always had this thing about how she wasn't good enough for me."

"You know, Jared, guilt is a feeling that almost all survivors of suicide experience, but it doesn't mean that you are responsible for Adrianna's death. Many couples fight. It comes with being in a serious relationship with someone. To take your life over a fight with your partner is not a healthy, rational response. It sounds like there were some other things going on with Adrianna that you didn't know about." You spend a little more time talking to Jared about mental illness, explaining that it prevents the brain from functioning properly, causes impaired judgment and mood disturbances. Jared listens attentively and you allow him some time to process what you have said. You sense that it is a lot for him to take in and you realize you will probably have to talk with him about this more in future sessions.

You continue, "I'm impressed at your openness, Jared. I'm sure it's not easy to talk about Adrianna's death and the feelings you have around it."

"No, it's not," Jared says. "I guess I keep hoping that if I don't talk about it, it will go away. But actually, this wasn't as bad as I thought it would be. I mean – I actually feel a little bit better."

"I'm glad. I think you are the kind of person who will make good use of counseling. I'm sure that if we continue to work together, we can help you find your way through this. What do you say? Should we set up another appointment?" you ask.

"Yeah. Let's do that."

4.3-1. What are some of Jared's strengths? What are some of your concerns for Jared?

4.3-2. In what ways could you help Jared with his emotional responses to the loss?

4.3-3. What additional information would you want to acquire regarding Jared's substance use? How could this behavior impact his grief process?

4.3-4. What do you make of Jared saying he doesn't want to be alone? How would you determine if this is a life-enhancing or life-depleting coping behavior?

4.3-5. How could you help Jared with his guilt feelings in life-enhancing ways?

4.3-6. What other resources might be useful for Jared?

REFERENCES

American Psychiatric Association [APA]. (2013). *Diagnostic and statistical manual of mental disorders* (5th ed.). https://doi.org/10.1176/appi.books.9780890425596

Bordere, T. C. (2019). Suffocated grief, resilience and survival among African American families. In M. H. Jacobsen & A. Petersen (Eds.), *Exploring grief: Towards a sociology of sorrow* (pp. 188–204). Routledge.

Bowlby, J. (1982). *Attachment and loss: Attachment* (Vol. 1). Basic Books.

Brodbeck, J., Berger, T., Biesold, N., Rockstroh, F., & Znoj, H. J. (2019). Evaluation of a guided internet-based self-help intervention for older adults after spousal bereavement or separation/divorce: A randomised controlled trial. *Journal of Affective Disorders*, *252*, 440–449. https://doi.org/10.1016/j.jad.2019.04.008

Brown, N. (2018). *Psychoeducational groups: Process and practice* (4th ed.). Routledge. https://doi.org/10.4324/9781315169590

Buddhist Funerals Guide. (n.d.). *Burial Planning*. www.burialplanning.com/resources/religious-funerals-guide/buddhist-funerals-guide

Burke, L. A., & Neimeyer, R. A. (2013). Prospective risk factors for complicated grief: A review of the empirical literature. In M. Stroebe, H. Schut, & J. V. Bout (Eds.), *Complicated grief: Scientific foundations for health care professionals* (pp. 145–161). Routledge.

Burke, L. A., & Neimeyer, R. A. (2014). Complicated spiritual grief I: Relation to complicated grief symptomatology following violent death bereavement. *Death Studies*, *38*(4), 259–267. https://doi.org/10.1080/07481187.2013.829372

Butler, E. A., & Randall, A. K. (2012). Emotional coregulation in close relationships. *Emotion Review*, *5*(2), 202–210. https://doi.org/10.1177/1754073912451630

Cole, A. H. (2021). *Counseling persons with Parkinson's Disease* [In press]. Oxford University Press.

Collins, N. L., & Feeney, B. C. (2004). Working models of attachment shape perceptions of social support: Evidence from experimental and observational studies. *Journal of Personality and Social Psychology*, *87*(3), 363–383. https://doi.org/10.1037/0022-3514.87.3.363

Corrigan, F. M., & Hull, A. M. (2015). Neglect of the complex: Why psychotherapy for post-traumatic clinical presentations is often ineffective. *BJPsych Bulletin*, *39*(2), 86–89. https://doi.org/10.1192/pb.bp.114.046995

Currier, J. M., Irish, J. E., Neimeyer, R. A., & Foster, J. D. (2015) Attachment, continuing bonds, and complicated grief following violent loss: Testing a moderated model. *Death Studies*, *39*(4), 201–210. https://doi.org/10.1080/07481187.2014.975869

De Leo, D., Dyregrov, K., & Cimitan, A. (2014). Helping with complicated bereavement. In D. De Leo, A. Cimitan, K. Dyregrov, O. Grad, & K. Andriessen (Eds.), *Bereavement after traumatic death: Helping the survivors* (pp. 125–136). Hogrefe Publishing.

Dykas, M. J., & Cassidy, J. (2011). Attachment and the processing of social information across the life span: Theory and evidence. *Psychological Bulletin*, *137*(1), 19–46. https://doi.org/10.1037/a0021367

Dyregrov, K., Cimitan, A., & De Leo, D. (2014). Reactions to traumatic death. In D. De Leo, A. Cimitan, K. Dyregrov, O. Grad, & K. Andriessen (Eds.), *Bereavement after traumatic death: Helping the survivors* (pp. 19–35). Hogrefe Publishing.

Dyregrov, K., De Leo, D., & Cimitan, A. (2014). Social support networks as a source of support. In D. De Leo, A. Cimitan, K. Dyregrov, O. Grad, & K. Andriessen (Eds.), *Bereavement after traumatic death: Helping the survivors* (pp. 65–80). Hogrefe Publishing.

Dyregrov, A., & Dyregrov, K. (2008). *Effective grief and bereavement support: The role of family, friends, colleagues, schools and support professionals*. Jessica Kingsley Publishers.

Exline, J. J., & Martin, A. (2005). Anger toward God: A new frontier in forgiveness research. In E. L. Worthington (Ed.), *Handbook of forgiveness* (pp. 73–88). Routledge.

Exline, J. J., & Rose, E. (2005). Religious and spiritual struggles. In R. F. Paloutzian & C. L. Park (Eds.), *Handbook of the psychology of religion and spirituality* (pp. 315–330). Guilford Press.

Felitti, V. J., Anda, R. F., Nordenberg, D., Williamson, D. F., Spitz, A. M., Edwards, V., & Marks, J. S. (1998). Relationship of childhood abuse and household dysfunction to many of the leading causes of death in adults: The Adverse Childhood Experiences (ACE) Study. *American Journal of Preventive Medicine*, *14*(4), 245–258.

Field, N. P., Packman, W., Ronen, R., Pries, A., Davies, B., & Kramer, R. (2013). Type of continuing bonds expression and its comforting versus distressing nature: Implications for adjustment among bereaved mothers. *Death Studies*, *37*(10), 889–912. https://doi.org/10.1080/07481187.2012.692458

Granqvist, P., & Kirkpatrick, L. A. (2013). Religion, spirituality, and attachment. In K. I. Pargament, J. J. Exline, & J. W. Jones (Eds.), *APA handbook of psychology, religion, and spirituality: Context, theory, and research* (Vol. 1, pp. 139–155). American Psychological Association. https://doi.org/10.1037/14045-007

Harris, R. (2009). *ACT made simple: An easy-to-read primer on acceptance and commitment therapy*. New Harbinger Publications.

Hart, O. V., Nijenhuis, E. R., & Steele, K. (2006). *The haunted self: Structural dissociation and the treatment of chronic traumatization*. W. W. Norton & Company.

Hayes, J. P., VanElzakker, M. B., & Shin, L. M. (2012). Emotion and cognition interactions in PTSD: A review of neurocognitive and neuroimaging studies. *Frontiers in Integrative Neuroscience*, *6*, 1–14. https://doi.org/10.3389/fnint.2012.00089

Hibberd, R. (2013). Meaning reconstruction in bereavement: Sense and significance. *Death Studies*, *37*(7), 670–692. https://doi.org/10.1080/07481187.2012.692453

Hidalgo, I. M. (2017) The effects of children's spiritual coping after parent, grandparent or sibling death on children's grief, personal growth, and mental health (Doctoral dissertation). https://digitalcommons.fiu.edu/etd/3467

Hopper, J. W. (2015). Harnessing the seeking, satisfaction, and embodiment circuitries in contemplative approaches to trauma. In V. M. Follette, J. Briere, D. I. Rome, & D. Rozelle (Eds.), *Mindfulness-oriented interventions for trauma: Integrating contemplative practices* (pp. 185–209). Guilford Publications.

Howarth, R. (2011). Concepts and controversies in grief and loss. *Journal of Mental Health Counseling*, *33*(1), 4–10. https://doi.org/10.17744/mehc.33.1.900m56162888u737

Hsu, M. T., Tseng, Y. F., Banks, J. M., & Kuo, L. L. (2004). Interpretations of stillbirth. *Journal of Advanced Nursing*, *47*(4), 408–416. https://doi.org/10.1111/j.1365-2648.2004.03119.x

Kosminsky, P. S., & Jordan, J. R. (2016). *Attachment-informed grief therapy: The clinician's guide to foundations and applications*. Routledge.

Levine, P. A. (2012). *In an unspoken voice: How the body releases trauma and restores goodness*. North Atlantic Books.

Levine, P. A., & Frederick, A. (1997). *Waking the tiger: Healing trauma*. North Atlantic Books.

Lipscomb, A. E., & Ashley, W. (2018). Black male grief through the lens of racialization and oppression: Effective instruction for graduate clinical programs. *International Research in Higher Education*, *3*(2), 51. https://doi.org/10.5430/irhe.v3n2p51

Mancini, A. D., & Bonanno, G. A. (2009). Predictors and parameters of resilience to loss: Toward an individual differences model. *Journal of Personality*, *77*(6), 1805–1832. https://doi.org/10.1111/j.1467-6494.2009.00601.x

Mikulincer, M., & Shaver, P. R. (2008). An attachment perspective on bereavement. In M. S. Stroebe, R. O. Hansson, H. Schut, & W. Stroebe (Eds.), *Handbook of bereavement research and practice: Advances in theory and intervention* (p. 87–112). American Psychological Association. https://doi.org/10.1037/14498-005

Mikulincer, M., & Shaver, P. R. (2009). An attachment and behavioral systems perspective on social support. *Journal of Social and Personal Relationships*, *26*(1), 7–19. https://doi.org/10.1177/0265407509105518

Mikulincer, M., & Shaver, P. R. (2014). *Mechanisms of social connection: From brain to group*. American Psychological Association.

Nagoski, E., & Nagoski, A. (2019). *Burnout: The secret to unlocking the stress cycle*. Ballantine Books.

Nguyen-Feng, V. N., Morrissette, J., Lewis-Dmello, A., Michel, H., Anders, D., Wagner, C., & Clark, C. J. (2019). Trauma-sensitive yoga as an adjunctive mental health treatment for survivors of intimate partner violence: A qualitative examination. *Spirituality in Clinical Practice*, *6*(1), 27–43. https://doi.org/10.1037/scp0000177

Parkes, C. M., & Prigerson, H. G. (2013). *Bereavement: Studies of grief in adult life* (4th ed.). Routledge.

Pearlman, L. A., Wortman, C. B., Feuer, C. A., Farber, C. H., & Rando, T. A. (2014). *Treating traumatic bereavement: A practitioner's guide*. Guilford Publications.

Pomeroy, E. C., Anderson, K. H., & Garcia, R. B. (2015). Bereavement and grief therapy. In K. Corcoran & A. R. Roberts (Eds.), *Social workers' desk reference* (3rd ed., pp. 675–684). Oxford University Press.

Pomeroy, E. C., & Garcia, R. B. (2018). *Direct practice skills for evidence-based social work: A strengths-based text and workbook*. Springer Publishing Company.

Pomeroy, E. C., & Holleran, L. (2002). Tuesdays with fellow travelers: A psychoeducational HIV/AIDS-related bereavement group. *Journal of HIV/AIDS in Social Services*, *1*, 61–77. https://doi.org/10.1300/J187v01n02_05

Porges, S. W., & Dana, D. A. (Eds.). (2018). *Clinical applications of the polyvagal theory: The emergence of polyvagal-informed therapies*. W. W. Norton & Company.

Puchalski, C., Ferrell, B., Virani, R., Otis-Green, S., Baird, P., Bull, J., & Sulmasy, D. (2009). Improving the quality of spiritual care as a dimension of palliative care: The report of the consensus conference. *Journal of Palliative Medicine*, *12*(10), 885–904. https://doi.org/10.1089/jpm.2009.0142

Rosenblatt, P. C. (2016). Cultural competence and humility. In D. L. Harris & T. C. Bordere (Eds.), *Handbook of social justice in loss and grief: Exploring diversity, equity, and inclusion* (pp. 67–74). Routledge.

Rosenblatt, P. C. (2017). Researching grief: Cultural, relational, and individual possibilities. *Journal of Loss and Trauma*, *22*(8), 617–630. https://doi.org/10.1080/15325024.2017.1388347

Rubin, S. S., Malkinson, R., & Witztum, E. (2012). *Working with the bereaved: Multiple lenses on loss and mourning*. Taylor & Francis.

Sangster, K. L., & Lee, A. C. (2017). Spirituality and traumatic loss: Pathways to health through spiritual classics and focusing. In N. Thompson, G. R. Cox, & R. G. Stevenson (Eds.), *Handbook of traumatic loss: A guide to theory and practice* (pp. 19–32). Routledge.

Sbarra, D. A., & Hazan, C. (2008). Coregulation, dysregulation, self-regulation: An integrative analysis and empirical agenda for understanding adult attachment, separation, loss, and recovery. *Personality and Social Psychology Review*, *12*(2), 141–167. https://doi.org/10.1177/1088868308315702

Scheidt, C., Hasenburg, A., Kunze, M., Waller, E., Pfeifer, R., Zimmermann, P., Hartmann, A., & Waller, N. (2012). Are individual differences of attachment predicting bereavement outcome after perinatal loss? A prospective cohort study. *Journal of Psychosomatic Research*, *73*(5), 375–382. https://doi.org/10.1016/j.jpsychores.2012.08.017

Shaver, P. R., & Mikulincer, M. (2011). Attachment theory. In P. van Lange & A. W. Kruglanski (Eds.), *Handbook of theories of social psychology* (Vol. 2, pp. 160–179). Sage Publications.

Shear, M. K. (2015). Complicated grief. *New England Journal of Medicine*, *372*(2), 153–160. https://doi.org/10.1056/nejmcp1315618

Shear, M. K., & Bloom, C. G. (2017). Complicated grief treatment: An evidence-based approach to grief therapy. *Journal of Rational-Emotive & Cognitive-Behavior Therapy*, *35*(1), 6–25.

Shear, M. K., Frank, E., Houck, P. R., & Reynolds, C. F. (2005). Treatment of complicated grief: A randomized controlled trial. *JAMA*, *293*(21), 2601–2608. https://doi.org/10.1001/jama.293.21.2601

Shear, M. K., Reynolds, C. F., Simon, N. M., Zisook, S., Wang, Y., Mauro, C., Duan, N., Lebowitz, B., & Skritskaya, N. (2016). Optimizing treatment of complicated grief: A randomized clinical trial. *JAMA Psychiatry*, *73*(7), 685–694. https://doi.org/10.1001/jamapsychiatry.2016.0892

Shear, M. K., Wang, Y., Skritskaya, N., Duan, N., Mauro, C., & Ghesquiere, A. (2014). Treatment of complicated grief in elderly persons: A randomized clinical trial. *JAMA Psychiatry*, *71*(11), 1287–1295. https://doi.org/10.1001/jamapsychiatry.2014.1242

Smid, G. E., Kleber, R. J., De la Rie, S. M., Bos, J. B., Gersons, B. P., & Boelen, P. A. (2015). Brief eclectic psychotherapy for traumatic grief (BEP-TG): Toward integrated treatment of symptoms related to traumatic loss. *European Journal of Psychotraumatology*, *6*(1), 27324.

Smith, A. J., Abeyta, A. A., Hughes, M., & Jones, R. T. (2015). Persistent grief in the aftermath of mass violence: The predictive roles of posttraumatic stress symptoms, self-efficacy, and disrupted worldview. *Psychological Trauma: Theory, Research, Practice, and Policy*, *7*(2), 179–186. https://doi.org/10.1037/tra0000002

Solomon, R. (2019, April). *The utilization of EMDR therapy with grief and mourning* [Presentation]. Compassion Works, Dallas, Texas, United States.

Solomon, R. M., & Rando, T. A. (2007). Utilization of EMDR in the treatment of grief and mourning. *Journal of EMDR Practice and Research*, *1*(2), 109–117. https://doi.org/10.1891/1933-3196.1.2.109

Speedlin, S., Milligan, K., Haberstroh, S., & Duffey, T. (2016). Using acceptance and commitment therapy to negotiate losses and life transitions. *Ideas and Research You Can Use: VISTAS 2016*.

Stang, H. (2016). Yoga for grief. In R. A. Neimeyer (Ed.), *Techniques of grief therapy: Assessment and intervention* (pp. 144–149). Routledge.

Stirling, F. J. (2016). Yoga and loss: An autoethnographical exploration of grief, mind, and body. *Illness, Crisis & Loss*, *24*(4), 279–291. https://doi.org/10.1177/1054137316659396

Stroebe, M. S., Boerner, K., & Schut, H. (2016). Grief. In V. Zeigler-Hill & T. K. Shackelford (Eds.), *Encyclopedia of personality and individual differences* (pp. 1–5). Springer.

Stroebe, M. S., Hansson, R. O., Stroebe, W., & Schut, H. (2001). Introduction: Concepts and issues in contemporary research on bereavement. In M. S. Stroebe, R. O. Hansson, W. Stroebe, & H. Schut (Eds.), *Handbook of bereavement research: Consequences, coping, and care* (pp. 3–45). American Psychological Association.

Stroebe, M. S., & Schut, H. (2010). The dual process model of coping with bereavement: A decade on. *OMEGA – Journal of Death and Dying*, *61*(4), 269–271. https://doi.org/10.2190/om.61.4.a

van der Kolk, B. A. (2014). *The body keeps the score: Brain, mind, and body in the healing of trauma*. Penguin Books.

van der Kolk, B. A., Stone, L., West, J., Rhodes, A., Emerson, D., Suvak, M., & Spinazzola, J. (2014). Yoga as an adjunctive treatment for posttraumatic stress disorder. *The Journal of Clinical Psychiatry*, *75*(06), e559–e565. https://doi.org/10.4088/jcp.13m08561

Wetherell, J. L. (2012). Complicated grief therapy as a new treatment approach. *Dialogues in Clinical Neuroscience*, *14*(2), 159–166.

Worden, J. W. (2018). *Grief counseling and grief therapy: A handbook for the mental health practitioner* (5th ed.). Springer Publishing Company.

Wortman, C. B., & Pearlman, L. A. (2016). Traumatic bereavement. In R. A. Neimeyer (Ed.), *Techniques of grief therapy: Assessment and intervention* (pp. 25–29). Routledge.

Zech, E., & Arnold, C. (2011). Attachment and coping with bereavement: Implications for therapeutic interventions with the insecurely attached. In R. A. Neimeyer, D. L. Harris, H. R. Winokuer, & G. F. Thornton (Eds.), *Grief and bereavement in contemporary society: Bridging research and practice* (pp. 23–35). Routledge.

CHAPTER 5

Expected and Traumatic Grief in Children and Adolescents

For many years, the conventional wisdom was that children do not experience grief. We now know that "anyone old enough to love is old enough to grieve" (Wolfelt, 1991). The impact of loss on children and adolescents is influenced by their chronological age and developmental stage because these factors shape youths' capacity to comprehend death, their emotional expression, and their understanding of the circumstances surrounding the loss. In addition, their necessary dependence on caregivers means that changes in the child's environment can dramatically impact their grief experience.

THEORIES OF GRIEF IN CHILDREN AND ADOLESCENTS

On the whole, the current frameworks and conceptualizations of grief refer to the experiences of adults. While these can provide a useful foundation, there are significant differences in the ways that children and adults experience loss and trauma. Exceptions to these adult-focused theories include Bowlby's work on attachment and loss and the newly developed Multidimensional Grief Theory (Kaplow et al., 2013; Layne, 2012). Multidimensional Grief Theory views a young person's grief through the distress experienced in the following areas: separation from the loved one, existentialism and identity, and the circumstances of the death. The theory maintains that there can be both beneficial and detrimental adaptations in each of these areas. This theory also acknowledges the role that numerous internal and external variables play in a young person's grief experience, including developmental stage, coping methods, reminders of the loss, secondary losses, caregivers, living circumstances, and culture (Layne et al., 2017).

The research on children's experience of grief and loss is still limited, though growing. The authors' strengths-based framework of grief and loss is applicable to all stages

DOI: 10.4324/9780429053634-5

of development. An explanation of how it can be applied to children is provided as follows:

1. Grief in response to the death of a loved one is a natural, expectable, and potentially health-producing process that aids the individual in adjusting to the absence of the loved one.

    While historically it was believed that children didn't have the capacity to grieve, we now know that grief is a natural reaction to loss for all ages. Children's grief may look different from that of adults, but it is equally useful in helping children adjust and adapt to loss.

2. The symptoms, emotions, and behaviors associated with expected grief reactions represent a process of healthy adaptation as defined by one's culture and are not inherently pathological.

    At each developmental stage, children have predictable reactions to the death of a loved one. Children may express a range of emotions that can aid them in processing the loss. While these reactions may be confusing to the child's caregivers, they may represent a healthy process of adjustment.

3. Mourners benefit by knowing that life-enhancing grief reactions facilitate healing within the mourner and are productive and beneficial.

    As with adults, children benefit by having their grief reactions validated. Adults can play a pivotal role in assisting grieving children with understanding that their grief can be a healthy process that can alleviate the pain they are experiencing. Children can also be taught life-enhancing methods to help them cope with the loss.

4. All persons have individual and environmental strengths that can assist them as they experience grief. The mourner benefits from the reinforcement of those strengths and the encouragement to consciously employ them during the grief process.

    Due to their developmental levels, children are often unaware of their own coping capacities as well as the environmental supports available to them. It is important for both personal and professional caregivers to teach children about their individual and environmental strengths and how to utilize them.

5. Environmental conditions can either help or hinder the mourner's ability to adapt to the loss and enhance the person's life.

    Environmental conditions that could impact a child's ability to adjust to loss include the caregiving system, the school and community environment, access to healthcare, and additional resources as needed.

6. Many symptoms of grief, though they may be uncomfortable, represent healthy coping mechanisms in that they facilitate the process of separation, adaptation to change, and integration of the loss.

    Some of the uncomfortable symptoms that are commonly seen in bereaved children include crying, fear-based behaviors, regression, and withdrawal. It is also true that children may not show visible signs of their grief, which can be confusing to caregivers. In both cases, children may be forming psychological safety nets in order to process the grief and move toward separation and adaptation to the loss.

7. Life-enhancing grief reactions to loss facilitate the process of adaptation and psychological separation from the deceased.

   In children, life-enhancing grief reactions can be facilitated by caregivers and helping professionals who are aware of children's needs for assistance with the grieving process.

8. Life-enhancing grief symptoms should not be discouraged. Rather, they should be allowed expression so long as they remain helpful to the mourner's process of adaptation.

   Caregivers can assist children with life-enhancing grief symptoms by providing structure, space to express emotions, encouragement, and reassurance.

9. Grief may be considered life-depleting when the symptoms it produces significantly interfere with the mourner's aspirations, competencies, and confidence. Life-depleting grief reactions are those responses and circumstances which act as impediments to the expected grieving process and interfere with the mourner's ability to live a fulfilling life.

   In children, grief may be considered life-depleting when it becomes an impediment to their normal development.

10. Life-depleting grief reactions thwart the process of adaptation and lead to entropy.

    Children's development can be seriously compromised when they are unable to cope with loss in healthy ways.

11. Life-enhancing and life-depleting grief reactions exist on a continuum of intensity.

    Children's reactions to loss can range from mild to severe. Some children may show no outward signs of grief, while others may display intense grief reactions. A child's grief reactions often vary over time and as the child progresses developmentally.

12. The experience of grief evolves over a person's lifetime and is experienced with varying levels of conscious awareness.

    Children re-experience the loss as they progress through the stages of development. At each stage of development their awareness and perceptions of the loss change.

13. The process of grief is fertile ground for communal or personal growth and the development or enhancement of the mourner's strengths.

    It is a common misconception that the death of a loved one will permanently scar children. Children have the capacity to be resilient and grow from their experience with grief.

(Pomeroy & Garcia, 2011)

DEVELOPMENTAL UNDERSTANDINGS OF DEATH AND GRIEF

Helping children and adolescents with loss requires knowledge of how cognitive development influences the ability to understand death. A complete and accurate understanding of death involves the ability to comprehend five core abstractions. First is the universality of death, which involves comprehending that all living beings die. The second concept involves the finality of the event and the realization that the deceased will not return to life. Third is the termination of the living being, including the person's thoughts, feelings, and physical functioning (Humphrey & Zimpfer, 2007). The fourth concept of death involves the ability to comprehend the reason for the death (e.g. accident, the aging process, illness, violence). The fifth concept of death relates to spirituality and the ability to mentally and emotionally conceptualize the post-death experience of the deceased. This involves ideas about the spirit of the deceased person which may include beliefs related to the afterlife, reincarnation, where the deceased's spirit dwells, or that there is no life after death. The cognitive, emotional, and social development of children determines their ability to fully internalize all of these concepts and, consequently, affects their response to the death of a loved one.

It is also important to note that most children experience intense pain in short bursts, rather than for lengthy periods of time. A child may be crying about their deceased loved one and abruptly switch to laughing and playing just a moment later (Dyregrov et al., 2014). Children need "time off" from their grief experience and an absence of grief-related symptoms does not indicate that the child has resolved all their feelings about the death. They often act out their feelings through play as this allows them to confront the loss from a safe distance (Landreth et al., 2005).

The following section summarizes the perspectives on death for neurotypical children in different age groups and how this impacts their experience of grief. There will be variations due to individual differences in development, neurological and cultural diversity, and the strength of the child's attachment to the deceased.

Age-Based Responses to Loss

From birth to 2 years, the loss of a significant adult can have a major impact on the infant's sense of security and well-being in the world. Attachment disorders can begin to develop during this time and can slow cognitive, emotional, and social development. Children of this age are sensitive to stress in their environment and changes in routine. The infant may display excessive crying, writhing, rocking, biting, and other anxiety-related behaviors. They may also exhibit disruptions in their sleeping and eating patterns. If they are not in familiar surroundings and with responsive caregivers, they can become withdrawn (Ferow, 2019). Feelings of abandonment can develop at this age and can lead to future relationship difficulties as an adult (Masterson, 1988).

Between the ages of 2–5 years old, children understand death to be a temporary state that can be reversed and often equate it with sleeping or being momentarily absent. Children of this age group may have tantrums and be difficult to soothe and exhibit regressive behaviors, such as excessive clinging and bedwetting (Pomeroy &

Garcia, 2011; Turner, 2020). They often engage in magical thinking and may believe that their thoughts or behaviors brought about the death of their loved one. They may believe that their loved one is still living and will physically return. Being explicit about the deceased (i.e. using the terms "dead" or "died") is extremely important in helping children of this age understand the permanence of the death (Turner, 2020). In this stage of development, children primarily use play to express their feelings (Pomeroy & Garcia, 2011).

Between the ages of 6–9, children begin to comprehend the biology of death and grasp its finality. They may display hyperactivity, aggression, and disruptive behaviors or, conversely, they may be withdrawn, sad, and forlorn. Fears associated with their own death or the death of a caregiver can arise and may be expressed in a reluctance to separate from them. Sleep disturbances, including nightmares, as well as regressive behaviors are not uncommon.

Children between the ages of 9–12 years old have a general understanding of death, though it may be distorted by inaccurate depictions of death in video games and other media. They are cognizant of the changes death causes in a family's life over which they have no control. While they are acquainted with basic feelings, they grapple with more complicated emotions that may arise with traumatic loss such as distrust, rage, vengeance, and forgiveness (Turner, 2020). As preadolescents, they may worry about their primary caregiver dying, fears that may be heightened by the physical and hormonal changes they are experiencing. Interest in the body, anatomy, and bodily functions increases at this age. When in a safe therapeutic environment, they may ask very precise and explicit questions about death, such as how long it takes someone to bleed to death, if death by suffocation is painful, or what happens to the physical body during the process of death (Turner, 2020). They may feel a strong need to control their feelings while at the same time have great difficulty doing so. Children during this stage can feel insecure and vulnerable due to the developmentally driven need to blend in with their peer group. Significant loss may create a sense of being different from peers and lead to feeling socially isolated, lonely, confused, scared, and guilty. A pervasive sense of self-consciousness, common at this age, can be amplified by the death of a loved one (Pomeroy & Garcia, 2011).

Adolescents, ages 13–19, are able to fully grasp the concept of death and its finality. The loss can provoke strong feelings of sadness, loneliness, confusion, fear, guilt, and anxiety. It may be difficult to identify grief reactions in adolescents because of their reticence to discuss topics that would make them feel vulnerable. They often resist expressing their grief out of a need to appear "strong," in control of their emotions, and to not be different from their peers. Some adolescents will mask their grief through risk-taking behaviors, such as reckless driving, alcohol and drug use, sexual promiscuity, defiance of authority, and self-injurious behaviors. These behaviors often represent a fervent need to avoid unpleasant emotions. Persistent avoidance can exacerbate depressive symptoms, such as lack of motivation, feelings of hopelessness, helplessness, worthlessness, and lethargy.

Adolescents can build strong walls of anger, withdrawal, denial, or numbing to protect themselves. Because it is also a very ego-centric stage of development, teens may feel closely connected to the cause of death and their inability to prevent it. They may become more easily distracted, experience sleeping and eating disturbances, perform better or worse in school, and display strong emotional lability. Like adults, adolescents may deny the reality of the loss for months or years following the death (Dyregrov et al., 2014). Despite these difficulties, adolescents can be very resilient and may eventually display greater maturity and growth as a result of the loss (Kilmer et al., 2014). Due to society's stereotype that adolescence is an inherently pathological stage of development, teenagers, in particular, respond positively to a strengths-based approach to grief and loss.

As children mature through subsequent developmental stages, feelings related to grief will resurface as they experience new understanding, recognition, and insight into the personal meaning of their loss (Hidalgo, 2017). Thus, they will periodically re-experience grief for many years after the death. For example, during birthdays, graduations, weddings, and other rites of passage, the loss of the loved one may be felt more intensely.

Fears Associated with Death

At all stages of development children often develop fears following a death. They may fear for their own death or the death of a caregiver (e.g. "When will I die?"; "Is Mommy going to die, too?"). They may worry about being alone at night, in an empty house, the house being robbed, being in a car accident, or having nightmares (e.g. "The boogeyman might come"; "I'm scared to go upstairs"; "I need you to stay with me"). In addition, children may have concerns about the intensity of their grief-related emotions and those of their caregivers (e.g. "If I cry, I won't be able to stop"; "I can't stand to see my mother crying"). Children and adolescents may fear that their friends and family members will treat them differently or withdraw from them due to the death (e.g. "No one will talk to me at school"; "They act like I'm weird"). Finally, they may develop safety-related fears that revolve around who will attend to their needs ("Who will take care of me?").

Explaining Death to Children

Given their cognitive limitations, it is important that death be explained to children in ways they can understand. Euphemisms commonly used to speak about death such as "passed away," "resting in peace," or "we lost her" can be confusing for children who often interpret these sayings literally. Anxiety may develop from these misunderstandings, such as when children develop fears of going to sleep after the death of their loved one was explained as "he went to sleep forever." Rather, precise descriptions that explain that the deceased does not have a heartbeat, does not use the bathroom, and cannot talk, think, or feel help children begin to more accurately grasp the concept of death. Caregivers also want to be mindful of how children interpret their spiritual beliefs to children. Hearing that "he's always watching you," for example, may bring comfort for some children and distress for others.

In addition to conveying accurate and age-appropriate explanations about death, it is generally believed that children benefit from honesty about the circumstances surrounding the loss, despite the tendency for caregivers to want to "protect" them from disturbing truths. This may be especially relevant in cases of suicide, homicide, and drug overdose. Children who are lied to about the circumstances of the loss may develop mistrust in their caregivers and consequently conclude that all adults are deceptive (Turner, 2020).

TRAUMA IN CHILDREN AND ADOLESCENTS

Traumatic experiences can impact children and teens cognitively, emotionally, physically, and behaviorally. Many times, the behaviors exhibited by traumatized children and adolescents are misinterpreted as oppositional, aggressive, attention seeking, closed off, or rude when, in fact, they represent biologically based trauma reactions, attempts at attachment, and efforts toward self-protection. Thus, compassionate responses to youth that are informed by knowledge of trauma reactions is essential so that caregivers and practitioners do not exacerbate these reactions and cause additional trauma.

Developmental Reactions to Trauma

In infants and children up to age 5, symptoms of trauma may manifest as irritability, fussiness, startling easily, and increased agitation. They may be difficult to soothe and have more tantrums than other children their age. They may exhibit extreme clinginess to caregivers and a hesitancy to explore their surroundings. For children this age, themes related to the trauma may appear repeatedly in their play or in conversation. For example, they may re-enact scenes from the loss event, bury their dolls, or have the characters in their play exhibit their fears. Additionally, some children will experience developmental delays. Frequent and severe trauma that is experienced at a young age can fundamentally impede important brain development and cause significant physical, emotional, and social delays. This is commonly referred to as developmental trauma and is beyond the scope of this book.

In children ages 6–12, traumatic experiences may cause them to become quieter and more withdrawn, or more defiant and combative. They may become upset more easily and talk frequently about scary thoughts and feelings. Traumatic experiences can hinder attention and concentration and make it more difficult for children to transition between different activities. They may eat more or less than they did before the trauma and suffer from somatic symptoms such as headaches or stomachaches. In addition, regressive behaviors such as thumb sucking and bedwetting may arise. It is as if they are instinctually pulled back to an earlier time that felt safer to them (Lokko & Stern, 2015).

Adolescents who experience trauma may talk about the trauma incessantly or, conversely, exhibit strong denial that it happened or that they are affected by it. They may be more likely to break rules or engage in risky behaviors, including substance abuse. They often experience disruptions in sleep and report continual feelings of fatigue and lethargy. In addition, traumatized teens often withdraw from their peers and seek comfort in isolation (Child Welfare Information Gateway, 2014). Beginning in early adolescence until about age 25, there are numerous structural, functional, and neurochemical changes in the brain. For this reason, trauma exposure during this time of life is believed to significantly impact the developing brain (Rosenzweig et al., 2017).

All of these behaviors represent instinctive responses to the trauma and attempts to secure protection from a felt sense of danger. They are not deliberate or planned and occur without consideration for possible ramifications on themselves and others (Child Welfare Information Gateway, 2014). Helping children and teens give voice to these fears and assisting their brains and bodies to recognize safe and adaptive responses in the present moment are fundamental goals of trauma interventions.

Protective Factors for Children Exposed to Trauma

Not all children who have been exposed to trauma will endure severe and life-changing challenges. Factors that influence the development of trauma-related symptoms in youth include:

- Age: Children will demonstrate more resilience in the face of trauma if they are older in age when the trauma began.
- Frequency: Children who experience a single incident of trauma fare better than those exposed to repeated traumas.
- Caregivers: The presence of healthy and supportive caregivers mitigates the negative impact of traumatic events.
- Internal resources: Intelligence, physical health, positive self-esteem, and other personal assets enable children to weather traumatic events more easily.
- Perception: The child's perception of the event, including their felt sense of danger and the degree of fear they experienced, can impact their capacity to manage, assimilate, and adapt to the experience in a life-enhancing way.
- Temperament: A child's general disposition can impact how they respond to a distressing event. For example, children who are by nature more sensitive than others may demonstrate greater difficulty (Child Welfare Information Gateway, 2014).

INTERSECTION OF GRIEF AND TRAUMA IN CHILDREN AND ADOLESCENTS

As compared with adults, the loss experience of children and adolescents has a greater probability of also being experienced as complex or traumatic. This is true for several reasons:

- The loss of a primary caregiver places children at greater risk of not having their physical or psychological needs met due to the centrality of attachment bonds to children's development. When the bond with a primary caregiver has been severed, this has the potential to interfere with healthy physical, mental, and emotional development. In addition, children's inherent dependency on adults makes them more vulnerable to feelings and experiences of powerlessness, a hallmark of trauma.

- Parents are the best allies for their children in times of trouble. However, the capacity of parents to attend to the unique needs of their grieving children may be hindered if the parent is also grieving or having trauma-related reactions.
- Children are attuned to their parents and primary caregivers. They may react not only to their own loss but to the painful feelings and increased levels of stress experienced by their surviving caregivers.
- Given the fact that routine is fundamental for a young person's sense of security, a transformation in the family's lifestyle can be extremely upsetting to children and create feelings of insecurity and instability.
- Children's coping skills are limited by their development, thus restricting their choices of adaptive responses. For example, young children often lack the capacity to express their thoughts and feelings in words or articulate abstract needs in a way that is clear to their caregivers.
- The age-appropriate limits in children's ability to impact their circumstances constricts the ways in which they can adapt to the loss. This potentially exposes them to more serious harm both environmentally and psychologically as well as heightened feelings of powerlessness. For example, a school age child can do very little to impact secondary losses such as a decline in the family's financial status.
- As with adults, exposure to distressing images, sounds, smells, and other experiences, such as a dying loved one or a mutilated body, can produce traumatic reactions.
- Due to their limited life experience, children will place their own age-related interpretations on the loss and the corresponding circumstances. This may include the idea that they are responsible for the death. If not corrected, this results in inaccurate conclusions about themselves and their world. For example, when Sammy was 7 years old, his brother died of cancer. When asked about the death by his counselor, he disclosed his belief that he was to blame for his brother's illness. He had reached this conclusion because of a moment when he was with his brother and he coughed without covering his mouth. Sammy's young mind applied the teaching he had received about how germs and sickness are spread to his brother's disease. He lacked the knowledge or life experience to understand that cancer cannot be transmitted in the same way as colds and flu.

For these reasons, many everyday events that are not disturbing to adults can be traumatic for children.

Furthermore, the precise origin of a child's traumatic reactions may not be readily apparent to adults. Even in situations where the cause of the trauma seems obvious, it may not represent the most upsetting moment for the child. Thus, a thorough assessment is essential. Practitioners, in conjunction with the child's caregivers, may need to piece together the events from the child's perspective in order to unearth the aspects that provoked the traumatic reactions. This is especially true with pre-verbal and very young children (APA Presidential Task Force on Posttraumatic Stress Disorder and Trauma in Children and Adolescents, 2008). Therefore, knowledge of how trauma impacts children and adolescents goes hand in hand with understanding how children comprehend and react to loss.

TRAUMATIC GRIEF

In addition to grief reactions, a loss that is traumatic in nature can induce the added symptoms that come with trauma, such as intrusive and disturbing images, negative beliefs about self and the world, hyperarousal, and nightmares. In addition, children and adolescents with traumatic grief are sensitive to both pleasant and unpleasant thoughts or situations that provoke memories of the deceased and how their loved one died. They experience three types of reminders that can cause distress. Trauma reminders are sights, sounds, smells, and places that are associated with the death. Loss reminders include people, locations, things, memories, or circumstances that remind the child of the person who died. Change reminders are the persons, locations, circumstances, or objects that highlight for children the changes that have occurred in their lives as a result of the death. For example, Clarita was 9 years old when her father was rushed to the hospital where he died from a heart attack. Clarita experienced agitation whenever she was exposed to an ambulance or was driven past a hospital (trauma reminder), when her grandmother took her to soccer practice instead of her dad (change reminder), and during baseball season which she had always enjoyed with her father (loss reminder).

Children and teens may also avoid thinking about their loved one because it leads to distressing thoughts associated with the disturbing aspects of the death. Because these reminders are nearly impossible to avoid, they may subconsciously respond by numbing their emotions. This can result in detachment from others, feelings of alienation, and interference with the natural process of grief (Mannarino & Cohen, 2011).

ASSESSING GRIEF IN CHILDREN AND ADOLESCENTS

In working with grieving children and adolescents, it is beneficial to gather information from a variety of sources in order to get valid information about the death, traumatic elements of the loss, and the problems the child has been experiencing. Therefore, interviews with parents or caregivers, the child's physician, the child's teacher or school counselor, and other adults who play an important role in the child's life (e.g. a grandmother who cares for the child after school) can be very informative. Even with older children and adolescents, the additional information gathered from such sources can be extremely valuable. In addition, it is judicious to assess any physical symptoms the child is exhibiting, such as encopresis or extreme lethargy, in collaboration with a physician. Medical origins of the problem should be ruled out before concluding that it represents somatic distress or regression associated with the loss.

When assessing children under the age of 13, play therapy techniques and astute observation of the child's imaginative play can provide rich information about the child's feelings about the loss and how they are trying to make sense of it. Additionally, games that encourage children to identify their feelings can both inform the assessment and provide therapeutic benefit to the child.

Older children and adolescents may be more able and willing to converse directly about their feelings. Often, a combination of some activity along with conversation is useful for establishing rapport with older children and making it easier for them to talk about difficult and emotional subjects. Frequently, adolescents will attend counseling reluctantly and only at the insistence of their caregivers. Thus, an extended period of time spent building the relationship may be necessary before they are willing to engage in activities and conversations that are relevant to their loss.

Grief Assessment with Children and Adolescents Using Standardized Instruments

Because there are few standardized instruments for measuring grief in children and adolescents, instruments that measure symptoms associated with grief and trauma must be used. Some common and relevant assessment instruments for this population are:

- Persistent Complex Bereavement Disorder (PCBD) Checklist – Youth (Hill et al., 2020)
- The Hogan Sibling Inventory of Bereavement (Hogan, 1990)
- The W. T. Grant Inventory (Clark et al., 1994)
- The Child Behavior Checklist (CBCL) (Achenbach & Edelbrock, 1983)
- The Piers–Harris Children's Self-Concept Scale (Piers, 1984; Kanoy et al., 1980; Mannarino, 1978)
- Hopelessness Scale for Children (HSC) (Kazdin et al., 1983; Fischer & Corcoran, 1994)
- Child PTSD Symptom Scale (CPSS) (Foa et al., 2001).
- Child Report of Post-traumatic Symptoms (CROPS) (Greenwald & Rubin, 1999)
- Child Trauma Screening Questionnaire (CTSQ) (Kenardy et al., 2006)
- Child Stress Disorders Checklist (CSDC) (Saxe et al., 2003).

STRENGTHS IN CHILDREN AND ADOLESCENTS

As stated in the strengths-based framework of grief and loss, all individuals are endowed with individual and environmental strengths. Children and adolescents are no exception to this rule. In fact, the numerous individual and environmental strengths of youth can be beneficial resources at a time when they are facing the adversity of a significant loss.

In an international research study called the International Resilience Project, researchers studied resilience in children and families from 30 countries around the globe. From this large-scale research project, Grotberg (1996) uncovered 26 strengths that were most frequently identified as contributing to resilience among children. Some of the individual strengths that were identified included a "sense of being loveable, autonomy, self-esteem, hope and faith and trust, and locus of control" in addition to possessing skillfulness with "communication, problem solving, and impulse control" (p. 6). Some of the environmental strengths, or resilience factors, that were identified included "trusting relationships, structure and rules at home, parental encouragement of autonomy, and role models" (p. 6). Many other strengths can be found in children and adolescents depending on their unique situations and personalities. From this study, Grotberg developed a practical method for classifying individual and environmental strengths and resources that children can readily understand. For environmental supports and resources that a child can access, Grotberg uses the term "I HAVE." For internal strengths she uses the term "I AM." These inner strengths include confidence, self-esteem, and responsibility. For social skills, she uses the term "I CAN," which refers to both interpersonal and problem-solving skills. These three components of resilience correspond to Erikson's stages of development, specifically trust, autonomy, identity, initiative, and industry. Children can be aided in consciously exploring the different components of resilience. For example, the more things a child can identify under the categories "I HAVE," "I AM," and "I CAN," the more equipped they will be to deal with the death of a loved one. Table 5.1 gives some examples of how a child's strengths can be viewed using Grotberg's components of resilience.

Using this paradigm, the counselor and the youth can effectively work together to identify and enhance the child's internal and external strengths and resources.

The list in Table 5.2 was created by 10-year-old Jessica and her counselor after the death of her older brother. During their sessions, the counselor and Jessica added to this list. By the end of their work together, the list was completed.

TABLE 5.1 Individual and Environmental Strengths for Children

Erikson's Stage of Development	Grotberg's Component of Resilience	Examples
Trust	I HAVE	• Caregivers with unconditional love for me • Appropriate role models • Caring mentors • People who structure my environment • People who help me stay safe • People who want me to be independent
Autonomy and Identity	I AM	• A loveable person • A caring person • A person who respects myself and others • A person who takes responsibility for my actions • Hopeful for the future
Initiative and Industry	I CAN	• Find someone to talk to about my feelings • Find solutions to my problems • Exhibit self-control • Talk to someone who can help me

TABLE 5.2 I Have, I Am, I Can

I HAVE	I AM	I CAN
A best friend	Determined to get through this	Ask Mom to spend time with me
Two parents that love me	A good friend	Tell people to stop asking me questions
A counselor	Kind to my parents, friends, and pets	Cry into my pillow
A girl scout troop	A person who tries hard and doesn't give up	Call my friend on the phone when I want to laugh
My own room	A person who will always love and remember my brother	Write in my journal
My puppy, "Jazz"	A creative person with a good imagination	Ask my teacher for help

At the end of each session, the counselor made a copy for Jessica to take home and post in her room. The counselor suggested that between sessions Jessica think about other things she could add to the list as well as keep a record of times that she used or practiced one of her strengths. As a result of this intervention, Jessica's resilience was strengthened and she was able to cope with the death of her brother and her parents' grief more effectively.

BOX 5.1 MOURNING RITUALS: MEXICAN AMERICANS

Many Mexican Americans place high value on their religious and spiritual beliefs, and this is reflected in their customs around death. For those who practice Catholicism, the mourning ritual begins with an open casket service one to two evenings before the funeral. During this service family and friends come to honor the deceased, and there is group recitation of the prayer of the Rosary for the soul of the deceased. Frequently, women host these events by leading the prayers, inviting family and friends, and providing food. A funeral mass is held at the church followed by a graveside service. The priest or deacon blesses the grave with holy water. It is customary to wear dark colors to this emotional occasion, and family members will travel from great distances to represent their familial connection with the deceased. Largely attended funerals validate the high regard held for the deceased, as well as the strength of family ties even beyond death (Hidalgo, 2017).

FAMILY-RELATED ISSUES

When a family member dies, the impact has a domino effect. Each family member has a unique response to the death according to their developmental phase, relationship with the deceased, personality, emotional make-up, and role within the family.

Most families naturally strive to maintain a homeostatic balance, or status quo. When a state of disequilibrium occurs as with a death in the family, family members will adjust roles, behaviors, and emotions in an attempt to restore the family balance. These adjustments can be explained on a continuum from life-enhancing to life-depleting. Children and adolescents are particularly vulnerable to these changes in the family. While each family situation is unique, there are some common themes that are often seen in grieving families.

The Overwhelming Strain of Grief

When the entire family is dealing with the destabilizing effects of grief, it can be more difficult for children to get the support they need from their caregivers. If surviving caregivers are unable to provide comfort and consistent discipline, children may struggle to manage their stress and regulate their emotions. The reinstatement of stability and security are crucial to preventing behavior problems, yet these are herculean tasks for bereaved caregivers who are overwhelmed with their own grief (Griese et al., 2017). Because children are often reluctant to share their feelings, their needs can easily go unnoticed. In addition, they may desire a respite from the grief reactions of other family members or feel the need to shield their caregivers from the pain they experience (Hidalgo, 2017).

In extreme situations the parent becomes so disabled by the loss that the roles of the parent and child are reversed, leaving the child with the responsibility of caring for the parent, emotionally or by assuming responsibility for activities of daily living, such as cleaning the house, buying groceries, or preparing meals. When the roles between parents and children become blurred, the child's feelings of safety and security are compromised. Furthermore, the child's own feelings of grief are undermined and may be sublimated or expressed in a life-depleting manner. Also vulnerable are children who lose a single parent or both parents. This results in numerous and complex secondary losses as they must adjust to living with different caregivers (Bergman et al., 2017).

The Toll of Trauma

The toll of grief that is also traumatic in nature can further strain families that are struggling to adjust to a loss. Depending on the circumstances, it may be that only one or all family members will have traumatic responses to the loss. The ripple effects, however, of even one person with symptoms of PTSD can impact all family members and increase their risk of PTSD (Horesh & Brown, 2018; Rabenstein & Harris, 2017). Parents may have traumatic reactions to seeing their children endure pain and suffering and by their knowledge of the trauma their child experienced (Rabenstein & Harris, 2017). Because children rely on their caregivers to help them manage stress and provide a safe environment that enables exploration and growth, they are greatly impacted by trauma-induced behavioral changes in other family members. This may include heightened anxiety and sensitivity, withdrawal, anger, and abusive behaviors as well as appearing disconnected or displaying extreme startle reactions or flashbacks. In addition, avoidance symptoms may make it difficult for the traumatized family member to participate in daily tasks and routines or be present to the children's activities (Rabenstein & Harris, 2017).

The circumstances surrounding traumatic grief can strain families' internal and external resources. Time, money, and energy may be diverted from family-strengthening endeavors to deal with legal proceedings, moving, changing schools, or managing tight finances. Relationships with other family members can be a source of support but if the stress becomes too high, family relationships can suffer from difficulties with communication, collaboration, and feeling close with one another (The National Child Traumatic Stress Network, n.d.). Without adequate support, these stressors threaten the child's fundamental need for safety and security in the home and with caregivers.

The Loss of a Sibling

The death of a sibling can have unique ramifications for families because the loss impacts parents and children differently. Once again, parents may be so consumed with their own grief that they may struggle to attend to the needs of the surviving children in the family. At the extreme end of this continuum, children learn to function without parental guidance, restrictions, or discipline. At the other extreme, parents may become overprotective of the remaining children and be highly anxious about their child's activities due to fear of losing another child. At either end of this spectrum, young people may begin to act out in an attempt to change their parents' compensatory behavior.

From the perspective of the child, a sibling's death comes with numerous secondary losses. Often it means they have lost a primary source of socialization as well as a mentor, companion, confidante, and playmate (Hidalgo, 2017). In addition, parents can inadvertently affect surviving children in the way they memorialize the child who died. Some siblings report feeling as though they can never measure up to the idealized image of the deceased child and feel trapped in the shadow of their sibling's legacy. They may struggle with developing their own identity apart from the deceased sibling. Others state that they wish they were the one that had died.

The life-depleting aspects of these family dynamics can be minimized when family members are able to openly and safely communicate their emotions and needs concerning the loss. In addition, families tend to fare better when the members understand and respect the individuality of each member's grieving experience. Parents who are able to recognize and cope with their own grief are available to assist their children in life-enhancing ways. Parents and children often need to mourn the loss separately, as well as together as a family. Some parents feel uncomfortable expressing grief in front of their children out of concern that a display of intense emotions will scare the children. Therefore, the challenge for grieving parents is to strike a balance between modeling the healthy expression of emotions while maintaining a sense of security in the home. Children benefit from reassurance that, despite the sadness of losing a family member, they will remain a family unit.

It is unrealistic to expect that families can successfully manage these challenges in isolation. They will benefit from a systemic approach that cares for the whole family and includes strong social supports, peer support programs, community resources, and at times, professional assistance (Griese et al., 2017). Strengths-based interventions are especially useful in working with families. Highlighting and supporting both the strengths of individual family members as well as those of the family as a whole lay the foundation for improved communication, understanding, and the ability to work together as a team.

SCHOOL-RELATED ISSUES

School is the major occupation of children and adolescents. It is where they are under pressure to function at their best intellectually, emotionally, behaviorally, and socially. When a death occurs in a family, children and teens are generally expected to return to school in a relatively short period of time. For some grieving children, school provides safety and comfort by allowing them to return to some semblance of routine and structure. For others, particularly adolescents, school can heighten the sense of loss, provoke anxiety, and be a stress-inducing environment that they want to avoid. There is some evidence that adolescents bereaved by a sudden loss experience difficulty in the school environment which may include lower academic performance, increased disengagement with the school, negative beliefs about teachers, and challenges with learning and concentration (Oosterhoff et al., 2018).

School counselors can be a valuable resource for children, adolescents, and families in bereavement. They are often viewed as safe professionals in the school, to whom the young person can turn when experiencing difficulties during the school day. They can serve as advocates for the family when negotiating with teachers about deadlines, workloads, and performance expectations of the student as well as alert family members to observations of students that are concerning (Hill et al., 2019). School personnel may be especially able to notice if students are isolating from their peers which can be a significant cause for concern. Many school counselors provide grief support groups for students in addition to referrals to relevant community resources. Because of the important role that social support plays both in academic functioning and in healing from loss, the school environment can be an important environmental strength for youth.

EMERGENCY CONSIDERATIONS

There are instances in which a young person's grief is severe enough that they may develop depression. Research confirms that bereaved children and teens are at an elevated risk of attempting suicide, even years after the loss (Guldin et al., 2015; Hill et al., 2019). Warning signs that an adolescent may be at risk of self-harm include social alienation and the feeling that they do not belong, the belief that they have no one to turn to, and the perception of being a burden to others (Hill et al., 2019). Due to a wish to avoid negative feelings and a lack of coping skills, youth may "act out" their feelings by harming themselves or "mask" their feelings with behaviors to keep adults from discovering their depression. Thus, it is very important that bereaved children and adolescents are assessed for suicidal ideation and behaviors.

As a result of their developmental stage some adolescents are more likely to engage in risk-taking behaviors. Bereaved youth may be especially drawn to dangerous activities motivated by their reactions to the loss. Risk-taking behaviors may represent a drive to conquer fears related to the traumatic death or to use thrill seeking as a way to distract themselves from the grief. They may abuse substances as a way to self-medicate, behave aggressively to avoid feeling helpless, assimilate unhealthy values or behaviors of the deceased in an attempt to feel connected with them, engage in suicidal ideation and reunification fantasies in an effort to alleviate separation distress, or become nihilistic and careless to manage their existential questioning. In addition, difficulty regulating their emotions and behaviors in response to loss and trauma reminders may dispose them to act impulsively (Layne et al., 2017).

BOX 5.2 MOURNING RITUALS: HINDUISM

While there is vast diversity in beliefs and practices among Hindu people, there is commonality in how they mourn the dead. Upon death, the body is bathed, rubbed with oils, and dressed. Cremation, which assists the soul's journey to the other world, must happen before the next sunrise. The next ten days are spent in prayer and meditation in order to facilitate the soul's transition. If these rituals are not carefully followed, the deceased will continue to be a bodiless spirit and will not become an ancestor. It is believed that the deceased observes the mourners during this time and detaches from its earthly life on the 11th day. Family and friends congregate on the 12th day to honor and remember their loved one (Hidalgo, 2017).

CULTURAL CONSIDERATIONS

The cultural background of the child and family must be taken into consideration when assisting children and adolescents with their grief. The family culture of grief (see Chapter 1) will have a prominent impact on how a child or adolescent perceives and experiences loss. Rituals surrounding the death are often family specific as well as culturally grounded. In some families, for example, it is believed that children should be protected from the negative experiences associated with death and grief and, therefore, children are excluded from rituals and discussions concerning the deceased. In other families, children are encouraged to be involved in all aspects of the death and memorialization of the deceased. These families talk openly about the death in the presence of children with no regard for their needs or feelings. Balancing these two extremes are the families who expose their children to some aspects of the grieving process while protecting them from other aspects that may overwhelm their coping abilities.

Because families often explain death to children in the context of their religious beliefs, practitioners need to have an understanding of the family's spiritual orientation and their views about death and the afterlife. Some families tell children that the loved one "went to heaven." Other families cope with loss with sayings such as "It was his time to go" or "God called him home." These spiritual explanations will be absorbed by children and may have either a positive or negative impact on their grief reactions. Practitioners play a role in mitigating any fears or misunderstandings engendered by these explanations while also being respectful of the family's beliefs.

It is important to communicate with the adults in the family about how the child has made sense of the death. Family members may be unaware of the child's reasoning abilities and how certain statements may be construed in the child's mind. When it is necessary to clarify a child's understanding of events surrounding the loss, practitioners should engage the family system in working with the child. This helps to ensure that the family's value and belief system is not invalidated.

INTERVENTIONS

Helping children and adolescents with grief involves creating safety in the therapeutic relationship, working with caregivers, psychoeducation, emotional regulation, processing the trauma, and mourning the loss. Play therapy techniques are often used to deliver interventions in a way that meets the child's level of development and at a pace that is tolerable for the child. Carter (2005) states that,

> Play therapy is effective for children dealing with traumatic grief since it gives them the opportunity to have control over the issues, to proceed at their own pace, and to experience the safety of projection and communicating in the language of play. (p. 123)

Creating Safety

As with adults, healing from grief occurs within the context of a safe, compassionate, and accepting relationship. Children naturally look to their primary caregivers for this, but when those caregivers are absent or are also struggling, professional assistance can be very helpful. When working with children, counselors use therapeutic play therapy skills along with appropriate pacing to establish a safe relationship with the child and help them remain within their window of tolerance (Turner, 2020).

For adolescents, an extended period of rapport building may be required before they are willing to be vulnerable. It is not uncommon for bereaved adolescents to spend the majority of their counseling session discussing school, peers, and other concerns and spend minimal time focusing on the loss. This is understandable given their need to manage multiple developmental challenges, in addition to grief. By taking a relational approach, the therapist creates an environment that supplements the teen with additional support that may not be readily available in their families. When issues surrounding the loss do arise, counselors are able to gently nudge teens to explore these because of the trust and safety that has been built into the relationship.

Working with Caregivers

Often a child or adolescent's response to grief and trauma are demonstrated and expressed through their behaviors. These behaviors can easily be misinterpreted by adults who are unknowledgeable about how this population responds to loss and trauma. For this reason, effective interventions often include educating the youth's caregivers and coaching them on how to care for their bereaved child. This may include providing information about how children understand death, age-appropriate ways to explain death to children, explanation of trauma responses, ways to help when children are experiencing strong emotions and concerning behaviors, as well as the importance of communicating to children that they are not the cause of the death or the family's subsequent difficulties. Because caregivers may also be struggling with their own grief reactions, connecting them with appropriate resources such as counseling and supporting them as they strive to provide a stable environment can be an essential component of helping children.

In addition to counseling, caregivers should be encouraged to help their children get ample nutrition, rest, and exercise as they are struggling to combat the stress of grief. Teens in particular may need encouragement to give attention to these matters. Caregivers can also support a grieving adolescent by encouraging participation in activities of interest, such as sports teams and student clubs. In one qualitative study of 253 adolescents, the researchers identified family, relatives, and friends as sources of support for grieving adolescents. In addition, a third of the adolescents surveyed felt that activities assisted them with the grieving process (Rask et al., 2002).

Psychoeducation

As with adults, children and teens benefit by knowing that their grief reactions are an expected response to their loss. Children may need assistance acquiring sufficient vocabulary in order to communicate their feelings and then be taught skills to help them manage those emotions. In addition, depending on their developmental stage, children will need assistance developing an accurate understanding of death and its causes. Particularly important is educating children to understand that they are not the cause of their loved one's death. There are many creative ways of delivering this information so that it meets the child's level of development and engages them in learning. It is preferable that these activities be enjoyable as play is a fundamental way that children acquire new information.

Emotional Regulation

Teaching children ways to manage overwhelming feelings is an important component of grief counseling. This often involves teaching specific skills that facilitate safe and healthy expression of emotions as well as stress-relieving activities. Physical movement and mindfulness exercises can be very useful in helping children improve their ability to regulate their emotions and reduce fear and anxiety. It is, of course, best to use language appropriate to the child's development and experience. Deep breathing, for example, can be described as smelling flowers (inhaling through the nose) and blowing out birthday candles (exhaling through the mouth). These activities are most effective when incorporated into the child's play or presented in the form of a game. One valuable resource for teaching emotional regulation to children is *Mindfulness Skills for Kids & Teens* by Debra Burdick (2014).

Processing the Trauma

A major aspect of helping children process traumatic events involves restoring safety in the child's environment. This necessitates working with caregivers to identify elements in the environment that evoke trauma responses and help children become desensitized to these. Some children will do this in their play by repeatedly re-enacting aspects of the trauma. For this reason, it is helpful to have toys available that facilitate this play such as toy ambulances, police cars, doctor kits, pill bottles, and other items that would be relevant to the child's experience of the loss event. Movement, art, and Eye Movement Desensitization and Reprocessing (EMDR) can also be useful in helping children and adolescents metabolize the overwhelming aspects of their experience.

Graduated exposure and role play of challenging situations can also help children learn to stay within their window of tolerance when confronted with triggers. For example, after his younger brother was killed, 7-year-old Kadeem became very anxious when getting dropped off at school and resisted separating from his mother. His therapist arranged for him and his mom to "practice" separating in her office. She instructed Kadeem and his mom to come up with a playful goodbye ritual (they designed a special handshake) and had Kadeem and Mom do this ritual at the door to the counselor's office. After Mom dropped Kadeem off at the pretend school, she left the office. With Kadeem's knowledge she was instructed to stand right outside the office door, while Kadeem and the counselor played school. A few minutes later, Mom would return to pick him up from school. They repeated this scenario several times, having Kadeem's mom stand farther away from the office each time until she eventually waited from her car in the office parking lot. In this way, Kadeem gained confidence that he could be okay when separated from Mom at school and that Mom would return for him.

Part of processing trauma may also involve helping children and teens identify and alter any cognitive distortions that developed from the loss event. These distortions can emerge as a result of fragmented memories or dissociation that often occurs with trauma. They may include negative evaluations of themselves and the world such as, "It's my fault," "I could have prevented it," "No one can be trusted," and "I'm not safe."

Mourning the Loss

Helping professionals have a unique role in assisting children and adolescents process the death of their loved one and support them as they mourn the loss by providing safe spaces for feelings that may be too uncomfortable to openly confront in their home environment. Children can be encouraged to tell the story of the loss, share memories of their loved one, and talk about how their life has changed as a result of the death. There are numerous ways these tasks can be folded into age-appropriate activities such as making memory boxes or scrap books, body maps, art projects, doll house play, puppet play, storytelling, and more. Likewise, activities such as writing letters to the deceased, releasing balloons with messages to the loved one, or designing jewelry that symbolizes the deceased's characteristics can engage children in nurturing continuing bonds with their loved one. Such activities can also prompt conversation about the deceased and the child's feelings that may be difficult to elicit otherwise. Even teenagers will participate in creative activities that allow them to express themselves and share their experience at a level that feels comfortable for them. One example is to have the adolescent decorate a box with the outside depicting what the teen presents to the world and the inside representing the teen's internal experience. Numerous activity ideas can be found on the internet as well as in books, including *Healing Activities for Children in Grief* by Gay McWhorter (2003) and *Creative Interventions for Bereaved Children* by Liana Lowenstein (2006).

STANDARD INTERVENTIONS

Trauma and Grief Component Therapy for Adolescents (TGCTA)

Developed by Saltzman et al. (2017), TGCTA is an evidence-based intervention shown to reduce PTSD, depression, and life-depleting grief reactions in bereaved, traumatized, and traumatically bereaved adolescents. In addition, research affirms that participants in TGCTA show enhanced connections with school and improved school behavior. The manualized instructions consist of modules that allow clinicians the flexibility to tailor the intervention to the needs of participants and provides assessment instruments to guide the customization. TGCTA has been used with a diverse population of youth both nationally and internationally. It can be delivered to individuals or groups and has been widely used in schools, residential treatment centers, clinics, and juvenile justice settings (The National Child Traumatic Stress Network, 2018).

Multidimensional Grief Therapy (MGT)

Though newer, and thus less researched, Multidimensional Grief Therapy (MGT) is an additional set of interventions based on Multidimensional Grief Theory. The activities in MGT are designed to decrease life-depleting grief reactions, promote life-enhancing coping mechanisms, and facilitate healthy adaptation to the loss. Elements of this intervention include psychoeducation about grief, identifying loss reminders, teaching coping skills, facilitating communication with caregivers, understanding the circumstances surrounding the death, and making meaning of the loss. Assessments are used to tailor the intervention to the unique needs of the youth.

GROUP INTERVENTIONS WITH CHILDREN AND ADOLESCENTS

Group interventions with same-aged children are especially powerful for bereaved youth because it allows them to find relief from the feeling of being different from their peers due to the loss. Group interventions may take many forms, including family counseling, counseling that involves groups of families, groups offered in the community, school-based groups, online support groups, and grief camps which assist youth with their grief in an outdoor setting. Important components of group intervention with children and teens include sharing the story of the loss, providing information about the grief process, validating and affirming grief responses, expressing feelings associated with grief, identifying life-enhancing coping mechanisms, addressing feelings of guilt associated with the loss, and memorializing the deceased (Garcia, 2017). Detailed curriculum and activities for conducting support groups for bereaved youth are available for practitioners. Lehmann et al. (2001a, 2001b, 2001c, 2001d, 2001e), for example, provide facilitators' guides and developmentally appropriate activities for children in preschool, elementary school, middle school, and high school.

CASES

CASE 5.1

Identifying Information:

Client Name: Hannah Holman
Age: 8 years old
Race/Ethnicity: White
Education level: Third grade
Members of household: Mother and sister, 19 years old

Intake Information:

Hannah's mother, Judith, called to request counseling for Hannah over the death of her father, Judith's husband, to cancer two months ago. Judith's voice quivers saying, "It's been hard for all of us. My husband was a really good man and a great father. I know Hannah is having a hard time and I'm not sure how to help her." You suggest a meeting with Judith alone before seeing Hannah. She is very agreeable to this and requests an appointment as soon as possible.

Initial Interview:

Judith arrives for the appointment on time and is rummaging through her purse while waiting for you in the lobby. You introduce yourself and hold out your hand to shake hers. She hurriedly finishes putting things back in her purse and shakes your hand saying, "I'm Judith. It's very nice to meet you."

As you walk with Judith to your office, you ask her if she had trouble finding the office building.

"Not really. I missed a couple of turns but I left the house early to give myself plenty of time. I've learned to do that since I've been so out of it lately," she says.

You and Judith enter your office and as you motion for her to take a seat, you say, "It wouldn't surprise me if you've been feeling out of it. You've had a lot going on."

"Yes, it's been….," her voice trails off as she dissolves into tears. You hand her the box of tissues.

"Thank you," she says, wiping her eyes and trying to pull herself together. "I'm sorry. I was going to try and not break down here today."

"It's perfectly okay for you to cry," you say.

"But," she says and then blows her nose, "I really want to focus on Hannah while I'm here."

"Okay," you say gently. "Why don't we begin with you telling me the reason you have decided to get some help for Hannah?"

"All right," Judith says. She takes a deep breath and seems ready to focus on her intended task of helping Hannah. "As I told you on the phone, my husband, Michael, died about two months ago. He got diagnosed with pancreatic cancer about nine months before his death. We're all having a hard time with it, but I'm especially concerned about Hannah. She was only 7 years old when Michael got sick and…well, she's trying so hard to understand it all. She keeps asking me questions about where her daddy is and why he died. Even though I feel like I've explained it all until I'm blue in the face. And she's been really weepy. She's just so young to lose her dad," Judith says with tears in her eyes. "I just want to do whatever I can to help her feel better."

"Of course, you do," you say. "And it is admirable that you are tending to Hannah's needs when you are in the midst of your own grief. Can you give me some examples of the weepiness that you see in Hannah?"

Judith answers, "Well, the other day she was playing around in the backyard and she fell and hurt her knee. It wasn't serious at all. It didn't even leave a mark, but she just burst into tears. She was sobbing! I hugged her tightly for a little bit and then she was suddenly okay again and ran off to play some more. Little insignificant things like that will set her off and she'll either start crying or become really whiny. The whining has been especially hard for me to deal with. I begin to lose my patience."

"Yes," you say, "I imagine that really tries your patience, especially when you are under so much stress already. What are some of the questions that she continues to ask?"

"She asks about cancer a lot. She wants to know what it is, if I'm going to get it, if she is going to get it, and on and on. She also asks about heaven a lot. The other day…" Judith pauses as tears run down her cheeks. "The other day she said she wanted to die and go to heaven. I nearly lost it! It scares me to hear her say things like that! Is she just wanting to see her daddy or is she so sad that she really wants to die?" Judith's voice is frantic now.

"Has she done or talked about doing anything to hurt herself?" you ask.

"No," Judith pauses as she tries to remember, "I can't think of anything."

"It is very likely that she is just expressing how much she misses her father," you say reassuringly. "But it's always a good idea to keep your antennae up for any signs that she is seriously trying to get herself to heaven or that she is severely depressed. Sometimes children will even do things to hurt themselves believing that it is a way to see their loved one. Usually, however, they don't understand the danger and permanency of their actions. This is certainly something I will evaluate and address when I meet with Hannah."

"Okay," Judith says. "I'm glad to have some help with this. I can barely hang on myself sometimes and I'm so afraid that I'm going to mess up with Hannah or miss something really important."

"The fact that you are worried about that and are taking some action towards your concern is a positive sign that you are paying close attention. It's a personal strength that you are aware of your own limitations. You are right when you indicate that this is too much to do alone. I commend you for seeking out assistance with this and I'm honored that you are trusting me to help you. Let's talk some more about the changes you have noticed in Hannah since your husband's illness and death," you suggest.

Judith explains that Hannah has been sleeping with her at night and has generally been clingier. She also said that Hannah has been complaining often of stomachaches. She is not aware of any changes in Hannah's school or social functioning, but she admits that she hasn't inquired about this to Hannah's teacher. She agrees to sign a form allowing you to consult with the teacher about how Hannah is doing in school.

You gather more information about Hannah, her strengths, interests, friends, and the kind of relationship she had with her dad. You also let Judith talk about the progression of her husband's illness. You learn that he died in their home under hospice care. You give Judith some printed brochures that discuss how children of different ages deal with grief and set up an appointment for you to meet with Hannah.

Initial Session with Hannah:

For your first session with Hannah, you enter the waiting room and find her snuggled up next to Judith on the couch while they look at a magazine. You squat down so that you are eye level with Hannah and introduce yourself. She nods at you but doesn't say anything. You compliment her on the purple jacket she is wearing and tell her that purple is your favorite color. She smiles, says it is her favorite color, too, and begins to tell you about her room in which everything is purple.

You bring Judith and Hannah into your office and address Hannah saying, "Hannah, I am a counselor and one of the things I do is to help families when someone they love has died. I've talked to many children who have lost a parent and they talk about feeling angry, confused, sad, and scared and some other big feelings that are sometimes hard to understand. You mom is bringing you here to see me so that I can help you with any of the feelings you may be having. I'll also be talking with your mom to help her know how to help you. Does that sound okay with you?"

Hannah nods. While you were talking Hannah would sometimes look at you and sometimes look at her feet and fiddle with her shoelaces. Your sense, however, was that she was listening closely.

"There is something else, Hannah, that I want you to understand – and this is very important," you say.

Judith gestures for Hannah to stop playing with her shoes and listen to you. Hannah looks at you and you continue, "In this room, you can say anything you want to say and you can have any feeling you want to have and you won't get in trouble for it. This room is a 'free zone'."

You expand on this idea for emphasis and Hannah nods her understanding.

As Judith gets up to return to the waiting room, Hannah hangs on her mother's arm and looks up at her, communicating that she doesn't want her mom to leave.

"You'll be okay, Hannah," Judith reassures her. "I'll be right down the hall if you need me." Reluctantly, Hannah lets her mother go.

You and Hannah chat about school, her pets, things she likes to do, etc. Then you supply Hannah with paper and colored pencils and ask her to draw a picture of her family. She draws a scene that includes her mother, herself, her big sister, and her pets. They are all smiling. In the top corner of the picture she draws her father and explains to you that he is in heaven.

"What do you think heaven is like?" you ask.

Hannah responds, "He isn't sick anymore and he's happy there."

"Do you ever wish you could go to heaven?" you inquire.

"Sometimes," Hannah says as she continues to draw.

"Why would you like to go to heaven?" you question.

"To see my daddy!" she says as if the answer should be obvious to you.

"I bet you miss your daddy a lot," you suggest.

Hannah nods.

"Have you ever tried to go to heaven?" you ask.

"No," she says. "Just thought about it."

Being sure to maintain a casual tone, you ask, "How would you get to heaven? Do you have any ideas?"

"Ummm.... I don't know," she says offhandedly.

"It would sure be neat to see your daddy again wouldn't it?" Hannah nods. "Would there be anything bad about going to heaven?"

"If I went to heaven then I couldn't see my mom," Hannah replies as she chooses a new color to use in her picture.

"That's right," you affirm. "We can't go back and forth can we?"

Hannah shakes her head and says, "Nope."

"It's hard to not have your daddy around, though," you comment gently.

Hannah nods and asks, "Can we do something else now?"

You then engage Hannah in a game in which each person moves their game piece around a board with feelings written on it. When a player lands on a feeling they are to name a time when they felt that way. During this game Hannah reveals that she feels scared when alone in her bed at night, happy when she goes to get snow cones with her big sister, angry at a classmate who teased her, and sad that her dad died.

When you land on the feeling "confused," you say, "Sometimes I feel confused about diseases like cancer and what makes people die."

Hannah seems to perk up when you say this and volunteers, "My dad had cancer."

"He did?" you ask.

"Yes," Hannah says. "He got real sick and had to have a special bed." She continues on, describing the hospital bed that her father had at their home and how it could be moved into different positions.

"Sometimes people believe that something they did caused their parent to die. Do you ever feel that way?" you ask.

"I played with his bed one time," Hannah says.

You try to clarify, "You played with the controls that made his bed go into different positions?"

Hannah nods but remains silent, making a design on the floor with the game pieces.

"Do you worry that moving Dad's bed made him die?"

Hannah shrugs as if to say, "I don't know." She then spies the chalkboard easel that you have in your office and asks to use it. She writes her name, draws some funny faces, and does some math problems as if she is playing teacher.

"Hannah," you say, "there is something very important that I want you to understand. Maybe you can write it on the chalkboard to help you remember."

"Okay," she says and readies herself for your dictation.

"Children do not cause cancer," you state confidently. You wait patiently and repeat this statement as needed while Hannah writes it on the chalkboard. When she is finished, you dictate one more sentence, "Moving hospital beds does not make people die." Again, Hannah copies this sentence and at your request reads what she has written back to you.

Your session time is up and you praise Hannah for all the sharing she did. She skips down the hall to reunite with her mother. While Hannah is in the restroom, you explain to Judith that you believe Hannah is at low risk for hurting herself and that her comments about going to heaven were probably her way of expressing how much she misses her father. You maintain, however, that she should be alert for additional statements or actions that may indicate otherwise. You also explain to Judith the tendency of young children to assume responsibility for the death and explain your suspicion that Hannah feels guilty about playing with the hospital bed. Judith seems surprised to hear this but agrees to look for opportunities to remind Hannah that she is not at fault for her father's death. You also suggest that Judith look for opportunities to help Hannah put words to her feelings and model this with her statements and behavior. You tell Judith that you will explore Hannah's worries and fears more when you meet with her again.

5.1-1. What are some of Hannah's responses to the loss of her father?

5.1-2. What aspects of her father's death could potentially feel traumatic to Hannah?

5.1-3. What kinds of coping skills could benefit Hannah? How could you teach her these in age-appropriate ways?

5.1-4. Do you think Hannah would benefit by having continuing bonds with her father? How might this look for someone her age?

5.1-5. What are some resources that could be beneficial to this family?

CASE 5.2

Identifying Information:

Client Name: Kelly Jackson
Age: 6 years old
Race/Ethnicity: African American
Educational Level: First grade
Members in Household: Mothers, Gina and Lachelle

Intake Information:

Gina called and told the intake worker that her daughter, Kelly, age 6, had recently been in a car accident in which her aunt, age 17, was driving. Kelly's 3-year-old sister, Octavia, died at the scene of the accident and there is concern about how this has impacted Kelly. Gina explained that she is in a same sex marriage and wanted to know how this would be regarded. After assuring her that they would receive total and complete acceptance, you recommend meeting first with Gina and Lachelle without Kelly. You explain that this will allow them to speak freely about their concerns and get to know you and how you work. Gina agreed to this and booked some time on your calendar.

Initial Interview:

Gina and Lachelle arrive at the Child Grief Center for their scheduled appointment. After greeting them in the waiting room, you escort them to your office and encourage them to find a comfortable place to sit.

"It sounds like you have been dealing with a very tragic situation," you begin.

Gina immediately gets tears in her eyes and reaches for a tissue. "Octavia was only 3 years old. We had her for such a short time. We're all in shock that she is gone. It's almost like this is just a bad dream and we'll wake up and find out it's not true."

"When did this happen?" you inquire.

Gina looks at Lachelle, and says, "Four weeks ago?"

"Yes, it's been a month, now," Lachelle replies. "The funeral was three weeks ago on Saturday."

"Okay, can you tell me a little about what happened?" you ask. "I imagine it's hard to talk about but it would help me know how to help Kelly."

Lachelle clears her throat and tells you about the night of the car accident. "My sister, Marie, is 17 years old. She's really my half-sister. My mother remarried after divorcing my father. Marie is 14 years younger than I am. Anyway, she was driving the car when a giant 18-wheeler pulled out in front of her at an intersection. It wasn't her fault. The truck driver had a red light and plowed through the intersection. Marie slammed on the brakes but hit the tail end of the truck. The car smashed into the truck on the passenger side. Octavia was sitting in the back seat on that side of the car. Marie hit the windshield and was knocked unconscious. When the ambulance arrived, Kelly was holding Octavia on her lap but we think she was already gone. The doctor said she died immediately upon impact. She didn't have a chance. Her door was completely pushed to the other side of the car. Kelly thought her sister would wake up. She kept saying, 'Octavia, it's going to be okay. Wake up!' Kelly has always felt like she's got to take care of Octavia, like she's the big sister and responsible for her little sister."

"I am so sorry," you exclaim. "I'm sure the past month has been a very stressful time for the whole family."

Gina stares out the window and sighs. "It's been the worst month of our lives. Octavia was such a happy and outgoing little girl and we all loved her so much."

"Tell me how Kelly has been coping with this situation," you suggest.

Lachelle shifts in her chair and looks concerned. "I don't know what's going on with Kelly. One minute she seems okay and the next minute she's throwing a temper tantrum or running through the house in tears. She seems all stirred up and in constant motion. She is having a real hard time being still."

"How has she been sleeping and eating?" you ask.

"Not well," Lachelle replies while Gina shakes her head.

"She's up three or four times during the night and is scared to sleep in her own room. She and Octavia shared a room so she's not used to sleeping by herself. Sometimes we let her get in bed with us, but sometimes we tell her she needs to stay in her own bed," Gina explains.

Looking very anxious, Lachelle says, "That's just one problem. She's going a million miles an hour all day long and hardly stops long enough to eat. You can't get her attention. She keeps moving and won't stop. She talks constantly and most of it is just chatter. We just don't know what to do. It's wearing us out, to be honest."

"I'm sure it is," you reply. "The loss of Octavia would be exhausting in and of itself and then trying to help Kelly on top of that must feel like an awful lot."

They both nod in agreement. "It really is," Gina confirms.

"How does Kelly understand what happened to Octavia? How have you explained it to her?" you inquire.

"We told her that Octavia has gone to heaven," Gina replies.

"We told her that Octavia wasn't coming back and that when the truck hit the car, she died," Lachelle adds.

"Okay, and has she talked about Octavia since the accident?" you ask.

"She hasn't mentioned her since the funeral," Gina says. "She seems to talk about everything in the world except Octavia."

"Except for that one night," Lachelle reminds her.

"That's right," Gina says. "There was one night, as I was putting her in her bed, she told me she used to talk to Octavia at night because Octavia was afraid of the dark. I told her that was because Octavia was just a little girl and I was proud of her for being a big girl and helping her sister. She told me she wished Octavia was still here and wondered if Octavia did something bad. I tried to reassure her that Octavia did nothing wrong and that it was just because the truck hit the car. It was an accident."

"Okay, are there any other concerns you have about how Kelly has been acting, thinking, or feeling?" you inquire.

They look at each other and Lachelle says, "Well she's having a lot of trouble at school. The teacher says she's having trouble sitting still and paying attention. She keeps jumping out of her seat and isn't doing her work. The teacher seems to understand, but I don't know how long she'll be able to put up with Kelly's behavior. I'm worried that she's going to have a hard time passing second grade if she can't do her work."

"Would you all be willing to give me permission to talk to Kelly's teacher?" you inquire.

"That's fine with us," both parents say in unison.

"Great. Thank you," you reply. "The behaviors you are currently seeing with Kelly, were they present before the accident?"

"No," Lachelle says. "This is a different kid. She's always been energetic, loved to play, friendly and all. Mostly easy going." She looks at Gina, "I mean she'd fuss sometimes but not like this."

"No, not like this," Gina adds. "That was usually just when she was tired or hungry. Like any kid. We rarely had to discipline her. Now, we are trying to figure out what to do. She's not as cooperative as she used to be."

You continue to gather information from Gina and Lachelle to inform your assessment. You also talk with them about how children deal with grief and trauma and answer their questions about your approach with children like Kelly.

"This is definitely a team approach," you explain. "You know Kelly better than I ever will and you are her best allies. Please communicate with me about what you are seeing at home so that we can make sure the counseling is helpful. And if you're open to it, I'll also do some coaching with you to help guide you in parenting Kelly right now."

"Yes, please!" Lachelle says. "We need that!"

"Yes," Gina agrees. "We are very open to that!"

Initial Session with Kelly:

When you enter the waiting room to meet Kelly for the first time, you see Lachelle picking magazines off the floor while Kelly proceeds to dump an entire box of Legos on the floor. Lachelle sighs.

"Well, hello," you say as you kneel down to get on eye level with Kelly. You introduce yourself and start some chit chat about playing with Legos. "I have some other things in my office that you might like playing with. Would you like to come see?"

Kelly nods and smiles.

"Let's clean these up," Lachelle says and the three of you work together to pick up all the Legos. You praise her for helping and show her the way to your office. As she skips down the hall, she asks questions about the office, who works there, if there is a bathroom, and so on. As you enter your office, Kelly looks around.

"Do you like to color, Kelly?" you ask.

"Yes," she says. You both sit at a small table and you each begin coloring on a piece of paper. "I like to draw rainbows," Kelly says, as she grabs numerous crayons looking for the right color. She continues talking about rainbows, coloring, and emptying the crayon box. When she has finished her picture you say, "Oh, I really like that! It's very pretty! Kelly would you draw me a picture of your family?"

"Okay," she says.

She begins drawing but gets distracted and spies the basket of puppets in the corner.

"Puppets!" she exclaims. "I like those puppets over there."

"Okay, do you want to go get one for you and one for me and we can play puppets?"

Kelly rushes over and pulls out two monkeys that have long arms and legs that wrap around the child. The legs can be attached with Velcro. "I'll take the girl monkey and you take the mommy monkey," Kelly says.

"How are you doing today?" you say through the monkey.

Kelly turns around in circles and says, "I'm fine. My name is Monica."

"Hi Monica, I have been talking to your parents," you say. "They tell me that you were in an accident."

Kelly jumps up and down with her monkey on her arm, "My aunt had a car accident and my sister got hurt."

"Oh, that must have been very sad," you say.

"Her name is Octavia and she's only 3 years old," Kelly says. "She's a little monkey – that's what her mommies say."

"I see. Can you tell me about Octavia?" you suggest.

"Octavia is an angel now – a little monkey angel," Kelly says. "And I'm an angel too, my name is Monica and I'm an angel on the ground and Octavia is an angel in heaven."

"Okay, so I bet you miss Octavia," you suggest.

Kelly put her arm around the monkey and begins twirling in a circle. "What's that?" she says pointing to something on your desk.

"The stapler?" you ask. In an instant, Kelly has thrown the monkey puppet on the floor and is climbing onto the top of your desk and stapling paper together.

"Let me give you some paper that you can staple down here," you say.

"Okay, I like to staple," Kelly says. She climbs off the desk and sees a game in the corner.

"Can we play that game?" she asks, pointing to the corner.

"Do you like to play games?" you ask.

Kelly goes over and pulls the top off the game. She opens the board and begins spinning the wheel around. She gets up and runs over to the other corner where there is a large ball.

"Can I play with this?" she asks.

"We can, but wouldn't you like to finish playing the game, first?" you suggest.

Kelly rubs her head and says "No, I don't feel like playing that game anymore." She grabs the ball and sits on the floor. You sit across from her on the floor and she begins rolling the ball to you.

"Kelly, can you tell me about missing Octavia?" you ask.

Kelly squirms around on the floor and says, "I miss Octavia because she is my sister and she's not here anymore and she just laid down on my lap and wouldn't wake up. I tried to wake her up but she just wouldn't. My mom said that's because she died and turned into an angel and went up to heaven."

"Okay, that must have been very sad when she didn't wake up," you suggest.

"I cried and cried," Kelly says. "And then we had a funeral and then we put her in the ground."

You ask Kelly questions about the accident, but she does not engage any further with you on this topic. As you continue to play together, you talk about things that help you get to know one another (e.g. favorite foods, favorite movies, what you like to do for fun, etc.).

As the session ends, you say "I enjoyed playing with you, Kelly. How would you like to come see me again?"

Kelly jumps up and says, "Yes, and remember, I am Monica not Kelly."

"Okay, you are Monica when we are playing monkeys, right?"

"Yup, can I play with that turtle next time?" Kelly inquires.

"Of course, next time you can play with the turtle," you say.

5.2-1. What additional questions would you ask Gina and Lachelle to inform your assessment?

5.2-2. In the initial session, what would you want Kelly's parents to know about how children experience grief?

5.2-3. What kind of information would you want to get from Kelly's teacher?

5.2-4. Given the circumstances surrounding Olivia's death, what are some toys you might want to have available during her sessions with you?

5.2-5. What are some activities that you could engage in with Kelly to help you assess her situation?

5.2-6. What kinds of interventions would be helpful to Kelly? How could you deliver these in an age-appropriate way?

5.2-7. What are some instructions that you could give to Kelly's parents to assist them with Kelly's behavior at home?

5.2-8. What are this family's strengths?

CASE 5.3

Identifying Information:

Client Name: Carlos Jimenez
Age: 4 years old
Race/Ethnicity: Hispanic
Educational Level: Preschool
Members in Household: Grandfather, grandmother, and two cousins, ages 8 and 10

Intake Information:

Mr. Jimenez calls and asks if someone can help his 4-year-old grandson, Carlos. He explains that Carlos has been living with them since his father (Mr. Jimenez's son) died, two months ago. Carlos's parents were divorced and the mother, he explains, has had no involvement with Carlos. Now the grandparents have sole custody.

Initial Interview:

You decide to meet with Mr. and Mrs. Jimenez for an initial interview before meeting with Carlos. They meet you in the waiting room and greet you warmly. Mr. Jimenez moans as he rises from his chair to shake your hand and you notice that he uses a cane to walk.

On the way to your office, Mrs. Jimenez states, "Thank you so much for helping us with little Carlos. He has been quite a handful for us."

Mr. and Mrs. Jimenez sit down and you begin by saying, "Has he? Tell me more about what's going on." Mr. Jimenez explains that his son, Freddie, was an electrician and died of an accident at work caused by an equipment malfunction.

Mrs. Jimenez adds with tears in her eyes, "He just didn't come home from work one day." She explains that she kept Carlos while Freddie was at work and that he would pick him up at their house every day on his way home. When you ask about the family history, the Jiminezes tell you that Carlos's parents divorced when he was 18 months old. They indicated that the marriage was very rocky and that they had argued a lot in front of Carlos. The Jimenezes explained that Carlos has not seen his mother since the divorce and that she readily gave sole custody to Freddie. You empathize with the loss of their son and ask about their concerns for Carlos.

Mr. Jimenez responds, "Well, he has always been a very active kid. Always running and tearing up things – you know how boys are. But since my son died he has really been acting bad. He hits his cousins a lot, pulls their hair, gets into their things. He is always doing something to make them angry."

"And I've noticed," Mrs. Jimenez adds, "that he gets frustrated very easily. It doesn't take much to set him off."

"What does he do when he gets set off?" you ask. Mr. and Mrs. Jimenez inform you that Carlos is prone to yelling, kicking, throwing things, and being very defiant of their authority.

Mrs. Jimenez says, "I have raised several children and grandchildren but I have never had a child act like this. He is out of control!"

"Have you noticed any other changes in Carlos's behavior since his father died?" you ask. "Perhaps changes in his sleeping or eating? Or has he been sick more often?"

"He doesn't eat," Mrs. Jimenez says. "Even when I make his favorite dinner, he just picks at his food. It's also been real hard to get him to go to bed. He wants me to lay down with him until he falls asleep. Sometimes while I'm laying there with him he'll ask me when his daddy is coming back. I say, 'Carlos, I've told you that your daddy is not coming back. He loved you very much but God called him to heaven. You need to be a good boy so you can see your daddy again someday'." She pauses and tearfully says, "Then I go to my room and cry my eyes out!"

You empathize with the difficulty of losing a child and praise the Jimenezes for taking on the difficult task of raising their grandson while in the midst of their own grief.

"We're in over our heads," Mr. Jimenez says. "As you can see, I can't get around very well anymore and these kids.... We love them to pieces and would do anything for them, but they wear us out. Carlos is almost more than we can handle."

"It is certainly a big job that you have taken on and I'd be happy to help you help Carlos," you say. "I will meet with Carlos but I'll also continue to talk with you often. I can give you some suggestions of things that you can do at home to help Carlos. Because he is so young, your involvement will be very important. We'll have to work as a team."

Mr. and Mrs. Jimenez both nod in agreement. "That's fine." Mr. Jimenez says. Then he adds, "What do you think we should do when he misbehaves?"

You explain, "A child's behavior is often a good clue as to how they are feeling. His behavior may represent how he is feeling about losing his father. There is nothing wrong with the way he feels. The problem is that since he is only 4 he doesn't know many other ways to express himself. One thing we will want to help him with is to find better ways to express his feelings. I will work on this with Carlos and you can help him with it at home, too."

"Should we punish him when he acts up?" Mrs. Jimenez asks. "He's been through so much already and he's only 4!"

You explain to the Jimenezes that discipline provides security for children and should not be waived for Carlos, especially at a time when he is likely feeling insecure due to all the change he has experienced. You describe the difference between punishment and discipline and review some positive discipline techniques. You also talk about healthy outlets for Carlos's feelings and how to respond when he acts out. The Jimenezes seem pleased to hear that there is some hope that things can improve and that there are steps they can take to help their grandson. You arrange to see Carlos later in the week.

Initial Session with Carlos:

When you enter the waiting room for your first session with Carlos, you find him hopping up and down in front of Mr. Jimenez begging for a certain toy that he seems to want desperately. You greet Mr. Jimenez, and bend down so that you are on Carlos's level. Mr. Jimenez introduces you to Carlos.

You tell Carlos you are glad to meet him, and add, "You seem to be pretty excited about something!"

"I'm going to get a new Power Ranger!" he exclaims.

"Now, I didn't say you were going to get that!" Mr. Jimenez warns Carlos.

On the way to your office, Carlos goes into detail about the Power Ranger he desires. You engage him in talk about Power Rangers for a few minutes. You and Carlos sit on a mat on the floor and you allow him to play with Play-Doh while you read a book to him about death that is appropriate for his age level. You use different points made in the book as prompts to ask Carlos about his father. When you ask Carlos what happened to his dad, he replies, "He went to work and he got hurt and then he went to heaven."

"Do you miss your daddy?" you ask. Carlos nods. "What do you miss about your daddy?" you ask.

"Everything," Carlos says and starts pounding on the Play-Doh. "I don't want to live with my cousins. They're mean to me."

"They are? What do they do that is mean?" you ask.

"They're just mean," Carlos says as he tears the clay into pieces.

"When people are mean to me, it makes me really angry!" you say as you pound on the clay as Carlos did. Carlos stops and watches you closely. "And sometimes when I feel angry I want to hit something or yell or cry!" you say continuing to demonstrate angry feelings as you play with the clay. Carlos joins you again in beating on the Play-Doh. While you are both pounding the clay you ask, "What are some other things that make you feel angry, Carlos?"

"When people go to work!" Carlos says.

"Yeah! Especially when they go to work and they don't come back. That makes me really angry!" you say.

"Yeah, me too!" Carlos chimes in.

"And what else? What else makes you angry?" you ask. Carlos proceeds to pound and tear the clay while together you name some things that elicit anger such as, "when I have to move to a new house," "when my cousin takes my game," "when Grandpa won't buy me a toy," etc.

After the energy of this activity has subsided, you say, "Carlos, it is okay for you to feel angry. There is nothing wrong about that feeling. I talk to a lot of kids who lost a parent and they tell me they feel angry, too." Carlos is watching you and listening closely. You continue, "But let's see if we can come up with some ways that you can be angry that won't get you into trouble. For every idea we can come up with I'll give you a chip. When you get six chips, you can get a prize out of my prize box."

Carlos's eyes light up when you mention the prize box and he nods that he is ready to begin. You take out some checkers and together you and Carlos talk about healthy ways to express anger. After each idea, you both act it out and then give Carlos a chip. The ideas include counting to ten, taking deep breaths, doing an angry dance, screaming into a pillow, scribbling angrily on a sheet of paper, and kicking a soccer ball in the backyard. You praise Carlos for his participation and let him choose a prize. On an index card, you write down the activities that you and Carlos identified. You give the card to Mr. Jimenez when he joins you at the end of the session.

"Carlos," you say in Mr. Jimenez's presence, "the next time you get angry, get Grandpa or Grandma to look at your card and help you choose an activity that you can do."

Turning to Mr. Jimenez, you add, "You might even get him to draw or cut out pictures from magazines of these things or other things he can do when he is angry. We don't want to send the message that it is wrong to feel angry. We just want to help him find better ways of expressing his feelings."

"Okay," Mr. Jimenez says. "I'll tell my wife. Maybe we can do that some morning while his cousins are at school."

You affirm this idea and explain to Mr. Jimenez that focused attention from adults can be extremely valuable and healing for children. Carlos grins and cuddles up next to his Grandpa. Mr. Jimenez says, "You like coming here, mijo?" Carlos nods enthusiastically. Mr. Jimenez smiles and says, "Well, I think we have found a real nice person that can help you, Carlos." He seems pleased with how the session has gone and arranges another visit with you.

5.3-1. What additional assessment information would you want to obtain to help you serve this family?
5.3-2. What are this family's strengths?
5.3-3. What outside resources might be helpful to this family?
5.3-4. What are some additional issues you might want to discuss with Mr. and Mrs. Jimenez?
5.3-5. What are some additional activities that might help Carlos deal with his father's death?
5.3-6. Find three books on death and grief that would be appropriate to read with Carlos.

CASE 5.4

Identifying Information:

Client Name: Samar Kapoor
Age: 17 years old
Race/Ethnicity: Indian
Educational Level: 11th grade
Members in Household: Father, mother, sister age 13

Intake Information:

Mrs. Pahal Kapoor called the Center for Grief and Loss to arrange an appointment for her 17-year-old son, Samar. She stated that one of Samar's best friends died about two weeks ago and she is concerned about how this is affecting him. She says she was given your information by Samar's school counselor. Mrs. Kapoor agreed to come with her son to the first appointment.

Initial Interview:

You greet Mrs. Kapoor and Samar in the waiting room and explain that you will meet with them both for a few minutes and then you will talk to Samar alone. Mrs. Kapoor tells you to call her Pahal and they follow you to your office. You start the interview by asking Samar some non-threatening questions such as his age, grade in school, and favorite activity. You learn that he enjoys video games, music, and is in his high school marching band.

"Okay, so tell me what brings you here today," you say.

Pahal looks at Samar and sighs deeply. "Samar had a good friend who passed away recently and I think it's been very difficult for him."

"I'm sure it has been," you respond. "Tell me about your friend, Samar."

"His name was Ryan. We were friends since third grade," Samar replies as he slouches down in his chair, leaning his head on his fist.

"Wow, you've known him a long time," you comment.

Samar nods.

Pahal adds, "They were very close. Ryan was at our house a lot. They grew up together."

"What happened? How did he die?" you ask gently.

"It may have been an accident," Samar mumbles.

Pahal clears her throat and stares at her son. "It appears that Ryan probably killed himself. They found a note."

"I see," you say. "That's so hard."

Samar looks visibly shaken. He rubs his forehead and shifts in his chair, looking at the ground. "I should have known something was wrong. I could have stopped him," Samar says.

You look at Pahal who has tears in her eyes. She puts her hand on her son's shoulder. "Samar, there is no way you could have known. Ryan didn't tell anyone how he was feeling." Samar says nothing to this. Pahal takes a tissue and wipes her eyes. She rubs her son's shoulder gently and looks quite distraught. "Samar, it wasn't your fault that Ryan died," she says to him. "He didn't tell you what he was thinking. There's nothing you could have done." Pahal looks at you pleadingly and adds, "We don't really know a lot about what happened. His family is not sharing much. It's just really hard."

"Of course it is," you affirm. "That's very tragic. Pahal, are you seeing any changes in Samal since this happened?" you ask.

While looking at him, she says, "He seems pretty down. Understandably. He's not eating much. And it's been really hard to get him up for school in the morning. I'm worried it's going to affect his grades...or make him want to do what Ryan did."

You ask Samar about sleep and appetite. He tells you he doesn't feel hungry and wakes up frequently during the night. When you ask if he's been able to keep up with his school work, he shrugs and says, "Mostly."

"Is there anything else you'd like me to know, Pahal, before I meet with Samar alone?" you ask.

"I don't think so. I just want him to know we are here for him and we want to support him. We don't want this to get in the way of his future goals."

You validate her feelings of worry and explain to both of them that Samar's sessions will be confidential unless he agrees that you can share information with her or if you feel there is concern for his safety. They indicate that they understand this, and Pahal returns to the waiting room so that you can meet with Samar privately.

"This is pretty rough, isn't it?" you say gently. Samar nods, still looking at the floor. "How is it for you when your mom tells you Ryan's death isn't your fault?"

Samar takes some time to consider your question, then replies "I guess she's right. I just keep thinking back about the last time I saw him. Trying to look for clues or signs. I keep wondering what I could have done."

You let Samar talk about his recent interactions with Ryan. Looking back, he says he did seem a little distracted, but Samar didn't think much about it. "We're both in marching band, and he's a top student in his class. I just figured it was the regular stress. I just don't understand it!"

"It makes it even harder, doesn't it?" you say. "This was very unexpected and it sounds like you don't have a lot of information." Samar nods. You encourage him to continue talking as he seems to be trying to wrap his head around what's happened. You learn about the kind of person Ryan was, the rumors circulating about how he died, and a little about the memorial service. You validate the confusion he feels and how difficult it is to understand and accept the loss. You briefly do some teaching about mental illness and suicide. He asks a few questions, but mostly just nods in understanding.

"It's a lot to process on your own, so I'm really glad you're open to talking about it. I know it can feel kind of awkward to talk to a complete stranger about these things." After a pause, you add, "Have you had any thoughts of hurting yourself?"

"No. No, I wouldn't do that," he says.

"Okay, I'm glad that's the case. This will get easier, Samar. It just takes some time and a little effort," you say. You do some teaching about the grief process. "It's especially hard with suicide, Samar. It's very common for family members and friends to ask themselves what they could have done to prevent it. It's important to remember that you have information now that you didn't have before, which makes it easy to be hard on yourself for not seeing something that wasn't there to see. Does that make sense?"

"Yeah. It does, I guess," Samar says.

"And it sounds like there were probably other things going on with Ryan that you didn't know about. Is that possible?" you ask.

"Yeah, I guess so," Samar replies.

You ask Samar if he has any questions for you and if he would feel okay about coming to see you again. He agrees and you return to the waiting room to meet Pahal and schedule an appointment.

5.4-1. Considering the confidential nature of your interview with Samar, write a short paragraph summarizing what you would say to Pahal Kapoor at the end of this initial session.

5.4-2. What other information would you like to obtain in order to assist Samar with his grief?

5.4-3. What strengths do Samar and his mother possess?

5.4-4. What are some interventions that you might use in your work with Samar?

5.4-5. How could you be helpful to Pahal in parenting Samar right now?

5.4-6. Find a scholarly article on adolescent suicide and summarize the findings.

CASE 5.5

Identifying Information:

Client Name: Alyssa Johnson
Age: 12 years old
Race/Ethnicity: Chinese, adopted into white family
Educational Level: Seventh grade
Members in Household: Aunt, uncle, and 17-year-old cousin

Intake Information:

Veronica Hunt called the office to schedule an appointment for her 12-year-old niece, Alyssa. She reports that Alyssa has been living with her ever since her parents were killed in a car accident during a severe thunderstorm. Veronica stated, "I think Alyssa is very unhappy and having a really hard time with the death of her parents. She is going to need more help than I can give her." Her voice suggests that she feels very anxious and she indicates that she would like to bring Alyssa in as soon as possible. You arrange an appointment for Alyssa and explain to Veronica that you would also like to meet with her to get some background information. Due to time and schedule restraints you and Veronica agree that your initial session with her will be over the phone.

Initial Interview:

You call Mrs. Hunt at the scheduled time. She tells you that she is home alone and is able to talk freely. "Tell me more about Alyssa's parents and how she came to live with you," you begin.

Veronica replies, "Ned and Diane, that's my sister and her husband, lived out of state. They adopted Alyssa from China when she was a baby. She was about 4 months old when they got her. About three months ago, they were driving home from work together and got caught in a severe thunderstorm. We don't know exactly what happened, but the car slid off the road, rolled over and landed in a ditch that had become flooded." Veronica's voice sounds shaky. "They were found dead at the scene."

"So, this was very sudden and unexpected," you say using the tone of your voice to demonstrate your empathy with the loss.

"Yes, it was very unexpected," Veronica says and takes a deep breath. "Poor Alyssa was home alone, expecting her parents to come in at any moment. It wasn't until 10 o'clock that evening that she found out what had happened."

"How did she find out about the deaths?" you inquire.

"Some people from the police department came to the house and told her. Then she had to stay at a shelter there until we could move her up here to live with us," Veronica answers.

"Oh, I bet that was difficult for her. For how long was she at the shelter?" you ask.

"The soonest flight I could get was not until two days later. After I got there we stayed at the house with Alyssa, had the funeral, packed up her things, and brought her here with us."

"I see. And how long has she been living with you now?" you ask.

"It's been about two months."

"Okay. And tell me what is going on with Alyssa that concerns you," you prompt.

Veronica explains that Alyssa has been noticeably unhappy. She explains that prior to her parent's death, Alyssa was characteristically cheerful, outgoing, and full of energy. Since the move, however, Veronica says Alyssa tends to mope around, saying little and being very lethargic. When you ask about school, Veronica explains that Alyssa had to transfer to a new school mid-semester. She says that Alyssa is very bright and normally earns good grades but lately her grades have plummeted and she is even failing one class.

"This isn't like her," Veronica says. "I know we lived apart, but I talked to my sister at least twice a week and I know Alyssa very well."

When you ask about how Alyssa has adjusted socially to her new school, Veronica says, "I don't think she has made any friends. Well, she has friends but none that are really close, you know? You know how kids this age have their cliques. I think it's been hard for her to become a part of any group of kids. She has missed a lot of school, too. She gets headaches and says she feels too bad to go. At first I was letting her stay home but now I'm wondering if she's just trying to get out of going."

You inquire about Alyssa's health as well as changes in sleeping and eating habits. Veronica says that she is not aware of any major sleep changes but added that Alyssa has awoken three to four times in the middle of the night screaming from a bad dream. As for her eating, Veronica says, "That girl can eat! It seems like every time I see her she is putting food in her mouth! I don't know if she was always like that or if that is something new for her."

Upon further inquiry you learn that Alyssa tends to eat a lot of junk food. You explain to Veronica that the headaches could be caused by a number of things, including her grief. You suggest that Veronica try to help Alyssa eat more nutritious foods, as this could help the headaches as well as feelings of depression, and suggest that Alyssa see a doctor to rule out any medical issues. Veronica indicates she will follow through with your suggestions. She also readily agrees to give you permission to contact Alyssa's doctor.

You are interested in knowing about the kind of relationship Alyssa has with her aunt. You begin exploring this by asking, "Tell me about how it has been to have Alyssa living with you now. I imagine that this has been quite an adjustment for you, too."

"Well, it has. It's been a big change for my whole family. And it's been hard because I've lost my sister, you know? I'm grieving, too! But we love Alyssa and, though I hate it that her parents died, there is no way I wouldn't have her here with us. I know she will always miss her parents, but we just want the best for her and we'll do whatever we need to do to get her through this."

"I understand," you say. "The situation is overwhelming for everyone with the grief and all the changes it has brought. Alyssa is lucky to have a family that is so dedicated to her. I am sure that you are being a tremendous help to Alyssa even though you may not see that right now."

"Well, I hope so," Veronica says. "She does talk to me a little and she has cried with me a couple of times. I just tell her over and over that we love her and she will have everything she needs."

You praise Veronica for responding this way to Alyssa's sorrow. You also commend her for seeking assistance with Alyssa and explain that you will continue to communicate with her regarding Alyssa's needs.

Initial Session with Alyssa:

You meet Alyssa and Veronica in the waiting room and introduce yourself. Alyssa gives you a soft smile.

After they are seated in your office you introduce the idea of counseling to Alyssa saying, "Alyssa, I have visited with your aunt a little bit and she has told me about your parents' death and about your move here. Your aunt will be bringing you here to meet with me because I have helped a lot of people who are dealing with the kind of changes you are going through. I think if we work together we can help you manage all the feelings you are having and help you to feel better. How does that sound to you?" Alyssa nods her head in agreement. You explain the limits of confidentiality and both Veronica and Alyssa indicate that they understand.

Veronica turns to Alyssa and says, "I want you to talk to your counselor, Alyssa. She is a good person and if you talk to her she can help you."

"Okay," Alyssa says.

"I'll wait for you in the waiting room," Veronica says as she leaves your office.

You show Alyssa some lanyards you have made and ask if she'd like to make one. She smiles and agrees. You spend some time teaching her how to weave the strings so that they form the lanyard. As you each work on your own lanyard, you talk with Alyssa about things she likes to do and her favorite subjects in school. You also ask her about ways that her current school is different from her former one. She tells you that the teachers at her current school tend to give more homework and that there seem to be more fights at her current school.

"Those are big changes," you say. "Has it been hard for you to get used to your new school?"

"Yes," Alyssa admits. "I wish I could go back to my old school."

"Tell me what you miss about your old school," you prompt.

Alyssa proceeds to tell you about some of her former teachers, school activities and about the friends she left back home. She finishes with a deep sigh.

"It must be really hard to leave your home, move to a new place, go to a new school, and have to make new friends," you say. Alyssa nods indicating that this is true. You continue, "And on top of that, you lost both your parents. How has that been for you?"

A tear runs down Alyssa's cheek. She looks at the floor and is silent.

After a moment, you say gently, "It hurts a lot, doesn't it?" Alyssa nods as the tears continue to run silently down her face.

"You must really miss them," you venture.

Again, Alyssa nods. She wipes her tears with the back of her hand. You gently prompt Alyssa with more questions but her answers are short and general. You deduce that putting words to her emotions seems to be an overwhelming task for her so you say, "I have an activity we can do, Alyssa, that might help you sort through some of these feelings. Want to give it a try?"

"Okay," she says.

You ask Alyssa to sit on the floor with you and provide her with construction paper and glue. You then instruct her to create something that represents how she felt when she learned about her parents' deaths. You explain that she might use different colors to represent different emotions and that she can fold or tear the paper into any shape that she desires. Before beginning, you guide Alyssa in a brief relaxation exercise that involves deep breathing. You sit silently while Alyssa works on her creation. When she is finished you ask her to tell you about what she has created. She explains her picture, which depicts a small child that is lost among several large and menacing looking trees. Rain is coming down through the trees as is lightning that is pointed directly at the child. As Alyssa tells you the story about her parents' deaths you gently prompt her to describe the feelings she had. She indicates feeling alone, lost, confused, and fearful. You listen empathetically to Alyssa's story while validating and normalizing all of these responses.

When she is finished, you say, "You really shared a lot today, Alyssa. Thank you for telling me your story. How was it for you?"

"It was okay," Alyssa says without hesitation. "It feels kind of good to get it all out."

"I'm glad you feel that you can talk in here. What do you think about coming to see me again?" you ask.

"Yes, I'd like that," she answers.

As you and Alyssa clean up from the activity, you talk about the kind of music she likes and other more light-hearted things. Upon returning to the waiting room, Alyssa smiles brightly when she sees her aunt. You and Veronica arrange for subsequent visits for Alyssa.

5.5-1. What additional information would you try to obtain as you work with Alyssa?
5.5-2. Considering Alyssa's developmental stage, her adoption, and the circumstances surrounding her loss, what concerns do you have for Alyssa?
5.5-3. Periodically, you will want to visit with Veronica to coach her on how to help Alyssa. What are some possible recommendations you might suggest?
5.5-4. What other kinds of activities might you initiate with Alyssa to help her with her grief?

Follow Up Session with Alyssa Johnson:

Alyssa continues to meet with you once a week on a regular basis. Sometimes she will talk about her parents, show you pictures of them, talk about the kind of people they were and what she misses about them. On other days, she evades the subject and you spend the session playing board games and talking about school and other things. You have communicated several times with Alyssa's aunt, Veronica, to get updates on how Alyssa is doing at home and at school. She reports that Alyssa seems to have developed a close friend and often spends a lot of time communicating with her over the phone or computer. Her school attendance has also improved. Alyssa's grades, however, are inconsistent. She will sometimes have high B's and A's and at other times have C's and F's. Veronica has reported that they have had to discipline Alyssa for not doing her homework or for rushing through it.

When you enter the waiting room to retrieve Alyssa for your next session, Veronica asks if she can talk to you for a moment first. You agree, take a moment to say hello to Alyssa, and walk with Veronica back to your office. Veronica begins talking as she enters the room.

"Something happened last night that I need to tell you about," Veronica says.

"Sure," you respond. "Have a seat and tell me what's going on."

"Last night we were all at the dinner table – me, my husband, Alyssa, and my 17-year-old daughter, Brittney. Brittney started arguing with me and my husband about her curfew and things got pretty heated. The whole time Alyssa just sat there looking at her plate and eating her food. Brittney was complaining that we weren't giving her enough freedom and she started talking about how she can't wait to move out and not have to deal with us anymore when Alyssa suddenly started yelling at her. She said, 'I wish you *would* move out of here. You think your life is so tough because you can't get every little thing you want! You're a spoiled brat and I'm sick of hearing you whine all the time!' Then she stormed off. A few minutes later we heard this crash. She had gone into Brittney's room and pushed everything off her dresser and tore one of the posters off the wall. Now you need to understand, we have never seen Alyssa act like that before. She has always been mild mannered and quiet and, except for the issues with her homework, she has never given us any trouble."

"That does seem a little out of character for Alyssa doesn't it? What happened next?" you ask.

"Yes, very out of character!" Veronica responds. "So, after I got over my shock, I went to Alyssa's room where she was with the door shut. I could hear her crying and screaming, 'It's not fair! It's not fair!' I tried to go in, but she had the door locked. I knocked and pleaded for her to let me in, but she never did. About 30 minutes later, I heard the crying stop and the room was very quiet. I think she must have cried herself to sleep. I'm really worried about her. I've never seen her like this. I know she's been sad, but I've never seen her get angry like this! It really alarms me because it is so unlike her!"

"Have you all talked about this since it happened?" you ask.

"I tried to talk to her this morning but she wouldn't say much. I told her I expected her to apologize to Brittney and she said that she would. I hope she will talk to you," Veronica says.

"I hope so too and I'm glad that you told me all of this," you say. "I wonder if she's been keeping a lot of feelings bottled up and it finally spilled over."

"Maybe that's it. I never knew she had a problem with Brittney. Brittney's been really good about helping her adjust to things and they've always gotten along fine," Veronica says.

"This might be more about her grief than it is about Brittney. Is there anything else going on that you think I should know?" you ask.

"No, that's it really," Veronica says. "Just let me know if there is something my husband and I should be doing. She's kind of a mystery to us, you know. We can tell that she's unhappy, but she doesn't want to talk about it much – at least not about her parents. I spend a lot of time wondering what's going on in that head of hers. And I don't know if we should give her a consequence for this behavior or not. I don't want her to think it's okay to do that, but I know she's going through a lot. I'd really like your thoughts on that."

"I will definitely try to offer you some guidance on this. Let's see how things go in the session today and I'll get back to you on that," you say.

Veronica thanks you and returns to the waiting room where Alyssa sits listening to music through headphones. She seems to be lost in her own world until you get her attention. With a sheepish look on her face, she takes off her headphones and walks with you to your office.

After the two of you make small talk for a while, you say gently, "Alyssa, your aunt told me you had a rough night last night."

Alyssa looks at the floor and nods.

"Can you tell me what happened?" you ask.

After a few moments of silence, Alyssa says, "I got really angry at my cousin."

"Okay. What were you angry about?"

"She just drives me crazy," Alyssa says. She continues with a litany of complaints about Brittney saying that Brittney "always" complains, is "always rude," plays her music too loud (music that Alyssa "hates"), talks too long on the phone, stays in the bathroom too long, and is a "slob."

"She really does make you angry, doesn't she?" you reflect. "It must be hard to live with all of that."

"It is!" Alyssa agrees.

"From what your aunt tells me, it sounds like last night you really showed her how angry you were," you say.

"Yeah, I tore up some of her stuff," Alyssa says.

"How do you feel about having done that?" you ask.

"I feel bad," Alyssa says genuinely. "I know that wasn't right. But she just makes me so mad!"

"It sounds like you exploded! Like a volcano that had been building up to an eruption," you suggest.

Alyssa nods.

"I didn't know you had so much anger towards Brittney," you say.

"I haven't always been so angry with her," Alyssa says.

"I wonder if there are other things you feel angry about," you say.

Alyssa is silent for a moment. "Yea, I guess there are."

"Let's make a list of all the things you feel angry about," you suggest.

Alyssa agrees to this idea and together you write down everything she is angry about, prompting her when necessary with topics such as school, friends, home, and her aunt and uncle. Alyssa mentions that she gets angry at people who talk badly about their parents.

"Do you think that was why you got so angry with Brittney last night?" you ask.

"Yes," she says.

You validate Alyssa's feelings and talk to her further about the relationship between her anger toward her friends who have parents and her own parents' death. Alyssa tells you that she is sometimes jealous of her friends for having both their parents alive and she thinks they should appreciate their parents more because they could die in an instant. You validate these feelings and explain that going through hard times often changes how we think of things and that in this way she is probably maturing faster than many of her friends. Then you suggest, "Now, let's make a list of things you can do when you feel angry that won't hurt you, won't hurt anyone else, and won't get you into trouble."

Alyssa agrees and together you begin brainstorming healthy ways to express anger.

5.5-5. What are some things that could go on Alyssa's list of healthy ways to express anger?

5.5-6. How do you view Alyssa's "negative" behavior, using the strengths-based framework for grief and loss?

5.5-7. What are some of this family's strengths?

5.5-8. What guidance would you offer Veronica and her husband on how to respond to Alyssa's outburst?

REFERENCES

Achenbach, T. M., & Edelbrock, C. S. (1983). *Manual for the Child Behavior Checklist and the revised Child Behavior Profile*. University Associates in Psychiatry.

APA Presidential Task Force on Posttraumatic Stress Disorder and Trauma in Children and Adolescents. (2008). Children and trauma: Update for mental health professionals. PsycEXTRA Dataset. https://doi.org/10.1037/e539742009-001

Bergman, A., Axberg, U., & Hanson, E. (2017). When a parent dies – a systematic review of the effects of support programs for parentally bereaved children and their caregivers. *BMC Palliative Care*, *16*(1). https://doi.org/10.1186/s12904-017-0223-y

Burdick, D. (2014). *Mindfulness skills for kids & teens: A workbook for clinicians & clients with 154 tools, techniques, activities & worksheets*. PESI Publishing & Media.

Carter, S. (2005). Puppets in the treatment of traumatic grief. In G. L. Landreth, D. C. Ray, D. S. Sweeney, L. E. Homeyer, & G. J. Glover (Eds.), *Play therapy interventions with children's problems: Case studies with DSM-IV-TR diagnoses* (2nd ed., pp. 122–123). Jason Aronson.

Child Welfare Information Gateway. (2014). *Parenting a child who has experienced trauma*. U.S. Department of Health and Human Services, Children's Bureau. www.childwelfare.gov/pubPDFs/child-trauma.pdf

Clark, D. C., Pynoos, R. S., & Goebel, A. E. (1994). Mechanisms and processes of adolescent bereavement. In R. J. Haggerty, L. R. Sherrod, N. Garmezy, & M. Rutter (Eds.), *Stress, risk, and resilience* (pp. 100–146). Cambridge University Press.

Dyregrov, K., Cimitan, A., & De Leo, D. (2014). Grief in the family. In D. De Leo, A. Cimitan, K. Dyregrov, O. Grad, & K. Andriessen (Eds.), *Bereavement after traumatic death: Helping the survivors* (pp. 49–64). Hogrefe Publishing.

Ferow, A. (2019). Childhood grief and loss. *The European Journal of Educational Sciences, special edition*. https://doi.org/10.19044/ejes.s.v6a1

Fischer, J., & Corcoran, K. (1994). *Measures for clinical practice: A sourcebook* (2nd ed.). Free Press.

Foa, E. B., Johnson, K. M., Feeny, N. C., & Treadwell, K. R. H. (2001). The Child PTSD Symptom Scale: A preliminary examination of its psychometric properties. *Journal of Clinical Child Psychology*, *30*(3), 376–384.

Garcia, R. B. (2017). Using grief support groups to support bereaved students at school. In J. A. Brown & S. R. Jimerson (Eds.), *Supporting bereaved students at school* (pp. 115–129). Oxford University Press.

Greenwald, R., & Rubin, A. (1999). Brief assessment of children's post-traumatic symptoms: Development and preliminary validation of parent and child scales. *Research on Social Work Practice*, *9*, 61–75.

Griese, B., Burns, M. R., Farro, S. A., Silvern, L., & Talmi, A. (2017). Comprehensive grief care for children and families: Policy and practice implications. *American Journal of Orthopsychiatry*, *87*(5), 540–548. https://doi.org/10.1037/ort0000265

Grotberg, E. (1996, July 24–28). *The international resilience project: Findings from the research and the effectiveness of interventions* [Paper Presentation]. The 54th Annual Convention of the International Council of Psychologists, Banff, Canada.

Guldin, M., Li, J., Pedersen, H. S., Obel, C., Agerbo, E., Gissler, M., Cnattingius, S., Olsen, J., & Vestergaard, M. (2015). Incidence of suicide among persons who had a parent who died during their childhood. *JAMA Psychiatry*, *72*(12), 1227. https://doi.org/10.1001/jamapsychiatry.2015.2094

Hidalgo, I. M. (2017). *The effects of children's spiritual coping after parent, grandparent or sibling death on children's grief, personal growth, and mental health* (Doctoral dissertation). https://digitalcommons.fiu.edu/etd/3467

Hill, R. M., Dodd, C., Oosterhoff, B., Layne, C. M., Pynoos, R. S., Staine, M. B., & Kaplow, J. B. (2020). Measurement invariance of the Persistent Complex Bereavement Disorder Checklist with respect to youth gender, race, ethnicity, and age. *Journal of Traumatic Stress*. https://doi.org/10.1002/jts.22560

Hill, R. M., Kaplow, J. B., Oosterhoff, B., & Layne, C. M. (2019). Understanding grief reactions, thwarted belongingness, and suicide ideation in bereaved adolescents: Toward a unifying theory. *Journal of Clinical Psychology*, *75*(4), 780–793. https://doi.org/10.1002/jclp.22731

Hogan, N. (1990). Hogan Sibling Inventory of Bereavement. In J. Touliatos, B. Permutter, & M. Strauss (Eds.), *Handbook of family measurement techniques* (p. 524). Sage Press.

Horesh, D., & Brown, A. D. (2018). Editorial: Post-traumatic stress in the family. *Frontiers in Psychology*, *9*. https://doi.org/10.3389/fpsyg.2018.00040

Humphrey, G. M., & Zimpfer, D. G. (2007). *Counselling for grief and bereavement*. SAGE.

Kanoy, R. C., Johnson, B. W., & Kanoy, K. W. (1980). Locus of control and self-concept in achieving and underachieving bright elementary students. *Psychology in Schools*, *17*, 395–399.

Kaplow, J. B., Layne, C. M., Saltzman, W. R., Cozza, S. J., & Pynoos, R. S. (2013). Using multidimensional grief theory to explore the effects of deployment, reintegration, and death on military youth and families. *Clinical Child and Family Psychology Review*, *16*(3), 322–340.

Kazdin, A. E., French, N. H., Esveldt-Dawson, K., & Sherick, R. B. (1983). Hopelessness, depression, and suicidal intent among psychiatrically disturbed inpatient children. *Journal of Consulting and Clinical Psychology*, *51*, 504–510.

Kenardy, J. A., Spence, S. H., & Macleod, A. C. (2006). Screening for posttraumatic stress disorder in children after accidental injury. *Pediatrics*, *118*(3), 1002–1009.

Kilmer, R. P., Gil-Rivas, V., Griese, B., Hardy, S. J., Hafstad, G. S., & Alisic, E. (2014). Posttraumatic growth in children and youth: Clinical implications of an emerging research literature. *American Journal of Orthopsychiatry*, *84*(5), 506.

Landreth, G. L., Ray, D. C., Sweeney, D. S., Homeyer, L. E., & Glover, G. J. (2005). *Play therapy interventions with children's problems: Case studies with DSM-IV-TR diagnoses* (2nd ed.). Jason Aronson.

Layne, C. M. (2012). *Integrating developmentally-informed theory, evidence-based assessment, and evidence-based treatment of childhood maladaptive grief*. Symposium presented at the International Society for Traumatic Stress Studies, Los Angeles, CA.

Layne, C. M., Kaplow, J. B., Oosterhoff, B., Hill, R. M., & S. Pynoos, R. (2017). The interplay between posttraumatic stress and grief reactions in traumatically bereaved adolescents: When trauma, bereavement, and adolescence converge. *Adolescent Psychiatry*, *7*(4), 266–285. https://doi.org/10.2174/2210676608666180306162544

Lehmann, L., Jimerson, S., & Gaasch, A. (2001a). *Grief support group curriculum facilitators handbook*. Brunner & Routledge.

Lehmann, L., Jimerson, S., & Gaasch, A. (2001b). *The mourning child grief support group curriculum: Denny the Duck preschool version*. Brunner & Routledge.

Lehmann, L., Jimerson, S., & Gaasch, A. (2001c). *The mourning child grief support group curriculum: Middle childhood version*. Brunner & Routledge.

Lehmann, L., Jimerson, S., & Gaasch, A. (2001d). *The mourning child grief support group curriculum: Early childhood version*. Brunner & Routledge.

Lehmann, L., Jimerson, S., & Gaasch, A. (2001e). *The mourning child grief support group curriculum: Teens together version*. Brunner & Routledge.

Lokko, H. N., & Stern, T. A. (2015). Regression: Diagnosis, evaluation, and management. *The Primary Care Companion for CNS Disorders*. https://doi.org/10.4088/pcc.14f01761

Lowenstein, L. (2006). *Creative interventions for bereaved children*. Champion Press.

Mannarino, A. P. (1978). Friendship patterns and self-concept development in pre-adolescent males. *Journal of Genetic Psychology*, *113*, 105–110.

Mannarino, A. P., & Cohen, J. A. (2011). Traumatic loss in children and adolescents. *Journal of Child & Adolescent Trauma*, *4*(1), 22–33. https://doi.org/10.1080/19361521.2011.545048

Masterson, J. F. (1988). *The search for the real self: Unmasking the personality disorders of our age*. Free press.

McWhorter, G. (2003). *Healing activities for children in grief*. Author.

Oosterhoff, B., Kaplow, J. B., & Layne, C. M. (2018). Links between bereavement due to sudden death and academic functioning: Results from a nationally representative sample of adolescents. *School Psychology Quarterly*, *33*(3), 372–380. https://doi.org/10.1037/spq0000254

Piers, E. V. (1984). *Revised manual for the Piers-Harris Children's Self-Concept scale*. Western Psychological Services.

Pomeroy, E. C., & Garcia, R. B. (2011). *Children and loss: A practical handbook for professionals*. Oxford University Press.

Rabenstein, S., & Harris, D. L. (2017). Family therapy and traumatic loss. In N. Thompson, G. R. Cox, & R. G. Stevenson (Eds.), *Handbook of traumatic loss: A guide to theory and practice* (pp. 179–200). Taylor & Francis.

Rask, K., Kaunonen, M., & Paunonen-Ilmonen, M. (2002). Adolescent coping with grief after the death of a loved one. *International Journal of Nursing Practice*, *8*(3), 137–142. https://doi.org/10.1046/j.1440-172x.2002.00354.x

Rosenzweig, J. M., Jivanjee, P., Brennan, E. M., Grover, L., & Abshire, A. (2017). *Understanding neuro-biology of psychological trauma: Tips for working with transition-age youth*. Research and Training Center for Pathways to Positive Futures, Portland State University.

Saltzman, W. R., Layne, C. M., Pynoos, R. S., Olafson, E., Kaplow, J. B., & Boat, B. (2017). *Trauma and grief component therapy for adolescents: A modular approach to treating traumatized and bereaved youth*. Cambridge University Press.

Saxe, G., Chawla, N., Stoddard, F., Kassam-Adams, N., Courtney, D., Cunningham, K., Lopez, C., Sheridan, R., King, D., & Kind, L. (2003). Child stress disorders checklist: A measure of ASD and PTSD in children. *Journal of the American Academy of Child & Adolescent Psychiatry*, *42*(8), 972–978.

The National Child Traumatic Stress Network. (2018). *TGCTA: General information* [PDF file]. www.nctsn.org/sites/default/files/interventions/tgcta_fact_sheet.pdf

The National Child Traumatic Stress Network. (n.d.) Introduction. www.nctsn.org/trauma-informed-care/families-and-trauma/introduction

Turner, R. (2020). Playing through the unimaginable: Play therapy for traumatic loss. *International Journal of Play Therapy*, *29*(2), 96–103. https://doi.org/10.1037/pla0000116

Wolfelt, A. (1991). A child's view of grief [Video]. Center for Loss and Life Transition, Fort Collins, CO.

CHAPTER 6

Expected and Traumatic Grief in Older Adults

With all of us, the experience of loss and trauma is shaped by the environment in which these events occur (recall the discussion on the P-I-E perspective in Chapter 3). This is especially true for older adults as their grief experience is influenced by their interactions with family and friends, the circumstances of their living situation, their interactions with the healthcare system, and how they are regarded by the larger society. As with all ages, responses to grief among the elderly range from mild to severe, expected to complex, and may be life-enhancing or life-depleting. It is important, however, that practitioners be aware of the many variables that are unique to older adults and thereby influence their course of grief. This chapter outlines some of these factors, including how practitioners can be effective. Special attention is given to the strengths that this population brings to their journey with grief.

INFLUENCES ON THE GRIEF EXPERIENCE OF OLDER ADULTS

Multiple Losses

One circumstance that is especially relevant to bereavement for older adults is the experience of having multiple losses. Elderly persons disproportionately experience death, including spouses, siblings, and peers (Worden, 2018). In addition to these losses, there are numerous personal losses that accompany the aging process. These include being out of the workforce, changes in health status and physical abilities, and for some, the ability to live independently. Because loss is a common occurrence of old age, it is often mistakenly assumed that the elderly are immune from the impact of grief or can manage the grief process more easily than younger persons (Lekalakala-Mokgele, 2018). While prior experience dealing with loss can help develop coping skills and resilience, the death of a loved one remains an extremely stressful life event and numerous losses over a short time span can overwhelm a person's capacity to grieve. In addition to the grief that comes with multiple types of losses, the death of so many of one's contemporaries (life partner, friends, siblings) prompts older adults to confront their own mortality, causing significant anxiety for some individuals (Lekalakala-Mokgele, 2018; Worden, 2018).

DOI: 10.4324/9780429053634-6

Older adults who live far away from their adult children may face a decision about relocating closer to family in order to receive adequate care and support. While there are certainly benefits to this, leaving one's home and community presents an additional adjustment and may be experienced as a secondary loss. Moving can be especially difficult when leaving places that contain memories of the deceased (Worden, 2018). In addition, there is some evidence pointing to increased mortality rates for senior citizens who are required to leave their homes after the death of a spouse (Spahni et al., 2016).

Social Disconnection and Isolation

Generally, the number of social relationships decreases with age, and over 40% of older adults live alone (US Census Bureau, 2019). While some older persons are active and contributing members of their community with strong social support networks, many experience loneliness and a dearth of social contact. A lack of social connection is known to have a significant impact on physical and mental health (Holt-Lunstad, 2017; Saeri et al., 2017) and this is compounded for older adults who are also grieving the death of a life partner, or other close relation (Perng & Renz, 2018).

Adapting to the death of a life-long spouse is generally thought to be one of the most difficult transitions older adults will face. As compared with their married peers, elderly widowed persons experience a greater amount of depression and feelings of isolation as well as decreased life satisfaction (Spahni et al., 2016). Among groups that experience grief, both elderly persons and bereaved spouses have a greater prevalence of complex grief reactions (Eckholdt et al., 2017). The death of a spouse in the older years can be especially difficult because of the roles spouses have in each other's lives and the deeply ingrained attachment bonds they developed (Worden, 2018). In addition, the degree of centrality that the deceased played in the surviving spouse's identity and life narrative is a particularly powerful risk factor that can make the adjustment especially difficult (Eckholdt et al., 2017).

Limited Access to Care

The effects of aging bring both practical and psychological challenges to getting one's needs met. Physical limitations can impinge on the ability to independently care for ourselves. For example, older adults who can no longer safely drive or navigate public transportation on their own will have to find ways to get to medical appointments, the grocery store, and social engagements. In addition, because loss in old age is expected, older persons may not be recognized as needing support with their grief, leaving it up to them to request assistance. For some, this loss of independence means they are having to learn to ask for help which may feel new and uncomfortable. Unfortunately, psychotherapeutic help is not widely used by older adults (Bartels et al., 2014; Böttche & Knaevelsrud, 2017), and there are several barriers that complicate their access to services. Frequently, it involves coordinating with other providers, caregivers, and family members and may also entail overcoming limitations with finances and transportation (Bartels et al., 2014; Böttche & Knaevelsrud, 2017).

Additionally, many older adults are reluctant to acknowledge and express psychological distress to others. Generational differences predispose some older persons to hold stigmatized views of therapy and perceive the need for such services as a sign of personal weakness (Bartels et al., 2014; Böttche & Knaevelsrud, 2017). They may only avail themselves of counseling at the insistence of concerned family members. Consequently, their internal pain often manifests as somatic complaints prompting them to seek relief from their primary care physician (Thorp et al., 2011; Hashim et al., 2013; Perng & Renz, 2018). Doctors, however, typically receive little, if any, training on grief and caring for the bereaved (Ghesquiere et al., 2013).

Some older adults also carry a great deal of concern about being a burden to their adult children and other family members. They may feel compelled to present an appearance of strength, though internally they are suffering deeply (Lekalakala-Mokgele, 2018). This is especially concerning as numerous studies, including some that focus specifically on the elderly, suggest that perceived burdensomeness is a risk factor for suicide (Chu et al., 2017; Jahn et al., 2015; Cukrowicz et al., 2011; Hill & Pettit, 2014). This perception adds to the difficulty for older adults to ask for help and for family members to recognize their suffering (Hashim et al., 2013). This may be especially pertinent when the entire family is grieving a loss and others in the family are also needing care and support. For example, when a grandchild dies, the grief experience of grandparents is often overlooked as most of the attention and support is understandably directed at the child's parents (Worden, 2018). In addition, bereaved grandparents often feel tasked with being strong for their children and therefore hide their own feelings from the family's view (Lekalakala-Mokgele, 2018). When an adult child dies, grandparents often step in to care for their surviving grandchildren, and similarly feel they must present as strong and stable for the surviving family members (Lekalakala-Mokgele, 2018).

Biased beliefs, negative stereotypes, and ageism about the elderly further complicate the ability for elderly persons to access care that appropriately and respectfully addresses their needs. Beliefs that the elderly are physically, mentally, and socially inferior to their younger counterparts are prevalent across many cultures (Wilińska et al., 2018). This results in treatment that ignores and discounts their needs (Wyman et al., 2018). Contrary to a strengths-based approach, they are treated with less dignity and respect. Several studies have shown that ageist attitudes and behaviors regarding older persons are no less prevalent among healthcare providers, educators, and counselors. Often this manifests as treating them in a childlike manner, using baby talk when communicating, or allowing them limited control over decisions that impact their lives.

BOX 6.1 MOURNING RITUALS: CARIBBEAN BLACKS

The mourning rituals of Caribbean Blacks are influenced by both their Christian and indigenous origins. In this primarily matriarchal society, older women play a central role in carrying out the funeral rites and traditions which are performed to safeguard the bereaved from sickness and adversity, including death caused by an aggrieved spirit. Mourning rituals typically have a festive atmosphere, involve food, rum, dancing, and singing and may last throughout the night. Women organize the wake including preparing the body and making refreshments. As women arrive at the wake, they commence wailing with expressions of praise and gratitude for the deceased, a skill they are expected to cultivate. Beginning on the first or second Friday after the burial, a Novena is held to assist the soul of the deceased as it leaves the earthly realm. The Novena is a Roman Catholic custom consisting of praying over a period of nine consecutive days. The final day of the Novena concludes with music, dancing, and additional prayers until dawn.

There are also traditions performed at the one-year anniversary of the death. After praying in the church, the mourning women participate in a bathing ritual at the beach. Females who were close to the deceased walk, fully clothed and arm in arm, into the water. They submerge themselves and then help each other up three times. Upon completion of this ceremony all the women return to the home where those who have been in mourning don jewelry and brightly colored clothes. There are offerings of food and drink to the deceased and a festive evening of food, singing, and remembrance ensues (Hidalgo, 2017).

GRIEF REACTIONS AMONG OLDER ADULTS

Emotional, Mental, and Physical Responses to Loss

While most older adults are extraordinarily resilient in the face of loss, the context within which elderly persons experience grief, as outlined earlier, may make them more fragile grievers and more likely to develop complex grief (Lundorff et al., 2017; Perng & Renz, 2018). Research suggests that 20 to 30% of bereaved older adults develop co-occurring emotional problems such as depression, PTSD, complex grief, or substance use disorder (Robbins-Welty et al., 2018). Of particular concern with older adults is the impact of loss on their physical and mental health as the grief process may exacerbate existing health problems or usher in additional physical complaints and ailments (Lundorff et al., 2017; Perng & Renz, 2018). While a younger person may find the energy, no matter how difficult, to function adequately while grieving, an older person may become more easily depleted both physically and emotionally by the taxing process of grief, leading to an overall decline in health and well-being (Ghesquiere et al., 2013; Perng & Renz, 2018). Research indicates that both older males and females show an increased risk of mortality following the death of a live-in partner with the risk being highest during the first three months after the death (King et al., 2017). There is further evidence that older widowed adults experience more sleep problems, poor diet, and a decline in other health-producing behaviors (Miner and Kryger, 2017; King et al., 2017; Stahl et al., 2020; Vesnaver et al., 2016).

Older persons may be less likely to identify the connection between their physical, cognitive, and emotional symptoms and the grief they are experiencing (Robbins-Welty et al., 2018). Even among helping professionals, temporary diminished functioning in these areas can be misinterpreted as a sign of illness or the aging process, rather than reactions to the loss. Further complicating assessment are medications commonly prescribed to older adults that have depression and cognitive decline as side effects (Chonody & Teater, 2018).

It is important for practitioners to know that older adults are at high risk for suicide. According to data gathered in 2017, adults aged 85 years and older comprised the second highest rate (20.1) of suicide in the United States (American Foundation for Suicide Prevention, 2020) with bereavement being noted as a significant risk factor. This is particularly relevant during the six months following the death of a loved one (Conejero et al., 2018; Meichsner et al., 2020).

Financial Ramifications of Loss in Older Adults

The influence of socio-economic status and environmental conditions in which older persons live can shape how they die and how they experience grief. Given that most older adults have retired and are living on fixed incomes, concerns about finances are prevalent among this population. Multiple studies show that bereavement is associated with financial strain, especially for older adults. This may be a direct result from the loss of a spouse's income or because the surviving spouse was not the one who managed the couple's finances. Due to traditional gender roles, this has often been the case for older females (DiGiacomo et al., 2015; Ghesquiere et al., 2016). The added stress of financial insecurity along with having to suddenly manage this new responsibility has implications on the physical, emotional, and cognitive health of bereaved older adults (DiGiacomo et al., 2015). Anxiety over finances may explain some of the distress and depression that is experienced by older widowed persons during bereavement.

Grief and Neurocognitive Decline

Older adults who have some form of neurocognitive decline (NCD) (e.g. Alzheimer's or Parkinson's type) may become quite confused and experience further decline when a loved one dies (Meichsner et al., 2020). This can be very distressing for the bereaved as well as their caregivers. Little is understood about how grief is processed by people with cognitive impairment. Efforts to learn more about their experience are challenged by the fact that people with NCD have difficulty accurately communicating their thoughts and emotions. In addition, correctly interpreting the words used by people with NCD can be problematic. Consequently, there are no clear guidelines on how to care for bereaved persons living with NCD (Watanabe & Suwa, 2017).

Among the scant research on this population is a study by Watanabe and Suwa (2017) comprising 13 family and professional caregivers of persons with NCD who had lost a spouse. Using qualitative analysis, this study revealed that the process of mourning for people with NCD is related to the stage of their functional impairment. The findings concluded that as compared with later stages of Alzheimer's, those in the early stages of cognitive decline may be more able to understand and remember that their loved one died, though this may be challenged when they are in a different context. For example, after losing his partner of 45 years, an 80-year-old male with NCD was forced to move to his daughter's household. Though he understood that he was relocating because his partner died, he seemed to forget this after the move. He often asked about when his partner would return from the grocery store. According to this study, as cognitive and memory impairment progresses, so does the difficulty with which people with NCD can discern that their loved one has died. It can take one to two years for them to recognize the death of their loved one and preserve it in their memory. They may experience surprise when told about their loved one's death and relive the emotional reaction that comes when learning of the death for the first time. In the most advanced stages of impairment, bereaved persons with Alzheimer's may have no ability to comprehend the concept of death, though they may display agitation.

Watanabe and Suwa's (2017) research suggest that the typical model for mourning, which involves accepting the reality of the death, may not be applicable to this population because they are forced to begin a changed life before comprehending the permanence of the loss. Thus a new model for understanding their grief process needs to be developed along with recommendations for how to care for them. For bereaved persons with NCD, confusion can be decreased with compassionate use of reality orientation techniques which involve making changes that help orient the mourner to the present circumstances. Examples include talking about the deceased using photographs, mentioning the death often, and encouraging participation in mourning rituals, including visiting the graveyard (Watanabe & Suwa, 2017).

The experience of caring for persons with NCD is extremely taxing both physically and psychologically. As cognitive functioning declines there are a cascade of losses that elicit grief reactions (Quinn, 2018). A gradual chipping away of the person the caregiver once knew occurs, as their personality and cognitive capacity changes. The added difficulty that comes when a loved one dies exponentially compounds this strain on caregivers as they attempt to manage their own grief while also shouldering the unconventional mourning process of the family member with NCD. Therefore, it is critical that caregivers receive relevant information and support in order to mitigate feelings of helplessness, hopelessness, and becoming burned out. This should include, when possible, respite care so that caregivers are able to sustain their capacity to provide care over time.

TRAUMATIC GRIEF IN OLDER ADULTS

Though the population of older adults is rapidly increasing, little research has been done on how trauma affects this population and what interventions would be most efficacious (Böttche et al., 2012; Dinnen et al., 2015). The few studies that are available focus on trauma resulting from wars and natural disasters. As discussed in previous chapters, the death of a loved one is experienced by some as trauma and may result in depression, anxiety, and an over-reliance on prescription drugs and alcohol (Meichsner et al., 2020), complicating the natural process of grieving. Several studies suggest that the death of a loved one who played a critical role in the survivor's identity are associated with complex grief reactions including PTSD (Boelen, 2017; Eckholdt et al., 2017). It may also be the case that latent trauma incurred earlier in life is triggered by the stress of bereavement (Böttche et al., 2012). One study suggests that older male adults with PTSD are at a 70% higher risk for dementia and older female adults are at a 60% higher risk compared to those without PTSD (Flatt et al., 2018). Based on these findings, it can be presumed that older adults who have experienced complex grief, depression, or PTSD are at a significantly higher risk for developing NCD.

Among older adults with PTSD, there is some evidence to suggest that symptoms of avoidance are more common than hyperarousal symptoms and represent an adaptive response to hyperarousal (Böttche et al., 2012). There may be an increased reluctance among older adults to dredge up traumatic memories after a lifetime of avoiding them. Symptoms of traumatic grief in older adults can be easily overlooked and mistaken by both providers and patients as the physical, sensory, and cognitive impairment that comes with aging (Dinnen et al., 2015). Additional research is needed to support effective interventions for traumatic grief in older adults.

ASSESSMENT OF GRIEF IN OLDER ADULTS

Learning about the social and environmental context of grief with elderly individuals is essential to effective assessment and intervention. In addition, there are many assessment instruments that can be used to evaluate both the primary and secondary symptoms that come with loss. While grief in older adults can be measured using the same instruments as with younger adults (see Chapter 3), additional instruments that measure health-related concerns, depression, loneliness, social support, and cognitive problems can also be very informative. Giving particular attention to the onset of symptoms and underlying medical conditions is also useful, as is working collaboratively with the client's physician. The following is a sample of the variety of measures that are available:

- The Satisfaction with Life Scale (Diener et al., 1985)
- The Geriatric Depression Scale (GDS) (Brink et al.,1982)
- The Register – Connectedness Scale for Older Adults (Register et al., 2010)
- Mini Mental Status Exam (MMSE) (Folstein et al., 1975)
- The Loneliness Rating Scale (LRS) (Scalise et al., 1984)
- The Multi-Dimensional Scale of Perceived Social Support (MSPSS) (Zimet et al., 1988)
- The RAND 36 Item Health Survey (SF 36) (Ware & Sherbourne, 1992).

BOX 6.2 MOURNING RITUALS: TRADITIONAL JUDAISM

In Judaism, as it is traditionally practiced, the body is treated reverently as it is prepared for burial. It is covered with a sheet and laid on the floor with the feet positioned in the direction of the door to help the soul leave the earthly world. The windows in the home are opened and a lit candle is placed close to the head to light the soul's journey. Vessels containing water (representative of life) are emptied to declare a death in the home. The body is ritualistically washed and placed in a plain coffin made of wood to represent the belief that all are equal in God's view. Observers remain with the body for 24 hours as stipulated by Jewish law until burial takes place. Prior to the funeral, mourners tear their shirt to symbolize the suffering caused by grief.

Following the funeral, shiv'ah begins. During this seven-day period the mourner abstains from work, television, listening to music, and sex. They wear the previously torn clothes and perform only basic hygiene. Mirrors are covered and a candle is lit in memory of the deceased. During shiv'ah the mourner's needs are provided for by friends and visitors from the community. It is customary on Yahrzeit, the anniversary of the death, to visit the gravesite and mark the visit by placing a small stone on the grave (Hidalgo, 2017).

CULTURAL CONSIDERATIONS

In addition to the cultural dynamics outlined in Chapter 1, practitioners must be mindful of the role that ageism plays in the lives of the elderly. The myths, clichés, and prejudicial views of older adults so permeate society that they are regarded as truths instead of stereotypes and largely go unrecognized. Elderly persons are commonly portrayed as inept, crotchety, physically and sexually unappealing, feeble, debilitated, having faulty memory, being poor drivers, and being incapable of learning or changing. These depictions are evident in disparaging jokes made at their expense in movies, television, memes, cartoons, and birthday cards. These limiting and negative beliefs are so pervasive that they have become socially acceptable views. The continual perpetuation of negative beliefs about aging generates, for many, apprehension about growing older and fuels the multibillion dollar industry of antiaging products and procedures designed to hide the "flaws" that come with growing older (Chonody & Teater, 2018).

Ageist views are harmful to older adults and lead others to infantilize them, disregard them, and discriminate against them in many areas, including employment and healthcare. In addition, perceived injustices caused by ageism have been correlated with poor health and decreased life expectancy (Luo et al., 2012). Some elderly persons will internalize these negative stereotypes leading to feelings of helplessness and hopelessness (Raina & Balodi, 2014). Elderly persons who are members of other oppressed groups will experience the cumulative effect of oppression due to their multiple stigmatized identities. For example, Ama, a 73-year-old Cherokee woman who is lesbian, encounters numerous barriers and limitations due to systemic oppression against those groups. Ama's capacity to manage these intersecting identities may influence how she adjusts to growing older (Fredriksen-Goldsen & Muraco, 2010).

Also relevant to the discussion about older adults is how they are influenced by the time during which they lived. Each generational cohort experiences defining events, cultural shifts, and social changes that shape the perspective of its contemporaries. Consistent with a person-in-environment framework (see Chapter 3), understanding the historical and social context of an older person's developmental years can provide valuable insight into assessing and addressing their needs. For example, historical events such as the Great Depression, World War II, and the Vietnam War played an enormous role in molding the values of those who experienced them. Likewise, discriminatory policies such as sodomy laws, Jim Crow, the Mexican Repatriation, the Chinese Exclusion Act, as well as restricted opportunities for women had far-reaching effects on the opportunities, beliefs, and attitudes of those who lived during those times. Additionally, views on aging, death, and bereavement are also influenced by a person's generational context.

TABLE 6.1 Generational Characteristics

Generation	Characteristics*
The Greatest Generation (1901–1927)	Traditional values, resilience, frugal, need for a sense of purpose
The Silent Generation (1928–1945)	Rule-oriented, hardworking, loyal, conformist, patriotic, respect for authority
Baby Boomers (1946–1964)	Optimistic, personal gratification, individuality, independent, youth-oriented, focus on health/well-being
Generation X (1965–1980)	Skepticism, value having fun, seek a work–life balance, self-reliant, global focus
Millennials (1981–2000)	Pride in accomplishments and contributions to society, realistic, civic engagement, optimistic, interested in health/well-being
Generation Z (2001–2020)	Still in development

Source: Chonody & Teater, 2018, p. 21

*A great deal of diversity exists within a particular generational group and older people have the ability to change, re-examine their perspective, adopt different ideals, or create a different set of values.

When working with elderly clients, the family's grief culture (see Chapter 1) may be especially relevant if the elderly person's care and living arrangements depend on the family's relationship and resources. Values, beliefs, and attitudes influenced by generational differences may result in conflicting perceptions of what would be helpful to the bereaved older adult. Practitioners, therefore, should consider the entire family as the "client," rather than focusing solely on the bereaved elderly individual.

It is important to remember that older generations are extremely diverse not only with regard to culture, but also in regard to physical functioning, mental competence, emotional expression, engagement with others, financial stability, and access to healthcare (Chonody & Teater, 2018). A common assumption about older adults is that they are narrow-minded and unwilling to change. Many elderly persons, however, have a love of learning, and an openness to new ideas and experiences. They may also be a treasure trove of wisdom gained from their lived experience.

INTERVENTIONS

Research supports the use of psychotherapy with older adults (Haigh et al., 2018). The same interventions of strength building, trauma processing, and mourning the loss (Wortman & Pearlman, 2016), as discussed in Chapter 4, are useful when working with bereaved elderly persons. However, due to different generational views on counseling, some older adults feel uncomfortable with the idea of therapy and ashamed to be in need of mental health services. It is important, therefore, to provide a conducive and inviting milieu that lowers the client's anxiety about entering a counseling relationship. It may be helpful for practitioners to create a therapeutic setting that feels less formal and has the tone of a relaxed "chat." Displaying deference to the client's life experience and using humor may also help engage older adults and reduce any feelings of intimidation. Some may appreciate being referred to as Mr. or Mrs. as it communicates inherent respect.

Life Review

In addition, life review, also referred to as reminiscence therapy, has been shown to be especially effective with elderly persons (Sharif et al., 2018). Life review is grounded in developmental theory, with the final stage being the achievement of integrity. This technique involves the retelling of past memories and experiences and is believed to promote adaptation to the process of aging. It facilitates discussion of emotionally difficult topics, evaluation of negative experiences, and the recollection of positive experiences that restore a sense of efficacy and the feeling that one is a valued member of society (Sharif et al., 2018; Worden, 2018). The ultimate goal of life review is to assist older adults in generating a sense of meaning and value in their lives (Sharif et al., 2018). For bereaved elderly persons, reviewing past memories and experiences related to their deceased loved one enables mourners to integrate the loss into their world schema and is compatible with the task of making meaning from the loss (Westerhof & Slatman, 2019). There is also evidence to indicate that life review is effective in helping older adults with post-traumatic stress (Sharif et al., 2018). Life review techniques can be used in both individual and group counseling settings.

Complicated Grief Treatment (CGT)

Complicated Grief Treatment (CGT), as discussed in Chapter 4, has proven effective with older adults. In fact, it is the only intervention studied exclusively with this population. When compared with Interpersonal Psychotherapy used to treat depression, CGT with older adults showed statistically significant improvements in relieving severe grief symptoms. Furthermore, the improvements were maintained six months following the intervention. Contrary to concerns that older adults would be unable to withstand the revisiting exercises in CGT which use exposure strategies akin to those used in treating PTSD, the research indicated this method was found to be highly appropriate for older adults and was well tolerated. CGT has also proven effective in treating grief due to traumatic loss (Shear et al., 2005, 2014, 2016). CGT has been successful when working with individuals, groups, and in internet-based therapy (Meichsner et al., 2020).

Group Interventions with Older Adults

As with other populations, group interventions can be very helpful to bereaved older adults. In addition to providing emotional support with the loss, groups provide needed social support and outside activities for bereaved older adults who are already vulnerable to intense loneliness and isolation (Worden, 2018). Some groups may provide structured and specific focus on aspects related to the loss while others may be more informal in nature and focus primarily on providing opportunities for social interaction. Grief support groups are often hosted by churches, senior living communities, hospitals, community clinics, senior centers, and hospice organizations. Facilitators of these groups can also serve as a conduit between participants and community resources.

A Strengths-Based Approach

All of the techniques used to assist older adults with loss can be enhanced with the added perspective of the strengths-based framework of grief and loss. This is a particularly relevant approach as older adults tend to hold a forgotten place in mental healthcare and society at large. An important facet of the strengths-based approach is to establish a relationship based on respect and cooperation between the older client and the therapist (Pomeroy & Garcia, 2018). The manner in which helping professionals interact with older adults is heavily influenced by their own personal beliefs, expectations, and apprehensions about aging (Raina & Balodi, 2014). Practitioners, therefore, must practice self-awareness, being especially mindful of patronizing approaches, impatience, feelings of frustration with their elderly clients, or attitudes of futility about helping older adults (Raina & Balodi, 2014). Instead, when using a strengths-based approach, practitioners assume a collaborative stance that includes appreciation and respect for the wisdom and life experience the older client brings to the therapeutic work (Pomeroy & Garcia, 2018). Furthermore, practitioners support older clients in tapping into the reservoir of strengths they have accumulated over the course of their life and facilitate the development of life-enhancing responses to the loss. For example, an exploration of previous adverse events, including prior losses in clients' lives, can lead to discoveries about how they persevered. Using these coping skills as reference points, practitioners can reinforce the client's ability to successfully adjust to the many changes that accompany the loss. In addition, practitioners can help by affirming and mobilizing the client's environmental strengths to support healthy adaptation to the changes that occur because of the death.

CASES

CASE 6.1

Identifying Information:

Client Name: Luis Sanchez
Age: 74 years old
Race/Ethnicity: Mexican American
Marital Status: Widowed
Educational Level: High school graduate
Occupation: Retired Air Force

Intake Information:

Juanita Ruiz called the hospice center and asked to speak to a bereavement counselor. She stated that her father, Luis Sanchez, has been very depressed and lonely since his wife, Maria, died approximately three months ago. Juanita told the intake worker that her father finally admitted he wasn't doing well with the loss of his wife and agreed to try counseling. Juanita wanted an immediate appointment and stated, "I'm afraid if I wait too long, he'll change his mind about coming in."

Initial Interview:

You find Mr. Sanchez and his daughter Juanita in the waiting room talking softly to each other. You introduce yourself and they politely smile, shake your hand, and introduce themselves.

You ask, "Juanita, will you be joining us or will it just be you, Mr. Sanchez?"

Father and daughter look at each other and Mr. Sanchez asks Juanita, "Do you want to come in?"

"Well, okay," Juanita says. "But just for a little bit. I want to be sure there is plenty of time for you."

As you walk them to your office, you make small talk about the weather and offer them water to drink, which they both decline. They seat themselves on your couch, and look at you politely waiting for you to begin. You notice Mr. Sanchez is wearing a sweatshirt of the state's professional football team and you use this as a chance to make conversation for a bit.

"So, let me explain a little about who I am and what I do," you offer. "As a counselor I spend time with folks who have lost a loved one. Working in a hospice, we've realized that many families continue to need some support after their loved one has died. Grief is such a difficult experience and we've seen that people tend to do better when they have a place where they can talk about their loved one and how they are coping with all the changes they have experienced. Sometimes it can be particularly helpful to talk to someone who is not a part of the family. You may feel more freedom to say whatever you'd like. You can be assured, Mr. Sanchez, that our conversations will remain confidential unless I feel that someone's safety is in danger."

Mr. Sanchez and Juanita both nod in understanding. "I understand that your wife, Mr. Sanchez, and your mother, Juanita, died recently," you say.

Mr. Sanchez nods slightly, "Yes, that's correct. She died three months ago last Tuesday."

"How have you two been doing?" you inquire.

"It's been hard," Mr. Sanchez admits. "My wife was my best friend. We were married for 53 years."

"53 years? My goodness!" you say in admiration. "It must be very difficult for you to not have her around now."

"Yes, yes, it is," he says. His eyebrows are furrowed and he wears a forlorn expression on his face. "It's been hard for both of us," he adds and turns to Juanita.

Juanita says, "Yes, it has been hard. We both miss Mom a lot. She was a good mother and wife. I'm sad and everything but I'm doing okay. I'm mainly worried about my dad."

Mr. Sanchez looks at Juanita and smiles slightly. "I've got a wonderful daughter. She takes good care of me. And she took real good care of her mom when she was sick." He pats Juanita's knee.

Juanita continues, "Mom and Dad lived in the same house for 40 years. Since she died he has moved in with me and my husband for a little while. Our houses are just about five miles apart. It was just too hard for him to be in that house without her."

"Yes, I bet that was difficult," you empathize. "Is there anything specific that worries you Juanita?" you ask.

"I just know that he is hurting a lot," Juanita says while looking at her father. "I also believe that it may be affecting his health. We've got an appointment with the doctor later this week."

You inquire about Mr. Sanchez's health and learn that he has been more lethargic, is having tightness in his chest and is having gastrointestinal problems. Prior to the death, he was generally in good health.

"Have you been able to eat and sleep as you did before, Mr. Sanchez?"

"Honestly, no. I don't sleep," says Mr. Sanchez. "And I try to eat but I just don't have an appetite. Juanita, bless her heart, makes all these good meals, but food has lost all its flavor to me. It's like I can't taste anything."

"It could very well be that your physical symptoms are in response to your loss," you explain. "That is quite common for people who are grieving. You are wise, however, to see a doctor. We want to rule out any medical issues, and there may be some things the doctor can recommend to ease your symptoms. I'm glad you are trying to eat and it's good that you are helping him with this, Juanita. The stress of grief can be hard on our bodies and it's important to attend to our basic physical needs such as nutrition, rest, and exercise during this time." Juanita nods and indicates her intention to do whatever she can to help her father. "Juanita, is there anything else you'd like to say before I meet alone with your father?" you ask.

"No, I don't think so. I just hope he can find some ways to get through all of this. I'll do whatever I need to do to help him. I'll leave now so you two can talk some more. I'll wait for you in the lobby, okay, Dad?" Juanita stands to leave.

"Okay, mi hija," Mr. Sanchez says as he squeezes her hand.

After Juanita leaves, you turn to Mr. Sanchez, "What a wonderful daughter."

"Yes, I am very blessed to have her. I'm sure she gets tired of me," he says.

"It looks to me like she loves you very much," you say. Mr. Sanchez nods and after a pause, you continue, "This has really been devastating for you, hasn't it, Mr. Sanchez?"

"Yes, I guess you could say that. I miss Maria so much," he says with tears in his eyes. "I feel like there is this big black hole inside of me. Sometimes it makes me want to double over with pain."

"What was Maria like?" you ask.

"She was a good woman. You can see that in how she raised my daughter. We moved around a lot when we first got married. It seemed like just when we got settled somewhere the Air Force would move me again. She never complained, though. She just packed everything up and then made the house again. She always did what she could to make sure that wherever we were it felt like home."

With a little encouragement from you Mr. Sanchez continues to talk about his wife, the different places they lived and the course of her illness. "It sounds like she was a very special person," you say.

"Yes, she was," he reflects. He is quiet for a few moments and then asks, "How long does this last? I can't imagine ever feeling better again."

You answer gently saying, "I'm afraid it will probably last much longer than you'd like it to. When you've shared a lifetime with someone, as you have with Maria, it takes some time to adjust to her being absent." Mr. Sanchez nods in understanding. You continue, "Gradually, you will have more good days than bad days, although that may be hard to believe right now. You will probably always miss Maria, but with some time you will begin to get used to it."

"I hope so. I'm just so tired. I feel exhausted all day and then I lay down to go to sleep and suddenly I'm wide awake," he says.

"That must be frustrating," you reply. "What happens when you lay down to sleep?"

Mr. Sanchez shakes his head as he looks at the floor, "I just can't stop thinking about her, how I wish she were here."

"Yes," you say empathically. "Nighttime can be a hard time. Are you able to go back to sleep?"

"No, I'm up for most of the night." Sighing, he adds, "Sometimes I pray to God to please take this pain away from me. I've been reading the Bible hoping to find something that will make me feel better. Do you know of anything I can do? My parents' death was hard, but this… this is worse."

You validate the feelings that Mr. Sanchez has just expressed and let him know that you hear these sentiments often from people who have lost a spouse. "I'm glad you are trying to find some relief," you say. "I wish there was a short cut through grief. Sometimes we just have to let ourselves feel the pain. And take extra good care of ourselves in the process. If you let yourself express those emotions, over time they will eventually be less intense and less painful. I know that what you are experiencing doesn't feel good, but it is a healthy and expected response to losing Maria."

You discuss other actions that might help Mr. Sanchez, such as visiting his wife's grave, talking to her, going for short walks, and taking breaks from the grief by doing something pleasurable like seeing a movie. You also inquire about additional friends and family that Mr. Sanchez has as support. He reports that while he has friends he has known for years, since his wife's illness he has become quite isolated. He also says that many of their friends are couples and it feels awkward to be around them now that he is no longer part of a couple. You validate this experience and suggest that a future goal for him may be to find ways to get some social connection. You also tell him about the bereavement support group your agency is offering for older adults who have lost a spouse. He expresses interest in attending and says he will talk with his daughter about it.

"Thank you for meeting with me," he says with sincere gratitude.

"You are very welcome, Mr. Sanchez," you respond. "I'm honored to learn about Maria and to be a part of this experience with you. Would you like to come see me again?" Mr. Sanchez says that he would. You both return to the waiting room where you, Mr. Sanchez, and Juanita discuss the bereavement support group and schedule an additional session with you.

6.1-1. Find two academic articles about the effects on physical functioning and social functioning for older adults who have lost a spouse. Summarize the findings.

6.1-2. Mr. Sanchez was born in 1946. Do research on this generation and explain how the information you obtained might influence how you work with him.

6.1-3. What are some strengths-based questions you could ask Mr. Sanchez?

6.1-4. What types of interventions might be beneficial for Mr. Sanchez?

6.1-5. What are this family's strengths?

6.1-6. Find three resources in your community that could be helpful in building up Mr. Sanchez's social support network.

CASE 6.2

Identifying Information:

Client Name: Martha Robinson
Age: 73 years old
Race/Ethnicity: White
Marital Status: Single
Educational Level: College graduate
Occupation: Retired teacher

Intake Information:

Martha Robinson called the grief counseling agency and asked to speak with a female counselor. She stated that her younger sister, Anne, age 67, died of cancer. Martha stated that she was very close to her sister and felt at a loss following her sister's death. She thought that talking to a female counselor might help her "sort things out."

Initial Interview:

You meet Ms. Robinson in the lobby of the Center for Family Survival and observe a neatly dressed, gray-haired woman sitting in the corner of the room knitting a blanket. You walk over to her and extend your hand as you introduce yourself. "You must be Ms. Robinson," you say.

She puts down her knitting and shakes your hand saying, "Call me, Martha. Nice to meet you."

"That looks like a beautiful project you've got going there," you say about her knitting.

"Oh well, thank you. I'm trying to finish this afghan before the weather gets cold," she explains.

"It's very pretty," you comment. "How long have you been working on it?"

"Oh, quite a while now. I started it when Anne was sick in the hospital and I was just spending a lot of time sitting beside her bed. I decided I needed something to do and was sick of watching that blasted television all day long."

"Sounds like a good idea. I love the colors you chose," you say as you continue to admire her work. "Are you ready to come back to my office?" you offer.

Martha gathers up her belongings and stands. "Well, I still have about six more inches and the fringe to do, but I should have it done by winter," Martha says referring back to her afghan. "Do you knit?" she asks.

"I've done a little bit but I've never attempted to make an afghan. That's a really big project," you reply.

Martha enters your office and sits down. "You have a very nice little office. I like your pillows."

"Thank you. Can I get you a cup of water?" you reply.

"Sure, thank you," Martha replies.

As you pour water, you and Martha chat about the colors in your office and the colors she has used in her previous knitting projects. "I understand you are here because your sister died recently," you begin. "Tell me a little about how you've been doing."

Martha takes the water and sips on it. "Well, Anne was my younger sister by four years. I can't believe she died before me. I would never have expected that turn of events. But they found a tumor in her lungs about three years ago. She had surgery and we thought she was out of the woods, but then the cancer came back. She went through all kinds of chemotherapy and radiation treatments but in the end, it didn't really help. She fought really hard and went through so much. It's just very sad. I miss her so much. It was just the two of us and she lived with me after her husband died about seven years ago. It was just like when we were children. We did everything together. Went out to eat and to the movies. We grocery shopped together and really enjoyed each other's company. Both our parents lived into their late 80s, so we expected to live together for a long time. I'm the only one left in the family now. I kind of feel like an orphan!"

"I can imagine," you reply. "So you took care of Anne throughout her illness?" you comment.

"Yes, she was in and out of the hospital and treatment. She was sick for three years, although some of that time she was home and seemed to be doing better."

"How long ago did she die?" you ask gently.

"It's been almost six months now," Martha replies. "I feel like I should be getting on with my life, but I'm having a real hard time."

"Can you tell me more about that?" you ask.

"Well, I spent so much time in the last three years taking care of my sister, that I kind of lost contact with other friends that I used to see on a regular basis. It's funny how people just kind of disappear when you're dealing with illness in the family. It happened with my parents, too. I took care of them when they were dying. I guess it's kind of my job to take care of everyone. You see, I never got married and taught school for almost 40 years. I took care of all those kids and then I took care of everyone in my family and now they're all gone." After a pause, she continues with tears in her eyes, "It's kind of a lonely feeling. I'm not sure what to do with myself now."

"Yes, I'm sure it feels very lonely," you validate. "You've not only lost your sister, but you've also lost your role. Your occupation, so to speak, was a caregiver and now there is no one to care for. Does that sound right?"

"Yes, you're right. I think that's why I feel so lost," she says.

"That's understandable. When you think about your future, what comes up for you?" you ask.

"It frightens me, to be honest," she says. "Every day, I wonder how much longer I have and what will happen if I get sick. Who will take care of me? It's just me. I'm all alone. And Anne's treatment in the hospital was very expensive. Her insurance covered a lot of it, but there are some enormous bills to pay and I don't know how I'm going to do it."

"It sounds like you're feeling uncertain and insecure about what's next and how you will manage. Is that right?" you ask.

"Yes," she confirms. "I don't know why I'm finding it to be so hard. I should be able to figure it out. Goodness knows, I've helped everyone else figure it out!"

You validate the distress this must be causing for Ms. Robinson and spend some time talking about the expected effects of grief and how this loss may feel different than the other losses she has experienced.

"Well, that does make sense. I hadn't thought of it that way," she says.

After giving her some time to consider this, you say, "Tell me how you are spending your time these days."

Martha explains that lately she has had a hard time motivating herself to do things. She says she tries to work on settling her sister's estate and getting the medical bills paid but very quickly gets overwhelmed. "I end up spending a lot of time playing

Solitaire on the computer. I watch the news, take a lot of naps. I'm trying to finish this afghan."

You inquire about her eating and sleeping.

"Sleep is fine. Seems like all I do is sleep, to be honest. Eating? It's so hard to cook for just one person. I'll end up making myself a sandwich usually."

You validate the challenge of being alone and how this makes caring for herself more difficult. You briefly discuss the importance of nutrition as well as how she may need some additional social or mental stimulation.

"You're probably right," she agrees. "It's just I can't get myself to do anything."

"I know," you empathize. "Sometimes we have to push ourselves a little bit at the beginning and trust that we'll feel better once we get started. It's not easy, though. I also imagine that things feel really hard right now because it's been about six months since Anne died. Many people struggle around that time. The reality of the loss starts to set in."

Martha takes this in and adds, "It does feel really hard right now."

"Yes, and so it might help to think in terms of small steps you can take to help you through this time. Maybe it's getting a nutritious meal, drinking more water, or taking a ten-minute walk," you suggest.

Martha considers this and says, "Yes, a walk would be good. Though my bad knee has been acting up. I used to do water aerobics. They have a class at the senior center. I haven't been in a while, but I used to enjoy the exercise and the water and seeing some of my friends there."

"That would be a great thing to do. Does that feel like something that is do-able for you right now?"

"I think so," Martha says. "Yes, I'll try to get myself to a class this week."

"Okay, that sounds like a good plan," you say. "It probably wouldn't hurt to get a medical check-up, too. Have you seen your doctor recently? I just ask because grief can be very hard on the body and you are under a lot of stress right now."

Martha explains that she had been so busy caring for Anne that many of her medical needs got pushed aside. She agrees to schedule an appointment with her doctor.

"That's another really good small step," you say.

You and Martha talk more about the ways her life is different now and she states that she would like to see you again. You agree and arrange to see her again next week.

6.2-1. What are some of Martha's strengths?
6.2-2. What would you say to Martha when explaining the expected effects of grief and why this loss may feel different from previous losses she has had?
6.2-3. What secondary losses is Martha experiencing?
6.2-4. What additional information would you want to gather as you work with Martha?
6.2-5. What kinds of interventions could be helpful to Martha?
6.2-6. What are some community resources that could benefit Martha?

CASE 6.3

Identifying Information:

Client Name: Joseph Feingold
Age: 78 years old
Race/Ethnicity: Jewish
Marital Status: Married
Educational Level: College degree
Occupation: Owned and managed hardware store, now retired

Intake Information:

Mr. Feingold called to set up an appointment for bereavement counseling over the death of his life-long friend. "I think I'm okay, but my wife is insisting that I see someone," he explains. "Well, there's no harm in coming in," you say in response. "Sometimes people are surprised by how much it can help."

"Is that right?" Mr. Feingold says. "Okay. How does this work?"

You arrange a time for Mr. Feingold to come in and give him directions to your office.

Initial Interview:

"Mr. Feingold?" you say upon entering the lobby.

"That's me!" says a balding and plump older man as he rises from his chair.

He shakes your hand and smiles as he says, "Please call me Joe. Mr. Feingold is my dad!" You join him in laughing at his joke.

"Okay, Joe!" you say. "Come on in and let's chat for a bit."

You lead Joe back to your office and offer him a cup of coffee, which he accepts. To make the situation seem less formal you sit in a chair adjacent to the couch where he is sitting, as if you were in someone's living room.

"Well, Joe," you begin, "tell me how you're doing."

"Oh, I'm okay," Joe says as he leans back on the couch. "I really am. But everybody is getting all worried about me since my friend died."

"Tell me about your friend," you say.

"His name was Stuart Abrams. We had been friends for 70 years!" Joe says.

"70 years?" you exclaim. Joe seems pleased with your awestruck reaction.

"That's right! Hard to believe I'm that old isn't it?" he says laughing.

You laugh at Joe's sarcasm and ask, "So how did you and Stuart meet?"

"We went to grade school together and we've been friends ever since. He used to joke that we'd known each other for so long that my bad looks were rubbing off on him!" Joe laughs heartily.

"So he was a jokester, huh?" you say, encouraging Joe to talk more about his friend.

"Oh, was he a jokester! He was always cutting up, acting crazy and pulling pranks on people. He would have people pretty confused. They wouldn't be able to tell when he was joking and when he was serious." Joe leans forward and says smiling, "And to tell you the truth I think he liked it that way."

"Really?" you say, returning the smile.

"There was this one time, we had been out on the town and had spent all our money. I mean, we didn't have one cent. But Stu was hungry and he was craving apple pie. So we went and sat down in this diner like we were going to order like regular customers. Well, Stu starts talking to the waitress and gets into this big story about how we had just got back from fighting the war in Germany and about how he had been awarded two purple hearts. And that's Stu for you. He can't keep it simple and say he got one Purple Heart, he has to make everything bigger than life. You should have heard the fishing stories he would tell. You'd have thought he had caught the *Titanic*, the way he would tell it! Anyway, he goes into this long story saying he got wounded in France and barely escaped with his life. He says, 'When I was in the infirmary, I was convinced I was going to die and I kept thinking about what I'd like for my last meal. It was my momma's meatloaf, mashed potatoes, and her homemade apple pie.' So Stu goes on and on saying that thinking about that meal was what kept him alive and if it weren't for that he wouldn't be sitting there in that diner at that moment. 'Unfortunately,' he says, 'I never got that meal from my momma. She died of a brain tumor before I got home.' Well, by this time," Joe chuckles, "that poor waitress was in tears and do you know, we both got a huge meal of meatloaf, mashed potatoes, and apple pie on the house?" Joe laughs. "I tell you, Stu was something else."

You laugh at Joe's story, which seems to delight him and he continues to recall several humorous stories about his adventures with Stu. You learn that Joe and Stu played baseball together when they were young, double dated together in college, were the best men in each other's weddings, and went fishing together in their older years.

"It sounds like you two were very close," you say.

"We were. He was like a brother to me. I'm really going to miss him," Joe says.

"How did Stu die?" you ask.

Joe sighs. "He had a heart attack. He had been having some problems with his blood pressure and the doctor had been trying to get it regulated and they just were never able to get it stabilized. I wonder now if he was taking his medication like he was supposed to. When it happened, though… Oh, it was awful." He pauses and seems lost in his own thoughts. You wait silently and after a few moments Joe says, "We were playing poker like we always did on Thursday nights. All of a sudden, he starts making this face. Then he grabs his chest and starts shaking and then he fell over on the table." Joe now has tears in his eyes. "I kept saying, 'Stu, get up! Get up!' I thought he was joking!" The intensity in Joe's voice rises and he seems to be reliving the events of Stu's death. You lean forward and continue to listen intently while Joe continues. "Then I finally realized he wasn't joking and I tried to revive him, but it was too late." Joe is very still but you notice a small tear in the corner of his eye.

"What a horrible experience for you!" you empathize.

"I should have been able to save him," Joe says and then adds angrily, "That rascal!"

"Do you feel responsible for Stu's death?" you ask gently.

"Sometimes, I do," Joe says. "If I had just realized sooner that he wasn't joking, maybe I would have been able to save him."

"It sounds like Stu was hard to read sometimes," you suggest, "and from what you've told me about him, faking a heart attack sounds like the kind of prank he would do."

"Yeah, it was. It was exactly the kind of thing he would do. But still.... I was his best friend. I should have known he was serious."

"How long was it before you realized he wasn't joking?" you ask.

Joe is quiet for a moment as he considers your question. "It wasn't very long. Just a couple of seconds, really. It all happened so fast."

"It sounds like you did the best you could in that situation. Even if you had realized sooner that Stu wasn't joking he still may not have made it. You just happened to be present at the time, and so it can be easy to feel responsible." You pause for a moment. "I know that you wish it could have turned out differently, though."

"I sure do. I know what you're saying is true. My wife tells me the same thing and I know it in my head. Sometimes it's hard to believe it in my heart, though," Joe says.

"I understand. It may take some time before you are able to turn down the volume on your guilt feelings. It does often help to talk about it with other people who can remind you that you are not responsible. Also, sometimes it helps to simply change the kinds of words you use when you think about it. For example, instead of saying, 'I feel guilty that I didn't save him' you can say 'I regret that I wasn't able to save him.' Or instead of 'I should have been able to save him,' you can say 'I wish I could have saved him.' It's a small change but the words we use can carry a lot of meaning and innuendo."

Joe nods his understanding and says, "Okay. I'll try that."

"Of course, you know that grief isn't usually a short-term experience. I would expect you to have some sad feelings about Stu's death for a while."

"Yeah. I've lost both my parents, you know. I always thought that nothing would be harder than that. But this has been hard, too, even though it's very different."

"Yes, every grief experience is different," you respond. "You had a very unique relationship with Stu so I'm not surprised that this has been hard, though it may be difficult in a different way than it was with your parents' deaths."

"When you get to be my age, I suppose you have to start getting used to your friends dying," Joe reflects.

"From what I understand, that can be a very hard thing to get used to, though," you suggest.

"Well, I thank you for talking with me. I do enjoy telling those stories." Joe chuckles, "I think my wife is tired of hearing them!"

"I loved hearing your stories, Joe! I'd like to hear more if you're up to telling them," you say. You and Joe arrange to meet again in two weeks.

6.3-1. What did the therapist do to build rapport with Joe?

6.3-2. How do you interpret Joe's insistence that he is "okay"? What are some ways you could respond to this?

6.3-3. What potential concerns do you have for Joe? How would you assess for these in subsequent sessions with him?

6.3-4. Find an article on Life Review Therapy and write a short paragraph describing this therapeutic technique.

6.3-5. What are Joe's strengths?

CASE 6.4

Identifying Information:

Client Name: Glenda Perkins
Age: 61 years old
Race/Ethnicity: African American
Marital Status: Divorced
Educational Level: Bachelor's degree
Occupation: Paralegal

Intake Information:

Glenda calls and with a shaky voice asks to speak with a bereavement counselor. She explains that she is grieving the death of her 45-year-old son who passed away approximately four weeks earlier. Glenda tells you that she can't believe that her son is dead and that it wasn't natural for a parent to bury her own son. Glenda seems quite distraught on the phone and you schedule an appointment for the following day.

Initial Interview:

You find Glenda sitting in the waiting room with an unopened magazine on her lap. She is holding a ball of tissue in her hand and looks exhausted. After greeting her and telling her your name, she silently follows you back to your office. She sits down quietly in your office, stares at the floor and waits for you to begin the conversation. You place a cup of water on the table next to her chair.

"Oh, thank you," Glenda says in a whisper.

"How are you, Glenda?" you gently inquire.

Glenda sighs. "I'm feeling pretty down in the dumps right now. I feel like this must be a bad dream and I'll just wake up and it will be over."

"Do you feel up to telling me what happened?" you tentatively question.

"Well, about four weeks ago, I got a phone call from my daughter-in-law, Susan. It was about 6:30 in the morning and she never calls that early. I knew something must be wrong. Susan was pregnant so my first thought was something happened to the baby. I was awake when she called and was just sitting down with a cup of coffee. She sounded terribly upset. She said something awful had happened and she didn't know how to tell me. It startled me and I asked her to tell me what happened. She just kind of blurted out that Howard, my son, was dead. She said the police were coming and she didn't know what to do. I couldn't believe my ears. I kept asking, 'Are you sure? Are you sure?'" Glenda takes a deep breath and continues. "She said that Howard had gotten up in the middle of the night, went into the garage and...shot himself. She didn't hear the gun go off. Somehow, he silenced it because she didn't realize he was gone until the next morning. She went downstairs and when she couldn't find Howard, she went to the garage to see if he'd already left for work. Sometimes he left early so he could go to the gym first. She saw him slumped over in the front seat of the car. It must have been terrible for her to see him like that."

"Oh, Glenda," you say softly as you hand her the box of tissues. "This must be so upsetting for you."

"I've never been so upset in my entire life," Glenda exclaims. "I feel like my whole world has just come to an end. It was like everything just stopped. I just sat there frozen still trying to understand what Susan was telling me. I couldn't grasp it. I kept saying, 'You mean Howard's dead? My son, Howard? How could this have happened?' Susan kept trying to convince me that he was dead. She was crying and I was crying and we weren't making much sense. I finally got a hold of myself and told her I was on my way to her house. They live about 30 miles away from me, so I had to get in the car and drive over there. I can barely remember the drive. The Lord was looking out for me to get me there safely because I was in bad shape."

"I'm sure you were in bad shape," you reply. Glenda sighs and takes a few sips of water. You give her some time and then gently prompt, "So you made it to their house?"

"Yes, and the police were there, and they were taking pictures and investigating the scene. A woman police detective was asking Susan questions in the living room when I walked into the house. She jumped up and ran to me when she saw me there. I think she was really scared and needed my help."

"It sounds very traumatic," you suggest.

"Yes, it was the worst day of my life. You never think you'll bury your own child," Glenda says. "It was traumatic and such a shock," Glenda goes on. "I knew that Howard had had these depressions in the past, but I never thought he'd take his own life. It's been so hard especially with Susan pregnant and all."

"How is Susan doing with all of this?" you inquire.

"She's doing okay, I think. Her mother came to stay with her. She's six months pregnant and I think her mother is going to stay with her until the baby comes."

Glenda goes on to tell you how she planned on retiring in a couple of years, selling her condominium and moving closer to her son. These goals no longer seemed viable and she felt she had no plans for the future. In response to the hopelessness she expresses, you ask if she has had any suicidal ideation of her own and she indicates that she is not suicidal. As you talk, you learn that Glenda lives alone but has a pet Maltese puppy that her son had given her a year ago. Glenda is very attached to her dog and feels that it is symbolic of Howard's love for her. You decide that the complexity of Glenda's situation will require several sessions, so you decide to discuss how she is coping with her loss at the current time.

"Have you gone back to work, yet?" you ask.

"No, not yet. It's been a month, but I just haven't been able to face the idea of going back to work," Glenda replies. "I decided to come see you before making that decision. Besides, my boss has been very understanding and told me to take all the time I need. I've worked for him for 30 years and hardly missed a day of work. He's a lawyer and has gotten someone in there on a temporary basis while I'm out. I've been thinking about going back in a week or so."

"I'm glad you've taken the time off," you continue. "Losing a child is one of the most difficult challenges that can occur in life, and suicide makes it even more challenging. The grief process is going to take time and you will need to take care of yourself and your needs more than ever right now. I can see why you feel your future plans will need to change and that is something we can work on together, if you'd like. It's not something you need to do immediately. Right now, the most important thing is taking care of yourself."

Glenda nods in agreement. "You are the first person who really seems to understand how losing Howard has affected me."

"Is that so?" you ask.

"Yes," she says. "I think people feel very uncomfortable around me, like I'm contagious or something."

"That can't feel good. What do you make of that?" you inquire.

"I think it's because he killed himself. It's such a taboo, you know? They don't understand why anyone would do something like that. It's really looked down on."

"A death by suicide is definitely harder to understand and accept. And as you've experienced, it can leave survivors feeling very alone. Unfortunately, there is still a lot of stigma against mental illness in our society. It makes it very hard for people to get the support they need," you say.

"That's true. That's really true. I'm not sure I fully understand it myself," Glenda says as she takes in what you've said.

"Different communities and different cultures approach it differently. I wonder what it's like in your community? I'm guessing from what you've said, mental illness is not something that is discussed?"

"Oh, heavens no!" Glenda says. "No. We don't talk about it. I guess people just want to pretend it doesn't exist...I wish that were the case."

You provide more education about mental illness and suicide, carefully judging how much Glenda is able to digest at this moment and understanding you'll probably be reviewing this kind of information with her more in the future.

As the session comes to an end, you let Glenda ask any questions she has about you or the counseling process. When she asks about your experience helping others in her situation, you discuss your work experience and briefly mention that your knowledge also comes from personal experience with surviving suicide. This seems to provide her some reassurance. You arrange to meet again the following week.

6.4-1. What are some of Glenda's strengths? How could these strengths help her as she grieves the death of her son?

6.4-2. What additional assessment information do you want to gather in subsequent sessions?

6.4-3. Find a scholarly article that discusses bereavement for survivors of suicide. What are some common difficulties that family members might experience?

6.4-4. What would you say to Glenda when providing information about mental illness and suicide?

6.4-5. What are some of the potential secondary losses that Glenda might be experiencing?

6.4-6. What do you think about the therapist's personal disclosure regarding being a survivor of suicide? Do you agree with the decision to do this? Why or why not?

6.4-7. What additional questions could you ask Glenda to learn more about the cultural context of her grief?

Follow Up Interview with Glenda Perkins:

Glenda continues to see you weekly, although she has missed a few times due to illness. During your sessions she has extensively discussed the events surrounding her son's death, his funeral (including her feelings about seeing her ex-husband there), and she has told you more about Howard's history of depression, which had gone undiagnosed and untreated for most of his life. Since her son's death, she has had tremendous difficulty sleeping at night. Though her doctor has prescribed a medication to help with this, she tries not to take it often because of the side effects. You have noticed that Glenda has a tendency to worry a lot about many things. She has admitted that this is part of the reason she has difficulty falling asleep. As Glenda takes her seat in your office today, you inquire about her health as she had missed her last session due to a bad cold.

"I'm on the mend," she says. "I've still got a bit of a cough but nothing like it was."

"I'm glad you are feeling better and were able to make it in today," you say. "Tell me how things have been for you since we last talked."

"Well, I've been thinking a lot about the baby," she says. "You know, Susan is due next week."

"Oh, yes! How are you feeling about that?" you ask.

"Well, on one hand I am absolutely thrilled. I have been looking forward to being a grandmother for a long time. Howard and Susan waited so long to start having children that I'd almost given up on the idea. But now I will get to be a grandma and I couldn't be happier about that. But sometimes I also feel sad about it. This little boy – she's going to name him Nicholas Howard – I just feel so sad for him that he will never know his father. And I feel sad for Howard that he is missing out on a relationship with his son."

"It is kind of bitter sweet isn't it?" you suggest.

"Yes, it is. Just so many different emotions. And then I start worrying. Well, you know me – that's what I do best!" Glenda chuckles in a self-deprecating way.

"What are your worries, Glenda?"

"Well, I worry that Susan won't want me to be around the baby as much as I'd like to be. I mean, at some point, she will probably start dating again and find a nice man to be her husband and she deserves that. But where will that leave me? Will she still want me to be a part of her life and the baby's life? Maybe I'll just be a reminder of Howard and this horrible thing he did and she'll start to push me away."

"So you're concerned that you won't get to have a relationship with Nicholas?" you ask.

"Yes, or that I'll develop a bond with Nicholas but she will change her mind when she meets someone else and then I'll be forgotten and just kind of fall through the cracks."

"I see," you say to show your understanding.

Glenda continues, "And then there's my ex-husband Gary. Is he going to start coming around a lot to see the baby? Am I going to have to start dealing with him again? I can tolerate him for short periods of time – very short periods, mind you – but I really don't want to have anything to do with him. And I certainly don't want to have to share Nicholas with him. My time with Nicholas will probably be limited as it is!"

You notice that Glenda is tearful and she seems to be working herself into an anxious state. You say, "Okay. I hear that you have a lot of concerns about the future and how things will be once Nicholas arrives." Glenda nods. "And I see that you get really anxious when you think about these things," you say.

"I do. I'm terribly anxious. I just can't stop thinking about all of this and the more I think about it the more upset I get. I can work myself into a panic," Glenda explains.

"It sounds like you get stuck on all the negative possibilities and can't find any hope that some of this may turn out to be okay," you say.

"Yes, you're right. Maybe I'm just trying to prepare myself for another disappointment. I don't want any more surprises. I've had enough disappointments in my life," she says.

"Do you think that's part of the reason you worry so much? – to keep yourself from getting hurt again?" you ask.

"Probably. Or just not to be surprised. I guess I feel that if I know about it in advance I'll be better prepared and it won't feel so bad. Or if I expect the worst then I can't be disappointed," she adds.

"I can certainly understand how you get to that line of thinking. I'm concerned, however, about the toll that all of this worrying takes on you. It seems to me that it's doing you more harm than it is good. Am I off base about that?"

"No, I think you're exactly right," Glenda says. "It really does stress me out. I have trouble concentrating and I always feel so tense. I can't make myself stop, though. I've told myself to just wait and see what happens, but I don't get very far with that."

"Perhaps I can show you some things that may help," you say. "First of all, let's explore how realistic these worries are. Let's start with your concern that Susan will limit your relationship with Nicholas." You and Glenda then discuss the nature of her relationship with Susan, the kind of person she is and Susan's previous statements about how she wants Glenda to be involved with Nicholas, including inviting Glenda to be at Nicholas's birth. All of this evidence seems to make the possibility of Glenda's worry becoming true less likely. You then talk with Glenda about her concerns about her ex-husband. Again you help her assess what is likely to happen given the evidence that is available. You also discuss some possible actions Glenda could take should her worst fears about these situations come true. By the end of this discussion, Glenda appears more relaxed and displays more confidence around her ability to handle these issues. Since there is a little more time left in the session, you teach Glenda some coping skills that can help quell her anxiety. She agrees to practice these skills until the next session.

6.4-8. Identify three coping skills you could teach Glenda to help her manage her anxiety. Write out how you would explain them to her.

6.4-9. What additional interventions might you want to use with Glenda?

6.4-10. Identify three strengths-based questions that might be helpful to ask Glenda.

REFERENCES

American Foundation for Suicide Prevention. (2020, March 1). Suicide statistics. https://afsp.org/suicide-statistics/

Bartels, S. J., Pepin, R., & Gill, L. E. (2014). The paradox of scarcity in a land of plenty: Meeting the needs of older adults with mental health and substance use disorders. *Generations*, *38*(3), 6–13.

Boelen, P. A. (2017). Self-identity after bereavement: Reduced self-clarity and loss-centrality in emotional problems after the death of a loved one. *The Journal of Nervous and Mental Disease*, *205*(5), 405–408. https://doi.org/10.1097/nmd.0000000000000660

Böttche, M., & Knaevelsrud, C. (2017). Psychotherapy for post-traumatic stress disorders in old age. *Neurologist*, *88*, 1234–1239. https://doi-org.ezproxy.lib.utexas.edu/10.1007/s00115-017-0409-9

Böttche, M., Kuwert, P., & Knaevelsrud, C. (2012). Posttraumatic stress disorder in older adults: An overview of characteristics and treatment approaches. *International Journal of Geriatric Psychiatry*, *27*(3), 230–239. https://doi.org/10.1002/gps.2725

Brink, T. L., Yesavage, J. A., Lum, O., Heersema, P., Adley, M. B., & Rose, T. L. (1982). Screening tests for geriatric depression. *Clinical Gerontologist*, *1*, 37–44.

Chonody, J. M., & Teater, B. (2018). *Social work practice with older adults: An actively aging framework for practice*. SAGE Publications.

Chu, C., Buchman-Schmitt, J. M., Stanley, I. H., Hom, M. A., Tucker, R. P., Hagan, C. R., Rogers, M. L., Podlogar, M. C., Chiurliza, B., Ringer, F. B., Michaels, M. S., Patros, C. H., & Joiner, T. E. (2017). The interpersonal theory of suicide: A systematic review and meta-analysis of a decade of cross-national research. *Psychological Bulletin*, *143*(12), 1313–1345. https://doi.org/10.1037/bul0000123

Conejero, I., Olié, E., Courtet, P., & Calati, R. (2018). Suicide in older adults: Current perspectives. *Clinical Interventions in Aging*, *13*, 691–699. https://doi.org/10.2147/cia.s130670

Cukrowicz, K. C., Cheavens, J. S., Van Orden, K. A., Ragain, R. M., & Cook, R. L. (2011). Perceived burdensomeness and suicide ideation in older adults. *Psychology and Aging*, *26*(2), 331–338. https://doi.org/10.1037/a0021836

Diener, E., Emmons, R. A., Larsen, R. J., & Griffin, S. (1985). The satisfaction of life scale. *Journal of Personality Assessment*, *49*, 71–75.

DiGiacomo, M., Lewis, J., Phillips, J., Nolan, M., & Davidson, P. M. (2015). The business of death: A qualitative study of financial concerns of widowed older women. *BMC Women's Health*, *15*(1). https://doi.org/10.1186/s12905-015-0194-1

Dinnen, S., Simiola, V., & Cook, J. M. (2015). Post-traumatic stress disorder in older adults: A systematic review of the psychotherapy treatment literature. *Aging & Mental Health*, *19*(2), 144–150. https://doi.org/10.1080/13607863.2014.920299

Eckholdt, L., Watson, L., & O'Connor, M. (2017). Prolonged grief reactions after old age spousal loss and centrality of the loss in post loss identity. *Journal of Affective Disorders*, *227*, 338–344. https://doi.org/10.1016/j.jad.2017.11.010

Flatt, J. D., Gilsanz, P., Quesenberry, C. P., Albers, K. B., & Whitmer, R. A. (2018). Post-traumatic stress disorder and risk of dementia among members of a health care delivery system. *Alzheimer's & Dementia*, *14*(1), 28–34. https://doi.org/10.1016/j.jalz.2017.04.014

Folstein, M. F., Folstein, S. E., & McHugh, P. R. (1975). Mini Mental State: A practical method for grading the cognitive state of patients for the clinician. *Journal of Psychiatric Research*, *12*, 189–198.

Fredriksen-Goldsen, K. I., & Muraco, A. (2010). Aging and sexual orientation: A 25-year review of the literature. *Research on Aging*, *32*(3), 372–413. https://doi.org/10.1177/0164027509360355

Ghesquiere, A. R., Bazelais, K. N., Berman, J., Greenberg, R. L., Kaplan, D., & Bruce, M. L. (2016). Associations between recent bereavement and psychological and financial burden in homebound older adults. *OMEGA – Journal of Death and Dying*, *73*(4), 326–339. https://doi.org/10.1177/0030222815590709

Ghesquiere, A. R., Shear, M. K., & Duan, N. (2013). Outcomes of bereavement care among widowed older adults with complicated grief and depression. *Journal of Primary Care & Community Health*, *4*(4), 256–264. https://doi.org/10.1177/2150131913481231

Haigh, E. A., Bogucki, O. E., Sigmon, S. T., & Blazer, D. G. (2018). Depression among older adults: A 20-year update on five common myths and misconceptions. *The American Journal of Geriatric Psychiatry*, *26*(1), 107–122. https://doi.org/10.1016/j.jagp.2017.06.011

Hashim, S. M., Eng, T. C., Tohit, M., & Wahab, S. (2013). Bereavement in the elderly: The role of primary care. *Mental Health in Family Medicine*, *10*, 159–162.

Hidalgo, I. M. (2017). The effects of children's spiritual coping after parent, grandparent or sibling death on children's grief, personal growth, and mental health (Doctoral dissertation). https://digitalcommons.fiu.edu/etd/3467

Hill, R. M., & Pettit, J. W. (2014). Perceived burdensomeness and suicide-related behaviors in clinical samples: Current evidence and future directions. *Journal of Clinical Psychology*, *70*(7), 631–643. https://doi.org/10.1002/jclp.22071

Holt-Lunstad, J. (2017). The potential public health relevance of social isolation and loneliness: Prevalence, epidemiology, and risk factors. *Public Policy & Aging Report*, *27*(4), 127–130. https://doi.org/10.1093/ppar/prx030

Jahn, D. R., Cukrowicz, K. C., Mitchell, S. M., Poindexter, E. K., & Guidry, E. T. (2015). The mediating role of perceived burdensomeness in relations between domains of cognitive functioning and indicators of suicide risk. *Journal of Clinical Psychology*, *71*(9), 908–919. https://doi.org/10.1002/jclp.22190

King, M., Lodwick, R., Jones, R., Whitaker, H., & Petersen, I. (2017). Death following partner bereavement: A self-controlled case series analysis. *PLOS ONE*, *12*(3), e0173870. https://doi.org/10.1371/journal.pone.0173870

Lekalakala-Mokgele, E. (2018). Death and dying: Elderly persons' experiences of grief over the loss of family members. *South African Family Practice*, *60*(5), 151–154. https://doi.org/10.1080/20786190.2018.1475882

Lundorff, M., Holmgren, H., Zachariae, R., Farver-Vestergaard, I., & O'Connor, M. (2017). Prevalence of prolonged grief disorder in adult bereavement: A systematic review and meta-analysis. *Journal of Affective Disorders*, *212*, 138–149. https://doi.org/10.1016/j.jad.2017.01.030

Luo, Y., Xu, J., Granberg, E., & Wentworth, W. M. (2012). A longitudinal study of social status, perceived discrimination, and physical and emotional health among older adults. *Research on Aging*, *34*(3), 275–301.

Meichsner, F., O'Connor, M., Skritskaya, N., & Shear, M. K. (2020). Grief before and after bereavement in the elderly: An approach to care. *The American Journal of Geriatric Psychiatry*, *28*(5), 560–569. https://doi.org/10.1016/j.jagp.2019.12.010

Miner, B., & Kryger, M. H. (2017). Sleep in the aging population. *Sleep Medicine Clinics*, *12*(1), 31–38. https://doi.org/10.1016/j.jsmc.2016.10.008

Perng, A., & Renz, S. (2018). Identifying and treating complicated grief in older adults. *The Journal for Nurse Practitioners*, *14*(4), 289–295. https://doi.org/10.1016/j.nurpra.2017.12.001

Pomeroy, E. C., & Garcia, R. B. (2018). *Direct practice skills for evidence-based social work: A strengths-based text and workbook*. Springer Publishing Company.

Quinn, C. A. (2018). Dementia: A cause of complicated grieving. In G. R. Cox, R. A. Bendiksen, & R. G. Stevenson (Eds.), *Complicated grieving and bereavement: Understanding and treating people experiencing loss* (pp. 153–162). Routledge.

Raina, D., & Balodi, G. (2014). Ageism and stereotyping of the older adults. *Scholars Journal of Applied Medical Sciences*, *2*, 733–739.

Register, M. E., Herman, J., & Tavakoli, A. S. (2010). Development and psychometric testing of the Register – Connectedness Scale for Older Adults. *Research in Nursing & Health*, *34*(1), 60–72. https://doi.org/10.1002/nur.20415

Robbins-Welty, G. A., Stahl, S. T., & Reynolds III, C. F. (2018). Grief reactions in the elderly. In E. Bui (Ed.), *Clinical handbook of bereavement and grief reactions* (pp. 103–137). Humana Press. https://doi.org/10.1007/978-3-319-65241-2

Saeri, A. K., Cruwys, T., Barlow, F. K., Stronge, S., & Sibley, C. G. (2017). Social connectedness improves public mental health: Investigating bidirectional relationships in the New Zealand attitudes and values survey. *Australian & New Zealand Journal of Psychiatry*, *52*(4), 365–374. https://doi.org/10.1177/0004867417723990

Scalise, J. J., Glinter, E. J., & Gerstein, L. H. (1984). The multi-dimensional loneliness measure: The Loneliness Rating Scale (LRS). *Journal of Personality Assessment*, *48*, 525–530.

Sharif, F., Jahanbin, I., Amirsadat, A., & Hosseini Moghadam, M. (2018). Effectiveness of life review therapy on quality of life in the late life at day care centers of Shiraz, Iran: A randomized controlled trial. *IJCBNM*, *6*(2), 136–145.

Shear, M. K., Frank, E., Houck, P. R., & Reynolds, C. F. (2005). Treatment of complicated grief: A randomized controlled trial. *JAMA*, *293*(21), 2601–2608. https://doi.org/10.1001/jama.293.21.2601

Shear, M. K., Reynolds, C. F., Simon, N. M., Zisook, S., Wang, Y., Mauro, C., Duan, N., Lebowitz, B., & Skritskaya, N. (2016). Optimizing treatment of complicated grief: A randomized clinical trial. *JAMA Psychiatry*, *73*(7), 685–694. https://doi.org/10.1001/jamapsychiatry.2016.0892

Shear, M. K., Wang, Y., Skritskaya, N., Duan, N., Mauro, C., & Ghesquiere, A. (2014). Treatment of complicated grief in elderly persons: A randomized clinical trial. *JAMA Psychiatry*, *71*(11), 1287–1295. https://doi.org/10.1001/jamapsychiatry.2014.1242

Spahni, S., Bennett, K. M., & Perrig-Chiello, P. (2016). Psychological adaptation to spousal bereavement in old age: The role of trait resilience, marital history, and context of death. *Death Studies*, *40*(3), 182–190. https://doi.org/10.1080/07481187.2015.1109566

Stahl, S. T., Smagula, S. F., Dew, M. A., Schulz, R., Albert, S. M., & Reynolds III, C. F. (2020). Digital monitoring of sleep, meals, and physical activity for reducing depression in older spousally-bereaved adults: A pilot randomized controlled trial. *The American Journal of Geriatric Psychiatry*, *20*(10), 1102–1106. https://doi.org/10.1016/j.jagp.2020.02.013

Thorp, S. R., Sones, H. M., & Cook, J. M. (2011). Posttraumatic stress disorder among older adults. In K. H. Sorocco & S. Lauderdale (Eds.), *Cognitive behavior therapy with older adults: Innovations across care settings* (pp. 189–217). Springer Publishing Company.

US Census Bureau. (2019, December 19). American community survey 2014–2018 5-Year estimates now available [Press release]. www.census.gov/newsroom/press-releases/2019/acs-5-year.html

Vesnaver, E., Keller, H. H., Sutherland, O., Maitland, S. B., & Locher, J. L. (2016). Alone at the table: Food behavior and the loss of commensality in widowhood. *The Journals of Gerontology Series B: Psychological Sciences and Social Sciences*, *71*(6), 1059–1069. https://doi.org/10.1093/geronb/gbv103

Ware, J. E., & Sherbourne, C. D. (1992). The MOS 36-item short-form health survey (SF36): I. Conceptual framework and item selection. *Medical Care*, *31*, 473–483.

Watanabe, A., & Suwa, S. (2017). The mourning process of older people with dementia who lost their spouse. *Journal of Advanced Nursing*, *73*(9), 2143–2155. https://doi.org/10.1111/jan.13286

Westerhof, G. J., & Slatman, S. (2019). In search of the best evidence for life review therapy to reduce depressive symptoms in older adults: A meta-analysis of randomized controlled trials. *Clinical Psychology: Science and Practice*, *26*(4). https://doi.org/10.1111/cpsp.12301

Wilińska, M., De Hontheim, A., & Anbäcken, E. M. (2018). Ageism in a cross-cultural perspective: Reflections from the research field. In L. Ayalon & C. Tesch-Römer (Eds.), *Contemporary perspectives on ageism* (pp. 425–440). Springer.

Worden, J. W. (2018). *Grief counseling and grief therapy: A handbook for the mental health practitioner* (5th ed.). Springer Publishing Company.

Wortman, C. B., & Pearlman, L. A. (2016). Traumatic bereavement. In R. A. Neimeyer (Ed.), *Techniques of grief therapy: Assessment and intervention* (pp. 25–29). Routledge.

Wyman, M. F., Shiovitz-Ezra, S., & Bengel, J. (2018). Ageism in the health care system: Providers, patients, and systems. In L. Ayalon & C. Tesch-Römer (Eds.), *Contemporary perspectives on ageism* (pp. 193–212). Springer.

Zimet, G. D., Dahlem, N. W., Zimet, S. G., & Farley, G. K. (1988). The multidimensional scale of perceived social support. *Journal of Personality Assessment*, *52*, 30–41.

CHAPTER 7

Grief Reactions and Special Populations

While there are many commonalities among bereaved persons regardless of the type of loss they have experienced, there are also some deaths that are unique in the way they impact mourners and the adjustment process that follows. Counselors require specialized knowledge and understanding to be most effective with these unique situations. The types of losses detailed in this chapter provide only a small sample of the wide diversity of client conditions that are seen in practice. For example, the grief experience of survivors of natural disasters, criminal and terrorist acts, domestic abuse, and bereaved prison inmates are additional groups that require specialized knowledge and unique interventions. For some losses, there is an abundance of literature devoted to the specific dynamics that are relevant, while for others, there is a dearth of information available. When applicable, practitioners should seek additional knowledge and supervision when encountering these distinct circumstances. This chapter will provide a brief overview of relevant issues of grief as it relates to persons with developmental disabilities, LGBTQ populations, anticipatory grief associated with terminal illness, the death of a child, refugees, military veterans, ambiguous loss, and pet loss.

GRIEF AND PERSONS WITH DEVELOPMENTAL DISABILITIES

Despite popular and historical opinions, persons with developmental disabilities develop emotional attachments to others and therefore, they, like all of us, experience grief (Powell, 2019). Unfortunately, their grief experience has only recently come to be acknowledged and given attention in the literature. For a variety of reasons, persons with developmental disabilities are especially vulnerable to experiencing complex grief after the death of a loved one, caregiver, or friend (Mason-Angelow, 2017). In large part this is because they are frequently misunderstood and disregarded both by society and by the individuals on whom they rely to provide information and meet their needs (Thorp et al., 2018). Though this is changing, people with developmental disabilities are often not told about the deaths of their loved ones or given very limited information. They may be excluded from participation in mourning rituals or quickly moved to new living arrangements. Though this often stems from a well-intended desire to protect them from pain, it leaves them feeling disregarded and alone (Clute, 2015; Powell, 2019; Thorp et al., 2018). Additional factors that present complexities for

DOI: 10.4324/9780429053634-7

bereaved persons with intellectual disabilities are difficulties in communicating their thoughts and feelings, limited control over their lives, limited experience and guidance on managing their emotions, and significant secondary losses, such as having to suddenly relocate and adjust to new caregivers (Young, 2016; Clute, 2015). These obstacles are heightened for persons with profound disabilities due to intensified challenges in communication, mobility, and their ability to cognitively understand the events surrounding the death (Young, 2017). Out of concern that they will cause distress to those around them, persons with developmental disabilities may avoid bringing up the loss. Instead, their grief reactions become evident in changes in behavior that may include weeping, angry outbursts, hyperactivity, agitation, decreased motivation, withdrawal, as well as changes in sleeping and eating (Clute, 2015). Unfortunately, caregivers may attribute these symptoms to the mourner's disability rather than recognize them as responses to the loss (Mason-Angelow, 2017).

The strengths of this population have been woefully underestimated by society, even by those who work with them on a daily basis. Thus, practitioners can play a unique role in bringing their strengths to light. This includes, but is not limited to, advocating that they receive accurate information about the loss and be allowed to decide on how they want to be involved in mourning rituals and post-death decisions that will affect their lives (Thorp et al., 2018). Initial research suggests that attachment-based approaches to helping this population process their grief may be preferable to cognitive-based interventions, particularly for those whose challenges are severe (Young, 2016). This includes strategies for emotional regulation, such as breath and movement techniques (Young, 2017). Life review and the use of photos and memory boxes have also been shown to be helpful (Mason-Angelow, 2017; Thorp et al., 2018). In addition, it has been widely observed that many persons with developmental disabilities benefit from utilizing their spiritual and religious resources (Clute, 2015; Powell, 2019).

Advocates for this population promote greater inclusion of persons with developmental disabilities in all facets of life, including loss and grief, so that they can acquire healthy and useful skills for coping with adversity, and thus lessen the need for specialized interventions (Clute, 2015; Thorp et al., 2018). Finally, as with other groups, practitioners must recognize that each person with a developmental disability is unique and generalizations should be avoided. When possible, a thorough psychosocial grief assessment can provide valuable information and assist in planning interventions.

GRIEF AND LGBTQ POPULATIONS

Though positive changes are occurring, there is still significant social discrimination, stigma, and prejudice against LGBTQ (lesbian, gay, bisexual, transgender, and queer/questioning) persons and this influences how they experience grief (Casey et al., 2019; Nolan et al., 2019). Particularly relevant to the discussion of grief with LGBTQ populations is the concept of "disenfranchised grief," a term first coined by Doka (1989). Grief is disenfranchised when the loss of a meaningful and significant attachment is not recognized and validated by others and when the loss "cannot be openly acknowledged, socially validated, or publicly mourned" (Doka, 1989, p. 15). This is the experience of many partner-bereaved LGBTQ persons when family, friends, and institutions do not recognize or give credence to their relationship with the deceased. Particularly influential to the trajectory of positive or negative coping with the loss is the bereaved partner's relationship with the deceased's family, both at the time of death and in bereavement (Nolan et al., 2019). Despite being in long-term and legally recognized relationships many LGBTQ partners are disregarded by friends and family who were not fully accepting of the relationship. This withholding of emotional support may take the form of excluding the partner in planning and participating in mourning rituals for the deceased, minimizing the impact the loss has on the surviving partner, imposing expectations of when their grieving process should end, evading discussions about the loss, and not recognizing significant dates and anniversaries relevant to the relationship with the deceased. The dismissive nature of these responses puts LGBTQ mourners at greater risk of social isolation and life-depleting grief reactions (Ingham et al., 2016; Nolan et al., 2019). In contrast, a positive and affirming relationship with the deceased's family as well as social validation of the loss leads to more life-enhancing grief reactions (Nolan et al., 2019).

The life experience of transgender persons is often accompanied by many non-death losses, particularly when friends and family are not accepting of their gender identity. Bereaved persons who are transgender may face added social complexities when a member of their family dies. Relationships with family members may be strained because the family is not aware of their acquired gender or because the family rejected them upon learning about it. Thus, there may be feelings of great distress upon making contact with estranged family members. Support in the form of an allied family member or friend who serves as a liaison with the family can be especially useful during the mourning period (Whittle & Turner, 2007). More research on the needs of bereaved transgender persons is needed in order to capably serve this population.

LGBTQ mourners often struggle to find community support that allows them to be truly authentic and open about their relationship with the deceased and their grief experience. Bereaved LGBTQ persons who have not disclosed the nature of the relationship to others face the decision of being open about the relationship and risk rejection and discrimination or keep the relationship private, thus limiting potential support and participation in mourning rituals. Bereavement support groups may or may not be hospitable depending on the cultural sensitivity and competence of the facilitator and the acceptance of other group members. Thus it takes tremendous courage for LGBTQ mourners to risk being vulnerable about their grief in these settings (O'Leary, 2019). Some older bereaved LGBTQ persons have found that support groups serving only LGBTQ members are more relevant to younger aged mourners. Grief support services, therefore, must be sensitive to heteronormative tendencies in grief groups (e.g. assuming all participants are grieving an opposite sex partner) and also remember that older LGBTQ mourners who have experienced more homophobia over their lifetime may be more hesitant to openly acknowledge their sexuality. All participants, therefore, should have the opportunity to retain their preferred degree of anonymity (Nolan et al., 2019).

It is important to recognize that there is tremendous diversity among LGBTQ persons. Practitioners must be mindful of implicit biases they may have concerning this population and refrain from making assumptions based on stereotypes. In addition, understanding the role of intersecting social identities and the practice of cultural humility is essential to providing quality services to LGBTQ mourners. For example, the experience of a Vietnamese transgender bereaved man will be unique to both his status in the country in which he resides as well as his cultural background.

BOX 7.1 MOURNING RITUALS: ISLAM

For Muslims, when an individual is on the brink of death they are placed flat on their back with their face toward Mecca (east). Perfumes are used to keep the room aromatic. Women in menstruation or anyone who is deemed unclean are not allowed in the room. The dying individual or family members read scripture from the Quran. The last words the dying person hears is the central statement of Muslim faith, the Shahadah: "There is no God but Allah and Muhammad is his prophet." These are also the first words spoken when a Muslim baby is born.

The corpse is immediately prepared for burial which traditionally occurs on the day of the death. This involves a ritualistic washing of the body performed by family members of the same gender as the deceased. According to tradition, the washing begins on the right side and at no point is the corpse completely uncovered. Islamic tradition prohibits embalming.

While Muslim culture permits mourning, it frowns upon open wailing and other such emotional demonstrations. Because of this, women are not allowed to follow a funeral procession. Though personal prayers are permitted, the Quran cannot be read near the corpse. Standing is required during these prayers and until the body is buried. Upon burial the body is removed from the casket and lowered into the ground. Attendants may speak softly to the deceased with directions about how to respond to the angels that will question the dead about his or her life. The face of the deceased is turned to face Mecca and the Shahadah is repeated. Dirt is placed loosely on the grave to allow the deceased to rise up when the angels arrive (Hidalgo, 2017).

ANTICIPATORY GRIEF AND TERMINAL ILLNESS

The experience of terminally ill patients and their family members is fraught with loss, beginning with notification of the diagnosis through to the moment of death. The progressive nature of a terminal illness, such as Alzheimer's or cancer, creates substantial and irrevocable changes in all aspects of the patients' and caregivers' lives, and each change elicits grief reactions. The losses experienced when a loved one is terminally ill are numerous. The loved one's role in the family is altered, plans made for the future are disrupted, and the family's lifestyle must change to focus on providing care to the patient. In addition, the relationship with the loved one changes due to their reduced physical and cognitive capacities, including the ability to communicate (Cheung et al., 2018). These changes are often accompanied with significant psychological distress, financial strain, increased physical demands of caregiving, long-term family disruption, and stressful decision-making regarding treatment and end of life planning (Coelho et al., 2018).

The terms anticipatory grief (AG), anticipatory mourning, and pre-death grief have been used when speaking of this experience, though there has been wide disagreement on how to conceptualize the phenomenon. Both the patient and family experience loss during this time, albeit from different perspectives. Coelho et al. (2020) define family caregiver anticipatory grief as "the family response to the perceived threat to the other's life and the subsequent anticipation of loss in the context of the end-of-life caregiving relationship" (p. 700).

The knowledge that a loved one will die must be delicately balanced with the fact that the loved one is still living. Caregivers are continually confronted with competing needs and desires which create tremendous psychological strain that must be endured over an extended period of time. For example, caregivers must confront the anticipation of death, while dreading the loss. They must adapt to changes in the relationship with their loved one, while also yearning to hold on to them even more closely. They take great efforts to shelter their loved one from emotional distress while also needing to honor their own needs and emotions. They must acknowledge the painful limits of their capacity to help while also finding a way to maintain a measure of control (Coelho et al., 2020). Given these numerous contradictions, it is no wonder that caregivers are overwhelmingly exhausted and emotionally depleted.

The experience of tending to loved ones with terminal illnesses also involves elements of trauma, separation distress, and difficulty in regulating emotions (Coelho et al., 2020). Traumatic aspects of the experience include contact with life-threatening conditions, disturbing images as the loved one's health deteriorates, and vicariously feeling their loved one's emotional pain. These experiences, in conjunction with the impossibility of predicting the course of the illness, leads to feelings of powerlessness and, in some cases, hopelessness. Some family members respond to this situation with hypervigilant behavior and overwhelming emotions while others may become numb and desensitized (Coelho et al., 2020).

Suffering related to separation distress involves anticipating the death, obsessively wondering when and how it will happen, and experiencing changes in the nature of the relationship with the loved one. In response, caregivers may draw nearer to the loved one or distance themselves as a way to manage this change.

Emotional regulation is an additional challenge for caregivers as they are under tremendous physical, emotional, and mental strain. Caregivers often experience less sleep, changes in eating and digestion, and rapid heart rates. They may be prone to irritability, anxiety, intrusive thoughts, feelings of dissociation, and despair. Some feel abandoned by their loved one and their community and worry about being able to cope effectively. Some caregivers question their faith and life purpose (Coelho et al., 2020). Managing these various and extreme states is even more complicated when caregivers feel they must hide their true thoughts and feelings in order to shield others from their pain (Coelho et al., 2020; Worden, 2018).

Often caregivers manage their discomfort with the impending separation and death of their loved one with periods of denial and hope. "Influenced by the current death-avoidant sociocultural norms, caregivers avoid thinking and talking about this painful reality and sustain hope in order to keep functioning and caring for the ill person" (Coelho et al., 2018, p. 54). This may interfere with tending to important end of life matters such as reconciling past conflicts, expressing forgiveness, honoring the loved one's final wishes, and being able to say goodbye (Coelho et al., 2018; Koenig Kellas et al., 2017). It also helps explain why family members often feel the death came too quickly, despite knowledge that it was expected. This is particularly true for loss due to cancer (Coelho et al., 2018).

Interventions for Anticipatory Grief

The challenge for practitioners working with anticipatory grief in caregivers is to accomplish goals that often appear contradictory. They try to help family members engage in the grief process and move toward acceptance of the loss while also discouraging premature detachment from the loved one before death occurs. Practitioners must be patient, understanding, and empathetic when caregivers demonstrate denial about the reality of the illness and express hope for recovery. Simultaneously, practitioners can gently encourage caregivers to think about their loved one's impending death so that "unfinished business" can be completed. This often involves helping the family reframe their goals for how to use the limited time with their loved one. The focus moves from curing to healing, extending life to enhancing quality of life. Practitioners can assess for anticipatory grief with attentive listening and astute observation on how caregivers are managing the ongoing changes with their loved ones. This includes checking to see if caregivers are avoiding social interactions or feeling restricted by their role in caring for their beloved. Based on this information, practitioners can provide interventions that capitalize on the family's strengths, mobilize additional resources, and teach life-enhancing coping skills (Coelho et al., 2018).

The intensity and complexity of what caregivers experience is largely hidden from view and often unacknowledged (Coelho et al., 2018). Caregivers may be unable or reluctant to pause, take time for themselves, and reflect on their experience. They may be hesitant to express feelings of anger, frustration, guilt, or resentment that are natural to the stressful job of caregiving. As one caregiver confided to her counselor, "Sometimes I just wish he would go ahead and die because I don't see how I can take it anymore. And then I feel like I'm the worst person alive." Practitioners can help by encouraging caregivers to accept outside assistance with caregiving, as well as naming and validating the losses that are being experienced. "This doesn't feel like a marriage anymore," remarked a woman whose husband had Alzheimer's. "All the care goes one way. I don't have a spouse. I'm his parent now."

It is especially helpful for families in this situation to receive psychoeducation pertaining to the course of the illness. Knowing what to expect as the disease progresses relieves the family from unnecessary alarm and reduces the uncertainty that contributes to the development of trauma symptoms. It also allows the family time and motivation to express love and appreciation for the patient and say "goodbye." The ability to say goodbye, even if they are not present at the time of death, has been shown to have positive outcomes for post-death bereavement (Otani et al., 2017). Thus, the anticipatory grief of caregivers requires as much attention as does post-death grief.

Efforts to determine if anticipatory grief impacts the bereavement experience after the death have yielded mixed results due to differing conceptual definitions and the numerous variables that impact the mourning process (Coelho et al., 2020; Worden, 2018). There is, however, some evidence to suggest that being able to process the experience of anticipatory grief in life-enhancing ways can positively impact the course of grief once the death transpires. Conversely, unresolved pre-death grief can give rise to life-depleting ways of dealing with complex grief after the death. Thus, assisting clients with anticipatory grief may lead to more positive outcomes after the death occurs (Moon, 2016).

GRIEVING THE DEATH OF A CHILD

Regardless of the mode of death or age of the child, multiple studies have indicated that bereavement due to the death of a child is more intense and longer lasting as compared with other types of bereavement (Vegsund et al., 2019). While sadness, yearning, anger, and guilt are expected reactions to loss, evidence shows that these are experienced more profoundly for parents mourning the death of a child (Morris et al., 2019; Zetumer et al., 2015). This can be explained by the fact that attachment bonds between parents and children are the strongest in human experience (Bowlby, 1980; Zetumer et al., 2015). Consequently, a child's death has numerous unique reverberations for the surviving parents.

There is substantial research showing that bereaved parents experience significant changes in their physical and mental health and are at an elevated risk for having complex grief reactions, anxiety, depression, PTSD, and suicidal ideation (October et al., 2018; Zetumer et al., 2015). Additionally, bereaved parents have a higher risk of developing physical illnesses when compared with their non-bereaved peers and are at a higher risk of mortality (Kim et al., 2019; October et al., 2018). This risk is even greater when the cause of death is traumatic in nature, for mothers as compared with fathers, and when children are minors (October et al., 2018).

Bereaved parents often experience a loss of self and life purpose when their role as caregiver and protector of their child is taken away. They are left feeling unmoored by the fundamental disruption in their plans, goals, and dreams for the future (Kim et al., 2019). Furthermore, because the expectation is that children will outlive their parents, the death of a child seems unnatural and challenges the assumptive worldview of these parents. This may account for the increased traumatic distress that is experienced with this type of grief (Zetumer et al., 2015). Surviving parents may experience great despair and guilt as a result of their perceived "failure" to protect their child and fulfill their roles as parents. Bereaved parents may also feel guilty about outliving their children or for occasions when they were less than ideal parents.

Bereaved parents commonly experience extreme anger when mourning their child. This anger is often intensified when the death was due to an accident or is perceived as being preventable. Parents may direct their anger toward doctors, other family members, the deceased child, themselves, or God. Anger may also be a result of the utter powerlessness that parents experience when a child dies. Practitioners should accept this anger without judgment and encourage parents to express it in constructive ways.

The traumatic impact of a child's death also disrupts the social functioning of bereaved parents in both the broader community and in relationships with family and friends (Vegsund et al., 2019). They often report feeling out of place or misunderstood by others. Even our language excludes them as there is no term for a parent whose child has died like there is for other losses (i.e. orphan, widow, widower) (Holloway, 2009). Bereaved parents often report having to deal with the awkwardness of others who are ill equipped to converse about their deceased child or their grief experience. For example, the common and innocent question of "How many children do you have?" can lead to discomfort for all parties. As one bereaved mother explained,

> I told her I have three kids. Then she asked their ages and so I told her that one of them died. While *I'm* trying to hold it together, *she* starts crying and stammering. You can tell she is totally freaked out. Then I'm in the position of trying to comfort *her*! What am I supposed to say? That it's okay? It's not okay! I could just say I have two kids but then I feel like garbage for denying the existence of my son.

Similarly, it can be difficult for parents to watch their child's peers grow up and reach milestones their deceased child will never experience. These factors cause many parents to experience isolation and despair (Morris et al., 2019).

The traumatic grief experienced by the death of a child can significantly impact marital relationships. While some grieving couples may become closer after their loss, for many, the stress experienced from the loss can be overwhelming and, if ignored or neglected, lead to further problems in the marriage (Salakari et al., 2014). Types of issues that typically arise between spouses include: depletion of energy to care for each other, differing styles of grieving, difficulty in attending to the daily needs of the household, feelings of abandonment by each partner, lack of communication in an effort to protect each other from painful memories and feelings, and avoidant or guilt-producing actions on the part of either partner. Misunderstandings often arise from these dynamics and drain the marital relationship of energy to cope with the loss.

Perinatal Loss

Perinatal loss refers to the loss experienced when a child dies due to miscarriage, stillbirth, or in the early weeks of life. Attachment to a child begins to develop the moment conception is verified, thus the grief experienced by parents of a perinatal loss is no less painful. The bereavement for these parents is unique in many ways, and they often do not receive acknowledgment or recognition of their loss by both society and their informal social support system.

With perinatal loss, the grief reactions of parents are largely influenced by the parents' perception of their unborn baby. Therefore, there may be a variety of responses to this kind of loss. For some, even though the loss occurs early in pregnancy it may be experienced as a devastating event (Krosch & Shakespeare-Finch, 2017). In addition to complex grief reactions, depression, and anxiety, perinatal loss is often accompanied with traumatic elements (e.g. exposure to traumatic images, enduring physical pain, and invasive medical procedures) and a significant number of parents will develop PTSD (Diamond & Diamond, 2014; Krosch & Shakespeare-Finch, 2017).

Parents grieving a perinatal death often experience significant challenges to their assumptive worldviews. The loss forces them to confront their beliefs about safety, fairness, and control and may also shake their beliefs in themselves (Black et al., 2015). Women may blame themselves or feel betrayed by their bodies (Leon, 2017). For women who faced fertility challenges or lesbian mothers who surmounted numerous social and practical obstacles to becoming pregnant, the enormity of their grief merits special consideration (Black et al., 2015). Studies indicate a correlation between the strength and prevalence of disturbances to core beliefs and trauma symptoms (Krosch & Shakespeare-Finch, 2017; Lindstrom et al., 2013; Triplett et al., 2012).

Support from family and friends for parents bereaved by perinatal loss may be weak or absent. In part, this is because perinatal deaths are typically witnessed and experienced only by the parents and healthcare providers. In addition, because family members and friends have no experience with the child, either before or after the death, they may view it as a medical event rather than the life-changing loss parents experience it to be (Leon, 2017). Thus, providing recognition of the loss can be very healing for bereaved parents.

Secondary losses that may accompany perinatal loss include the parents' plans for the future and their societal status as parents. Mothers, in particular, having lost the socially revered status of "expecting mother," often find it difficult to navigate their place in society. Because she does not have a baby, others do not identify her as a mother even though she feels that she is a mother. Being caught between "two incomplete rites of passage" (Markin & Zilcha-Mano, 2018, p. 22) leaves her feeling marginalized and misunderstood.

For these reasons, participating in rituals that recognize the loss can promote healing. In addition, many parents benefit from spending time with the body of their deceased baby before it is taken away. This, along with the opportunity to participate in memory-making activities, has become standard practice in many hospitals for parents who choose to participate (Steen, 2019).

Interventions for Bereaved Parents

Helpful interventions for bereaved parents include those outlined in Chapter 4 and can be done in individual, couple, and family counseling settings. There is great value in helping families understand and support the unique grief experience of every family member (Albuquerque et al., 2018). Counseling can also be used to address any distorted cognitions and guilt feelings parents have regarding their role in the child's death as well as validating and encouraging constructive expressions of anger.

Many bereaved parents are instinctively drawn to establishing continuing bonds with their deceased child. They may preserve objects that belonged to their child (Kim et al., 2019), wear jewelry symbolic of their child, or participate in activities in memory of their child. These externalized continuing bonds have been shown to be tremendously helpful to grieving parents (Albuquerque et al., 2018).

In addition, social support has been shown to be very helpful. The presence of positive support networks plays a substantial role in the course of grief for bereaved parents. This may take the form of family and friends or support groups with other parents who have lost a child. Such groups can provide great value in allowing parents the opportunity to talk freely about their deceased child without experiencing judgment or discomfort from others. This kind of support increases resilience and mitigates post-traumatic stress (Aho et al., 2018; Vegsund et al., 2019).

BOX 7.2 THE DEATH OF A CHILD IN THE KOREAN CULTURE

In the Korean culture, the parents of a deceased child are met with great scorn. Mothers, especially, are traditionally regarded as "sinners" for letting their child die. A child's death is a taboo topic in Korea, and bereaved parents are frequently rebuked and questioned about their capacity to care for a child. Consequently, bereaved Korean mothers often suffer from intense feelings of guilt and shame. Furthermore, Korean culture holds that children should not be grieved, a sentiment echoed in the Korean maxim, "Parents are buried in the ground, and children are buried in the heart." Thus, Korean parents who have lost a child are discouraged from expressing their grief which leads to feelings of isolation (Kim et al., 2019).

GRIEF AMONG REFUGEES AND FORCIBLY DISPLACED PERSONS

The number of people who have been forcibly displaced from their home countries is at an all-time high, reaching 79.5 million at the end of 2019 with a disproportionately high number of these being under the age of 18 (United Nations High Commissioner for Refugees, 2020). This escalation has highlighted our need for understanding the experiences of refugees and how to effectively serve them. Having faced persecution in their countries due to race, ethnicity, religious beliefs, nationality, political beliefs, or association with a particular social group, the stressors faced by this population are numerous and extreme. They include the death and disappearance of loved ones, separation from family, and exposure to violence, torture, and life-threatening injuries (Lacour et al., 2020). Along with the adverse conditions that prompt migration, they often face precarious living situations in their host country including uncertainty about the future and the difficult task of adjusting to a new culture (Kokou-Kpolou et al., 2020).

While the research on this population is continuously emerging, several studies have documented a high prevalence of traumatic grief among refugee and forcibly displaced populations that far exceeds that found in the general population (Killikelly et al., 2018). These conditions frequently coexist with anxiety, depression, and PTSD and may impede their ability to function in the environment (Bryant et al., 2020). Interviews with bereaved persons who have been forcibly displaced often reveal extensive somatic distress, and it is believed that this may be a cultural expression of their bereavement. This may also suggest that somatic grief reactions need to be given more consideration in how complex grief is conceptualized (Kokou-Kpolou et al., 2020). It is important, therefore, that assessment of this population includes asking about significant losses to avoid misdiagnoses and accurate identification of their needs (Steil et al., 2019).

Several factors contribute to the severity and complexity of the grief experience for forcibly displaced persons. Many are grieving losses that occurred by violent means, such as murder and torture, and some have witnessed their loved ones being killed (Bryant et al., 2020; Lacour et al., 2020). In addition to loss by death, the life of a migrant contains an accumulation of losses, including the loss of their country of origin, cultural belonging, financial stability, and housing (Killikelly et al., 2018). They have lost a sense of place and belonging in the world. This can be particularly impactful for children who face changing familial roles or are without any family.

In addition to the circumstances that force families to leave their homes, the conditions they face post-migration often complicate the mourning process. Many lack dependable social support systems and struggle to meet their basic needs of safety, secure housing, and employment (Killikelly et al., 2018). For some, these challenges can exacerbate their traumatic grief reactions and interfere with their ability to adjust to their current circumstances. For others, the energy needed to heal from their losses is instead directed toward adapting to the new environment (Bryant et al., 2020). An added complication for bereaved forced immigrants is that their circumstances often prevent them from performing culturally relevant death and mourning rituals. There are also reports that the bereaved experience distress about the spiritual well-being of their loved ones and worry if they had successfully transitioned to the afterlife (Kokou-Kpolou et al., 2020).

While there is an increased understanding of the needs of forcibly displaced persons, there are significant barriers to serving them. In addition to a lack of information about available services, many are reluctant to avail themselves of mental healthcare due to negative views of such services and fears of being considered mentally disordered. Concern about facing stigma from their community is also a powerful deterrent to accessing mental healthcare (Bryant et al., 2020). For these reasons, culturally sanctioned approaches may be favored, such as using a traditional healer, spiritual leader, or elder (Bartolomei et al., 2016). These barriers are further compounded by the large numbers of refugees and forced immigrants in need of mental health services as compared with the numbers of professionals available to provide services (Silove et al., 2017).

Numerous types of interventions have been used with this population including Cognitive Behavioral Therapy (CBT), EMDR, interpersonal therapy, psychoeducation, and art therapy. More research is needed to determine the efficacy of these interventions (Nocon et al., 2017). Some experts recommend giving more attention to identifying individual adaptive factors and structuring interventions to be both resilient and trauma based (Lacour et al, 2020). In addition, Silove et al. (2017) suggest that social programs for forced immigrants could be very helpful by providing a sense of belonging and connection, strengthening social networks, and encouraging self-supportive endeavors (Silove et al., 2017).

GRIEF AMONG VETERANS AND THEIR FAMILIES

The mental health needs of military service members and their families have received renewed attention in light of the thousands of soldiers deployed in in the Global War on Terrorism after 9/11. Only recently, however, has research emerged around the role that grief plays in the lives of those involved in war. In addition to high rates of anxiety, depression, and PTSD, military service members are at elevated risk of experiencing traumatic grief (Charney et al., 2018) as the death of a fellow service member during deployment is a common event and frequently occurs by violent means (Jacoby et al., 2019). As compared with other populations, the death of a combat buddy is correlated with a greater occurrence of complex grief, more severe PTSD, impairments in daily living, survivor's guilt, and lifetime suicide attempts (Simon et al., 2018). The impact of grief on military personnel is especially concerning in light of what is known about PTSD in this population: that treatment for PTSD is less effective for combat-related trauma versus interventions for PTSD among civilians. In addition, traumatic loss interferes with the ability to recover from PTSD even when using evidence-based interventions (Jacoby et al., 2019).

There are several aspects of the grief experience that are unique to military personnel. First, due to their shared experiences and interdependent relationships with each other, service members experience the death of a fellow soldier as a devastating loss. The death of a comrade is comparable to that of a close family member and soldiers often cite it as their most distressing war experience (Litz et al., 2018; Simon et al., 2018). Some bereaved soldiers also experience intense feelings of guilt for a comrade's death and irrationally conclude that they could have somehow prevented it (Yarvis et al., 2017). In addition, they may also view their service negatively and feel they are not worthy of recovering and enjoying their life since their fellow soldiers did not make it home alive (Jacoby et al., 2019; Lubens & Silver, 2019). Second, while grieving their comrades, service members are simultaneously making the difficult transition from active duty to civilian life which can strain their capacity to cope with their losses. Finally, further compounding these challenges is the fact that service members are often reluctant to seek help for mental health issues. The military culture is inculcated with the belief that doing so represents weakness and will destroy their careers (Weiss et al., 2017). Among those that do avail themselves of support, many find themselves working with providers who are unfamiliar with the unique aspects of military-related bereavement (Dooley et al., 2019).

Bereaved Military Families

Many service members who die during war leave behind grieving parents as well as spouses and young children. Bereaved military widows have been shown to experience a two to fivefold increase in depression, PTSD, and adjustment disorders after their spouse's death in addition to an increased use of mental health services (Cozza et al., 2020). Several factors contribute to the complexity of the grief these widows experience. These include the sudden and violent nature of the death, the young age of the spouse and children, and their limited access to consistent support systems due to frequent moves. Additionally, these families were typically already under tremendous strain from long and frequent separations from their loved ones during their deployments as service members (Cozza et al., 2017). Upon the soldier's death, these young families subsequently face numerous secondary losses such as having to move off base, change schools, and transition to a non-military identity and lifestyle. It can be more difficult for them to remain connected to military support systems, especially if they live far away from the military base (Cozza et al., 2017).

There are, however, protective factors unique to military families that can attenuate the difficulty of their grief experiences. These include the tangible resources and social support provided by military communities including assistance provided by military support services, and military survivor death benefits (Cozza et al., 2020). Peer support groups with others who have grieved a military loss have also been shown to be beneficial (Dooley et al., 2019). In addition, the pride associated with their loved one's death and high regard by the community for their beloved's sacrifice can be an important protective factor (Cozza et al., 2020).

Grieving Veterans who Die by Suicide

Unfortunately, military service families bereaved by suicide face greater challenges. This has become a significant concern in light of the marked rise in suicide rates in all branches of the military (Department of Defense, 2014; Harrington-LaMorie et al., 2018). Though substantial work has been done to curb the phenomenon, suicide is a leading cause of death among service members (Department of Defense, 2014). In addition to the traumatic nature of the loss, often with a family member discovering the body, several factors put these bereaved family members at risk of developing traumatic grief. In contrast with the honor given to "heroes" who gave their lives in service to their country, military deaths by suicide are often viewed as "dishonorable deaths" that bring shame to the deceased, their loved ones, and the military profession (Harrington-LaMorie et al., 2018). Service members who die by suicide are often not recognized with the same ceremony and reverence given to deaths that were more clearly associated with the line of duty. In these cases, the customary Line of Duty Investigations, which examine the circumstances surrounding the death and ultimately determine if the family will receive benefits, are often lengthy and painful processes that can exacerbate feelings of guilt and humiliation. The result is that family members often experience increased shame, isolation, and real or perceived limitations in the support that is available to them (Harrington-LaMorie et al., 2018).

Service members who die by suicide are also grieved by their fellow soldiers. A 2017 survey of Iraq and Afghanistan veterans revealed that 58% of veterans know a service member who died by suicide and 65% know one who has attempted suicide (Iraq and Afghanistan Veterans of America, 2017). Because these deaths are unexpected as compared to combat-related deaths, they can be harder to accept. Additionally, there is often guilt over failure to prevent the suicide (Lubens & Silver, 2019). Mourners who are grieving a death by suicide tend to have higher rates of suicidal ideation. More research is needed to determine if the suicides of comrades account for the high suicide rates among veterans (Lubens & Silver, 2019).

GRIEF AND AMBIGUOUS LOSS

Ambiguous loss is a category of loss first identified by Pauline Boss in 1999. The term is used to refer to situations where the finality of the death is uncertain. The person is physically absent but there is insufficient evidence to ascertain whether or not they are alive, such as with missing persons, man-made or natural disasters in which the body is never recovered, and military personnel who are considered missing in action.

Ambiguous loss creates traumatic and enduring grief that is difficult, if not impossible, to accept. Such losses are particularly complex because the survivors are unable to separate and begin the detachment process. They feel they must "hang on" and remain hopeful even after months and sometimes years of waiting for evidence that their loved one is either dead or alive. The continuous condition of "not knowing" indefinitely suspends the grieving process, obstructs the development of coping skills, and leaves survivors in a state of helplessness. These long and unending conditions that defy resolution make ambiguous loss one of the most complex types of loss (Boss & Ishii, 2015). Boss stresses that the struggles mourners experience in the face of ambiguous loss lie with the complexity of the type of loss being experienced, rather than with mourners themselves (Boss, 2016).

For unambiguous losses, society has constructed rituals that provide mourners with resources and social support that recognize the loss and facilitates the mourning of the deceased loved one. There is, however, no social recognition or protocol for how mourners of ambiguous losses should be treated by their community or proceed with living. Instead, they are often criticized for not finding "closure" and failing to move on with their lives. Additionally, ambiguous losses are accompanied by confusion about family roles, who is a member of the family and who is not. This "boundary ambiguity" causes significant stress for mourners as family members come to different explanations about the loss (Boss & Ishii, 2015; Boss, 2016).

Traditional grief interventions are often inadequate and off-putting for those bereaved by ambiguous loss. Because full resolution of the loss may never be possible, Boss suggests that the goal for intervention is to build the mourners' resiliencies and strengthen their capacities to live well despite the ambiguity (Boss, 2016). This includes supporting mourners to develop dialectical, or both-and, thinking that accepts both the absence and presence of the loved one and reminding them that "No one they love is fully present all the time; nor are they fully absent even after disappearance or death"

(Boss & Ishii, 2015, p. 285). An example of this dialectical thinking would be, "Our mother is always with us and she is also gone." In addition, practitioners can assist family members by clearly defining the loss as an ambiguous one and validating their feelings of anger, anxiety, distrust, confusion, depression, trauma, and other somatic symptoms as being directly related to the uncertainty about the loss. Having a name for their distress and recognizing that the ambiguity lies in circumstances beyond their control can bring some relief.

With ambiguous loss, each family member will need to construct their own way of coping and making meaning of the loss. Practitioners play an important role in helping family members communicate openly and respectfully about their divergent perceptions of the loss and their feelings related to the uncertainty. In helping families build resilience for living with the long-term tension and anxiety of ambiguity, they can be assisted to create new ways to make decisions, carry out their daily lives, support each other, and mourn what they have lost (Boss & Ishii, 2015).

PET LOSS

In the United States, about 57% of households own a companion animal (American Veterinary Medical Association, 2017–2018). Across the globe, pets, especially dogs and cats, have become integral members of the family unit and are regarded by many as surrogate children. Owners spend millions of dollars each year on pet food, supplies, medical care, and specialized services for their pets.

Pets provide numerous physical and mental health benefits to their owners, and many people form significant emotional attachment bonds with their pets. Built on daily and routine interactions, these relationships supply consistent feelings of security and non-judgmental positive affirmation. Thus, for relationships in which there was a strong attachment to the animal, a pet's death is experienced as a major disruption that causes significant distress and is grieved similarly to a human death (Messam & Hart, 2019; Spain et al., 2019; Testoni et al., 2017). Pets are often considered an important member of the family that have been with them through multiple transitions and developmental milestones. For some, animals make up for a lack of other social relationships as is true for pets that are the sole companion of single or elderly persons who live alone. In circumstances in which the pet is trained as a service animal for a person with disabilities, the pet and owner depend on each other to meet their respective daily needs and the reciprocity in the relationship creates an especially strong attachment (Messam & Hart, 2019). Consequently, the grief experienced by pet owners can be an immensely painful experience that should be regarded as a valid and legitimate response to the loss.

Though it is changing, social recognition of this loss is often in short supply, and mourners may feel surprised and embarrassed by their intense grief reactions. Dismissive comments from family and friends (e.g. "It was only a dog") make it difficult for bereaved pet owners to give themselves permission to mourn and seek support for the loss. This inability to grieve the death of their pet has been correlated with increased levels of stress, depressed mood, and severe grief. It can be extremely challenging to cope with the grief and trauma-related symptoms that come with this kind of loss (Adrian & Stitt, 2017).

Many owners will react with feelings of guilt upon the pet's death and feel that they are responsible. Some owners blame themselves for previous decisions made regarding the animal's medical care and failure to detect terminal conditions in their animals. Decisions to euthanize pets are frequently preceded by weeks of agonizing over the alternative options (Messam & Hart, 2019; Wong et al., 2017). The death of a pet can dramatically alter owners' daily routines and upset their emotional stability. Mourners' reactions vary from wanting to replace the pet immediately to desiring to wait for a period of time, to never wishing to own pets again because of the pain involved in losing them. All of these reactions are a component of the expected grief experience.

The death of a pet, while in and of itself it may be devastating, can also provoke feelings from previous losses. For example, a 40-year-old female client contacted a grief counselor due to the death of her 15-year-old toy poodle. While discussing the loss with the counselor, the client also disclosed that her husband died two years prior. Her husband had given her the dog on their first wedding anniversary. Thus, the dog's death held a deeper meaning that enveloped the loss of her husband, the loss of her marriage, and the loss of their happiness together. Therefore, practitioners need to be sensitive to the symbolic representation of other losses connected with the death of a pet (Messam & Hart, 2019). The results of a study by Adrian and Stitt (2017) suggest that the responses to pet loss may be an extension of grief from previous losses and can influence how mourners manage these losses. In addition, their findings suggest that the death of a pet can be a possible trigger for mourners who have symptoms of PTSD.

Practitioners should be mindful that cultural context and spiritual beliefs will influence an owner's approach to pet loss. Some cultures believe that animals undergo the same post-life transitions as humans and this in turn shapes their approach to the illness and death of a beloved animal (Testoni et al., 2017). In Japan, for example, euthanasia is considered to be a reprehensible act with most families providing palliative care for their pet in their home. In addition, a pet's death is marked with religious ceremonies, rituals around interring the animal's body, and memorializing the animal as are performed for humans (Spain et al., 2019).

Practitioners can help bereaved pet owners by acknowledging and validating the intensity of their loss. For owners who are struggling with the decision to euthanize their animal, compassionately delivered information about the animal's health can be very beneficial. In addition, veterinarians can provide helpful tools, such as the 5H 2M Scale, that trains owners to assess the pet's quality of life and take actions that bring comfort to the animal. Because grief over pet loss is less socially acceptable, mourners may need encouragement to engage in self-care activities, perform actions that memorialize their pet, and participate in counseling and support groups specifically geared toward this kind of grief (Messam & Hart, 2019). Veterinarians and the Humane Society are useful resources for counseling referrals, online memorial platforms, and books that provide comfort and information about pet loss.

CASES

CASE 7.1

Identifying Information:

Client Name: Angela Aguilar and her son Roberto
Age: 51 years old and 18 years old
Race/Ethnicity: Cuban American
Marital Status: Angela is married to Jose, age 58, diagnosed with Alzheimer's disease, early onset
Education Level: Bachelor's degree
Occupation: Librarian

Intake Information:

Angela Aguilar called the Family Guidance Center regarding her 18-year-old son, Roberto, who has been struggling with the changes he is seeing in his father who was diagnosed with Alzheimer's disease five years ago. Because Angela is the primary caregiver for Jose and he cannot be left alone, you have arranged to meet with them at their home.

Initial Interview:

Angela greets you at the door and welcomes you in. Roberto comes in from the other room. They both shake your hand but Roberto appears to be feeling somewhat shy and awkward in the situation. They invite you to sit with them in the living room.

"You've come at a good time," Angela says. "Jose is asleep right now so we should be able to talk easily." She offers you something to drink which you accept out of respect and politeness. You engage them in discussions about the family photos on the wall and use this time to build rapport. Angela looks eager to begin the conversation about their situation.

"Thank you for welcoming me into your home. Can you tell me more about how things are going for you all?"

"Terrible," Roberto mumbles.

"In what ways is it terrible?" you ask. Angela sighs deeply. Roberto squirms in his chair.

"Well, I wouldn't say terrible," Angela responds.

"How else would you describe it?" Roberto retorts. "It's always the same thing day in and day out. Dad is always asking you for something that he's forgotten and following you around the house. He paces back and forth and asks you the same thing five hundred times. He's not my dad anymore; he's like a little kid and it gets to me after a while," Roberto practically shouts.

"Mijo, keep your voice down! You'll wake him up!" Angela says in a loud whisper. "Your dad is doing the best he can and all of this strange behavior is part of the disease and you're just going to have to understand that, Roberto." Angela pushes her hair off her forehead and sighs loudly. You sense that she is feeling very tired and stressed.

"I DO know that," Roberto replies, "but it doesn't help. It's so irritating to always come home to this dad that I barely know anymore. It's like someone else has taken over his body. After he has asked me the same question five times, I feel like turning around and just walking out the door. I don't know how to communicate with him anymore. I hate it."

"What was your dad like before Alzheimer's disease entered the picture?" you ask.

"He would always ask me how my day was and if I had homework. Sometimes, he'd help me because, you know, before he got really bad, he was an education professor at Sunnybrook college. He knew everything about all kinds of subjects. Before he got his PhD, he taught high school Spanish and history. Dad would grade papers while I'd do my homework and then he'd check it for me. I used to have so much respect for my father, you wouldn't believe it. Besides that, he coached my baseball team the whole time I was in elementary and middle school. We'd always go out after the games and all my friends loved my dad. He knew them all and their families."

Roberto stops suddenly and you notice that he has gotten tearful. He looks shaken and maybe embarrassed by all he has just told you.

"So this has been a huge change for you," you say.

Roberto nods and continues, "All I can do now is try to keep my friends away from him so he won't feel embarrassed. My dad can't remember who they are anymore. How would that make you feel?"

"I think that must be a very difficult situation to live with," you suggest.

"Like I said, it's terrible," Roberto replies. Abruptly, he sits up straight and wipes his tears from his face. "I'm sorry. I don't mean to complain. It's just really hard."

"No need to apologize," you say. "It's expected that you would have lots of feelings around this. Do you talk about how you feel often?"

Angela chimes in, "No, he doesn't. That's why I called you. You need to talk about this, Roberto."

"I'm glad you are talking about it now. I'd like to hear more," you encourage.

With a deep sigh, Roberto begins again, "I just can't figure out what to do anymore. I know my mom wants me to be happy and continue on with my life, but it's like someone pushed the 'pause' button on our family and no one can make plans even for next week much less next year."

"What kind of things have you been putting on hold?" you inquire.

Angela looks at Roberto who remains silent and then at you. "Well, Roberto will graduate from high school at the end of this semester and we are trying to decide where he will go from there. He wants to go to college, but he's feeling like he should stay here and help me out with his father. I tell him that's not his job, but I think he feels guilty thinking about going away to school. Education is very important to our family, and I know his father would want him to go to college."

Roberto glances at his mother. "But Mom, you can't take care of Dad by yourself. Already you're trying to work, take care of the house, and bills, and me and Dad, and it's about to kill you. I see it in your face. You're tired all the time."

Roberto looks at you and says, "She never sleeps. She drinks coffee all day long. She's lost a lot of weight and she never gives herself a break. I'm worried about what will happen if *she* gets sick."

Angela looks at you with tears in her eyes. "Roberto is right. I have a lot on my plate right now. I'm constantly on the go. I feel like I can't sit down for a minute or I'll collapse. I have to make all the decisions now for me and Roberto and my husband. I'm afraid I'll let them all down. Jose has given us so much over the past 20 years, and I feel I need to be there for him whenever he needs me which is all the time these days. He can't tie his shoes or figure out how to get dressed. I have to be there to help him with everyday things that we all take for granted. My relief is when Roberto comes home from school and I go to work at the library. It's hard on all of us."

"I'm really struck by all the massive changes you are both describing. Everything is different for you now, and it's hard to predict how things will be in the future," you comment.

"It's hard to think about this disease getting any worse," Angela continues, "but the doctors tell us it will. It's hard to prepare for how things will work when Jose can no longer take care of himself at all. I think that's why Roberto is so fearful about leaving home for college, because we don't know how it will be for Jose in a year."

"Besides all the changes you are trying to adjust to, you've also experienced many losses since Jose got sick. In many ways, you've lost the man you once knew as your husband and father," you suggest. They both nod silently looking at the floor. "There are several ways I may be able to be helpful. There are a lot of emotions to process through, and my sense is you probably both need some space to talk about what you're experiencing." Angela and Roberto both nod in agreement. "And there are also some practical matters to sort through, such as how to care for Jose and make plans for the future. Does that sound like it would be helpful?"

"Yes," Angela says.

Roberto agrees and says, "I feel a little better just having the chance to get all that off my chest."

In the remainder of the session, you learn more about the intensity of Jose's needs, the demands of Angela's work, and how school is going for Roberto. You schedule an individual session with Roberto and one with Angela and then another family session following that.

7.1-1. What are the losses this family is experiencing?
7.1-2. What are this family's strengths?
7.2-3. What are possible goals for the second session with Angela? With Roberto? What are possible goals for the next family session?
7.1-4. Identify three local resources that could be helpful to this family.
7.1-5. Find a website that provides information for families caring for an Alzheimer's family member. What suggestions are offered that would be useful for Angela and Roberto?
7.1-6. What value conflicts is this family confronting? How could you help them navigate this being careful to not impose your own values?

CASE 7.2

Identifying Information:

Client Name: Julia Turner
Age: 35 years old
Race/Ethnicity: White
Marital Status: Single
Educational Level: Bachelor's degree
Occupation: Teacher

Intake Information:

Ms. Turner requested a counseling appointment related to the recent death of her Labrador retriever. She tells the intake worker that she would like the soonest appointment that is available because she has been feeling extremely depressed and anxious.

Initial Interview:

You go to the waiting room with the intake information to meet your new client, Julia Turner. An attractive woman with long blonde hair pulled back in a ponytail and sunglasses is sitting in a chair near the door. You notice that she has a white cane next to her chair. You approach her, ask her name, and introduce yourself. You suddenly realize why this woman is so upset about losing her dog. Julia follows you back to your office with your assistance.

"Julia, this is my office and there is a chair on your right next to my desk. Can I get you some water?" you ask.

Julia settles down in the chair and accepts a cup of water. "Thank you, it's hot out there today."

"Yes, I think the weather report said that it's going up into the 90s this afternoon," you reply. After a short pause, you resume the conversation. "Julia, I understand from the intake worker that you lost your dog recently. Was this dog your companion dog?" you inquire.

"Yes, she was my graduation present from college. My parents helped me get her and I've had her since I was 24 years old. Her name was Joy. She was my closest friend and guide through all these years. I don't know what I'm going to do without her."

"This must be tremendously sad for you. How old was Joy when she died?" you ask.

"She was almost 14 years old," Julia tells you. "She was my eyes and sometimes ears – my very best friend. I feel like I've taken a giant step backwards ever since she passed away." Tears are streaming down Julia's face.

"That's such a big loss," you say in validation. After a pause you add, "I have some tissues here if you'd like." Julia nods and you place the box of tissues in her hand. She takes some tissues and begins blowing her nose.

"You and Joy must have been very close," you respond. "How are you coping without her?"

"Not too well, actually," Julia replies. "Just normal living has been harder. I've had a guide dog for so long, I've had to re-learn how to get around without one," Julia explains. "You see, I'm a teacher at the School for the Visually Impaired and I have my own apartment near the school. For years, I have walked the mile or so to school every day and taught Braille and reading and spelling to visually impaired children. I love my job and Joy went to work with me every day. The children adored her, and she was an inspiration to all of them. I would tell them that someday they could have a dog, too. She gave me the confidence I needed to live independently from my parents and go about life like everyone else. I've made a lot of friends because of Joy. Now, I don't even want to get out of bed in the morning. I've been having a hard time sleeping at night and don't really care if I eat or not. Everything reminds me that Joy is no longer there. Sometimes, I find myself putting out my hand to grab the handle on her halter and it's not there. And then, I feel immobilized. I don't want to go anywhere or do anything. Even getting to school is going to be a nightmare and I'm dreading going back. I've lost my confidence along with my dog." Julia begins sobbing at this point in her story.

"I can see why this has rattled you so much, Julia. Joy was such an integral part of your life, wasn't she?" you inquire.

"Yes, she really was my guardian angel. She saved me on more than one occasion from stepping into traffic or tripping over an obstacle in my way. You can't imagine how much I had to trust her every move. I think I trusted Joy more than I've trusted most people. She was just the greatest dog in the world and she and I communicated in a way that most people will never experience. I just don't know what I'm going to do without her." Julia begins crying again, though her tears seem to be a little less intense.

"I can see why this has been so difficult for you. Do you have friends or family nearby that can help you out right now?" you tentatively ask.

"I have a good friend, Amy, who comes over every day. She said she'd walk to school with me when I go back. Amy is sighted and has always been there for me. She's known me forever, even before I lost my eyesight," Julia responds. "But I'm scared I'm just wearing her out. I'm afraid she'll just get sick of helping me and then I'll lose a human friend, too."

"So, you haven't always been blind," you carefully inquire.

"Oh no, I had a degenerative eye disease and didn't completely lose my sight until I was about 10 years old. Before that I had to wear these thick glasses, but I could still see. I remember what blue or yellow looks like and there's a lot of things I can remember before losing my sight," Julia tells you.

"Do you have brothers or sisters?" you question.

"I have one sister who is ten years older than me," Julia states. "She lives out of state and I hardly ever see her. She's got kids and doesn't visit often. I've gone out there to visit once or twice. We get along just fine when we see each other but, because of the age difference, we've never been that close."

"What about your parents? Are they still living?" you inquire.

"Oh yes, my parents live about 40 miles away. They have always been very supportive. They are getting older though, and are having some health problems.

I don't want to be a burden to them. They have been so proud of how independent I've become. I hate to disappoint them. My mom calls every day and is worried. She says I need to get another dog as soon as possible. She doesn't understand that I can't just snap my fingers and get another guide dog. It takes a while. It might be several months before a dog is available for me and then we have to spend a lot of time training together. And I don't know if I even want another dog, if I can't have Joy."

"Okay, so there's your mom and dad and Amy. Do you have friends at school, co-workers?" you ask.

"Oh yes, I've got several friends at school both sighted and visually impaired," Julia replies. "I just don't want to bother them with trivial things."

"Julia, I'm not sure that your friends would think that the loss of Joy would be trivial. I bet they understand how important your dog was to you. Don't you think?" you ask.

"Yeah, I guess. I've just been so down and out, I haven't felt much like calling or going out with them. I guess I just don't trust myself that I'll be okay and won't just burst into tears. I seem to be crying a lot lately."

"I can understand not wanting to lose control in front of people, though crying is a very appropriate response to what you're experiencing. It helps our bodies process the stress we're experiencing. Maybe your friends would understand your need to cry and be sad?" you suggest.

"Yeah, maybe. I think I just see myself as kind of a miserable person to be around these days. I'm usually so happy and upbeat and positive that this has really shook me to the core." Julia is beginning to look calmer and less uncomfortable as the discussion progresses.

"It sounds like you're being pretty hard on yourself, Julia. I think anyone in your situation would feel really undone by this. One thing to keep in mind is that you won't feel this way forever. I know it's kind of hard to believe. The grief process can take some time, but it won't always feel as intense as it does now," you say.

"Well, that's good to hear you say that. I just can't imagine a future without Joy."

"Yes, I hear that. And I also know, just in the short time I've gotten to know you, that you are someone who adjusts and adapts, even in the face of huge obstacles. Your current life and career are evidence of that. I'm not saying it will be easy or fun, but it seems to me you have what it takes to manage this challenge as you have managed other challenges in your life," you explain.

Julia considers what you've said. "Well, I can't argue with you there. I'm no stranger to struggle." You allow some time to let this sink in. Then she adds, "As hard as it might be to get used to a new service dog, I think I'll feel better once I have one. And, like I said, it will take a while before that can happen. Maybe by the time a dog becomes available, I'll be ready."

"That makes sense to me," you say. "In the meantime, maybe it's okay to depend on friends and family to help you get through this difficult period," you suggest. You allow Julia to talk more about why this loss feels hard and the struggles she has with daily living which seem to be as much about her grief reactions as they are about not having the extra guidance that Joy provided. You offer some guidance to help her feel less overwhelmed with it all.

"Maybe I could come back and talk to you again? I think just talking about it is helping me feel less hopeless," Julia responds.

"I think that's a great idea," you respond. "I would enjoy the opportunity to work with you more."

7.2-1. What are Julia's strengths?
7.2-2. What are your concerns for Julia?
7.2-3. What additional information would you like to obtain to help your work with Julia?
7.2-4. What kind of guidance would you provide Julia to reduce her feelings of overwhelm?
7.2-5. What additional interventions could be helpful to Julia?
7.2-6. Write three questions you could ask of Julia to help you better understand her experience as someone who is differently abled.
7.2-7. Write a summary of your second session with Julia.

CASE 7.3

Identifying Information:

Client Name: Moki Simmons
Age: 23 years old
Race/Ethnicity: Native American, Cocopah tribe
Marital Status: Married
Educational Level: High school graduate
Occupation: Customer service representative for a cell phone company

Intake Information:

Moki called the Grief Counseling Center and asked if there was counseling available for parents who had lost a newborn. She reported that about four weeks ago her baby daughter died just a few hours after being born. After arranging an appointment for her, she asked if it would be okay if her husband came with her. You told her that would be fine and she said, "I don't know if he will come or not, but I'll ask him."

Initial Interview:

You find Moki in the waiting room and introduce yourself. She gives you a slight smile and shakes your hand. After you are both seated in your office, you say, "Tell me a little about why you are here and what kind of help you are seeking."

"I had a baby about a month ago," Moki begins. "But she didn't make it."

"What was her name?" you inquire.

"Anna," Moki answers.

"What happened to Anna?" you ask gently.

"She had a heart defect. The doctors told us that she probably wouldn't live for very long and that there was nothing they could do." Moki pauses a moment and you wait for her to continue. "So, my husband and I just held her and talked to her.... She died in my arms."

"That sounds very difficult, Moki," you empathize. "How have you been dealing with Anna's death?"

Moki's eyes are wet with tears. "I have been so sad. I wake up in the morning and just lie in bed and cry. And I feel so tired all the time. Some days I don't even get out of my pajamas."

"This is not how you thought you would be spending this time is it?" you prompt.

"No, not at all. We came home to her nursery and her crib...." Moki is openly crying now. "But we didn't have a baby!"

You allow Moki to spend a few moments crying and then say, "What a disappointment for you! So many hopes and expectations that weren't able to be fulfilled."

"Yes. I had really been looking forward to being a mom. I feel like I've been cheated! I worked so hard during my pregnancy to make sure I did everything right," Moki says tearfully. "But it didn't matter!"

You validate Moki's sentiment saying, "It doesn't feel fair that you don't get to reap the rewards of all your hard work."

Moki nods. "No, it's not fair. We hardly got to have any time with her! Sometimes my arms ache because they are not holding my baby!"

"Yes," you say. "That is actually a common complaint from new mothers who have lost an infant."

"Really?" Moki responds with surprise. "It just doesn't seem right that this happened. I just don't understand what went wrong. I keep worrying that I did something. Maybe I ate something that I wasn't supposed to eat."

"Have you asked the doctors about that?" you inquire.

"Yes, I did," Moki answers. "They said nothing I did caused her death. But I can't stop wondering about it."

"Sometimes when something very random and tragic happens we try to find a way that it could have been prevented. The idea that we could have had some control feels less scary than the thought that something catastrophic can hit at any time. You are going through a lot right now so I hope that you can be gentle with yourself. It may help to keep reminding yourself of the medical evidence that the doctors presented to you. Some people will even schedule another visit with the doctor to review what happened from a medical standpoint. It can be hard to fully digest all of the information at such an emotional moment. Talking about your feelings as you are doing now also helps. Do you have supportive friends and family that you can talk to?"

"Not really. We just moved here about a year ago from Arizona for my husband's job," Moki explains. "My parents and my brothers and sisters are all in Arizona. Ever since I moved away our relationship has been tense, especially with my parents. They are really traditional, and it was hard for them that I moved so far away from the family. They were very nice when I first told them what happened but now they just seem kind of angry with me. Sometimes I think they blame me for what happened."

"What leads you to think that?" you ask.

"Well, just a couple of comments they have made here and there," Moki answers. "You see, in my culture, it is customary to use a midwife for giving birth. People are kind of suspicious about high tech medical practices – and that's how my parents are. But my husband, David, he's white and was really uncomfortable not using a doctor and having the baby at home. So we used a medical doctor and had the baby in the hospital."

"I see," you say. "It must be hard to deal with this without feeling the support of your family. Do you have any friendships that are supportive?"

"I have a few friends from my job, but we really only see each other at work. I haven't heard from them much since Anna died. I think it makes them uncomfortable. I had scheduled to have this time off as maternity leave and so I haven't been back to work yet," Moki explains.

"Unfortunately, many people don't know what to do or say to someone in your situation. It's too bad because at a time when you are most needing their support, they can't seem to give it," you say.

"Yeah," Moki agrees. "David's mom keeps telling me, 'You're young. You'll have more babies.' I guess they think that will make me feel better. But I want my little Anna!"

"Yes, of course you do," you say.

Moki sighs, pauses for a moment and then asks, "Do you think I should go back to work?" Moki asks.

"I'm not sure. That is something we might want to explore more together. It may be a good thing that you have some time to grieve without the responsibility of work. Also, your body is still adjusting to not being pregnant. All of those physical changes can affect your mood also. It's a very tender time for you right now. It's a time when you want to take particularly good care of yourself."

"Okay. That's good to know," Moki says. "I have been feeling like I should be doing better by now, or at least that others expect me to be doing better."

"How is your husband dealing with this?" you ask.

Moki pauses a moment before speaking, "I don't really know, to tell you the truth. I know that it was real hard for him at first. He doesn't say much about it. He has been pretty grumpy lately, though. He went back to work right away. Maybe he is trying to stay busy so he doesn't have to think about it."

"How did he respond to your suggestion that he come to counseling with you?" you inquire.

"He said he couldn't get away from work. I think if he had really wanted to, he could have," Moki says.

"How does he feel about you coming to counseling?"

"He thinks it's a good idea," Moki answers.

"I wonder if you might ask him again to come in with you," you suggest. "We can be sure to schedule the next session at a time that won't interfere with his work. Losing a baby is very hard for both parents but people show their grief in different ways. Talking about the differences and your expectations for one another during this time can prevent a lot of misunderstandings."

"Maybe if I put it to him that way he would. I don't know, maybe he really did have a work conflict that he couldn't get out of. We haven't been talking a whole lot lately," Moki says.

"That happens to a lot of couples when they are going through hard times," you reassure Moki. "All the more reason to get help for you as a couple in addition to you getting support individually."

Moki agrees with you and then asks, "What do I do in the meantime? How am I supposed to deal with this?"

You do some teaching about the grief process so that Moki has a realistic idea about what to expect from herself during this time. You also discuss the ways that a perinatal loss is different from other losses both for the parents and their friends and family. You then engage Moki in a discussion about ways that she can take care of herself. Together you come up with the following list: eating nutritious food, getting fresh air, exercise (once she has gotten approval from her doctor to do so), keeping chores and "to do" lists to a minimum, soothing baths, and reading a book about perinatal loss. You also inform Moki that some parents find it helpful to make a memory box for their infant in which they keep the baby's hospital bands, clothes, blankets she used, pictures, etc. You and Moki then make arrangements for a subsequent visit at a time that her husband will likely be able to come.

"Thank you so much," Moki says. "I'm glad I came to see you."

7.3-1. Identify some of Moki's strengths and explain how they might be helpful to her in her grief process.

7.3-2. Describe how you would conduct the session with Moki and her husband.

7.3-3. Identify three books or other written resources that might be helpful to Moki as she grieves her infant's death.

7.3-4. Write what you would say to Moki when discussing the differences between perinatal loss and other losses.

7.3-5. What are some resources in your community that might be helpful to Moki and her husband?

7.3-6. Write three questions you could ask Moki that would help you better understand her grief experience.

CASE 7.4

Identifying Information:

Client Name: Nora Alvarez
Age: 36 years old
Race/Ethnicity: Mexican American
Marital Status: Single
Education Level: High school graduate
Occupation: Seamstress

Intake Information:

Nora called the counseling center to request grief counseling over the death of her 3-year-old daughter, Josie. You learn from the intake information that Josie died suddenly by drowning.

Initial Interview:

Nora arrives for her appointment at the scheduled time. Her demeanor is subdued, though polite, and you sense a weariness about her.

After sitting on the couch in your office, you ask, "How can I help you, Nora?"

"My daughter, Josie, died six weeks ago," she says, her eyes filling with tears. She reaches for a tissue. You wait patiently. "It's so hard. I don't know how to handle it. I miss her so much." She puts her head in her hands and starts to sob quietly.

"I can see that your daughter's death is very painful for you," you say quietly.

Nora nods. After a few moments, she continues. "She was such a sweet girl. Only 3 years old. I don't know how to go on without her. I just feel so lost."

"The loss of a child can feel insurmountable. Many parents feel the deepest sadness and a sense of feeling lost as you describe," you empathize. "How did Josie die?"

Through heavy tears Nora tells you the story of Josie's death. She was at the house of Nora's brother and sister-in-law while Nora was running errands. They believe she followed the dog out to the back yard and fell in the pool. She wasn't found until several minutes later. 911 was called and they rushed her to the hospital. "By the time I got there it was too late," Nora says, "She was already gone." Nora continues to cry.

"So in an instant your life has turned upside down," you venture.

"Yes. I don't know up from down. I don't know what to do with myself. I feel this heaviness, this dark hole deep in my heart. It's the worst thing that I have ever experienced," she says through her tears. "I don't know how to get through this. This wasn't supposed to happen."

"No. As parents we never expect that we will outlive our children," you say softly.

"Yes! Exactly! This all seems so unfair and unnatural. I just want my daughter back!" she says, her voice rising a bit as the tears continue.

"You really miss her," you say. Nora nods and continues to cry. You sit with her quietly. When her tears subside a bit you ask, "Tell me about Josie. What was she like?"

Nora responds, "Josie was so sweet and precious. She was always singing and dancing, always making us laugh. She loved to be cuddled and read to. She was just such a joy." Nora's eyes seem to light up a little bit as she talks about her daughter. "She was about to start dance class and she was so excited! She talked about it non-stop. Always asking, 'Is today the day I go to dance class?' She always wanted to wear dance clothes." Nora reaches for her phone and pulls up pictures of Josie. As you look at the pictures you comment on how cute she is and on the sparkle in her eye.

"I just miss her so much," Nora says.

"I bet you do," you affirm. "How have you been managing since her death?"

"I cry a lot. Sometimes I feel like I will never be able to stop crying. I can't sleep. I lay down and I just can't stop thinking about her. I have pictures of her up all over my house. I haven't changed anything about her room. Sometimes I go in there, just trying to feel her. I know that may sound crazy..." Nora's voice trails off.

"Not crazy at all," you say. "I would expect you to be looking for some way to find some connection with her. The mother–child bond is a very strong one."

Nora nods in agreement and continues, "I can't concentrate and I feel so sluggish. I can barely make myself do anything."

"How are you feeling physically?" you ask.

"I'm just so tired. And my chest feels heavy, like there's ten ton weight on it. I don't see how I'm ever going to get through this," she explains.

"I know it must feel like it's just too much. It's a huge loss. I'm not surprised by anything you have described. Those are common and expected responses to a loss." You add, "The physical discomfort you describe is common, too. Many people have chest pains, or headaches, or changes in their appetite. It doesn't feel good but it is what we expect when someone is grieving such a significant loss."

"It is? I didn't know. I've been feeling like I'm losing my mind," Nora says.

"Yes, it feels crazy, but it's not. It's part of how your body is trying to adjust to the change. Have you had thoughts of hurting yourself, Nora?" you inquire.

"No, not really. Sometimes I wish I could just not wake up in the morning but I've got an elderly mother that needs me. I've got to stick around for her," Nora says. You discuss this feeling more with Nora and confirm that she is not currently at risk for hurting herself, though you plan to monitor this closely. "I just wish I hadn't left her that day. I feel so guilty. I should have just brought her with me. Then maybe I'd still have her..." Nora's voice trails off and she begins to cry again.

"I can understand wanting to go back in time. Do you remember your reasoning at the time for not bringing her with you?" you ask gently.

"I thought she'd have more fun at her cousin's house," Nora says. "It was going to be a lot of waiting in long lines. She would have hated it. It would have been stressful on both of us."

"Yes, those kinds of errands don't mix well with active 3-year-olds," you say. "I know this may be hard to take in, but you didn't do anything wrong, Nora. In fact, you made a very reasonable decision that was in the best interest of Josie. You had no way of knowing this would happen."

"No, I didn't," Nora says. "She has been at their house a lot. They have always been good about helping me out since I'm a single mom. And she loved going over there. She was so excited that morning...I just wish it hadn't happened."

Nora continues to talk about the specific circumstances that led to Josie's drowning. It seems that her sister-in-law was in the bathroom when Josie went outside. Nora says she understands it wasn't intentional or negligent and could have happened to anyone. She goes on to explain that her brother and his family are also heartbroken and have been very supportive.

"I know they feel just terrible about it," she says.

"That's admirable that you can be so understanding of them. I wonder if you ever feel angry?" you ask.

"Oh yes. I feel angry," Nora says. "But I don't stay angry at them for long. I really do get that it was an accident. But I feel angry at God that he let this happen, angry that she'll never get to go to dance class, angry at all the mothers who still have their kids. I know that's irrational, but..."

"But it's completely understandable," you affirm.

You allow Nora to talk more about her anger, validating her feelings. You gently turn the discussion to how she is managing her feelings and offer some suggestions for how she can manage them when they become overwhelming.

As the session draws to a close, Nora says, "I think I'm going to need to see you again. Probably for a long time."

"I'd be honored to work with you Nora," you say. "This is too much to try to do alone. When you're ready, we might also talk about you attending a support group, one that is specifically for parents who have lost a child."

"Yeah, okay," Nora says. "I'm open to that."

7.4-1. What are some of Nora's strengths?
7.4-2. What are your concerns for Nora?
7.4-3. What are some other ways you could respond to Nora's feelings of guilt?
7.4-4. What additional information would be helpful as you work with Nora?
7.4-5. How might Nora's single mother status impact her grief process?
7.4-6. What types of interventions might be helpful to Nora?
7.4-7. Identify three resources in your community that might be helpful to Nora.

CASE 7.5

Identifying Information:

Client Name: Amanda Wright
Age: 32 years old
Race/Ethnicity: White
Marital Status: Married
Educational Level: Bachelor's degree
Occupation: Bookkeeper for a small business

Intake Information:

Amanda calls the counseling center and asks about the kind of counseling that is available. She tells the intake worker, "I guess I need grief counseling...well, I don't know if you would call it that. My husband has been missing for two years." She goes on to explain that her husband disappeared while serving in the military and his body hasn't been recovered. "Have I called the right place? Can your agency help me?" she asks. The intake worker assures Amanda that her situation is appropriate for the services the agency provides and schedules an appointment for her to come in later that week.

Initial Interview:

You find Amanda in the waiting room. After introductions, you escort her to your office.

Once you are both seated, you begin the session saying, "Tell me what brings you here, Amanda."

Amanda sighs and begins, "My husband John was in the Air Force. He was assigned to some flying missions in Iraq. His plane went down but to this day they haven't found his body. He has been declared missing in action."

"For how long has he been missing?" you ask.

"It's been almost two years," Amanda responds.

"So for two years, you have lived without any contact from your husband and no evidence to indicate that he is alive or dead, is that right?" you clarify.

"You got it," Amanda says matter-of-factly. "They found the plane and they said it was pretty mangled. They said it is very unlikely for him to have survived the crash, but there's no physical body to prove it."

"That sounds so difficult, Amanda! How has this been for you?" you inquire.

She takes a deep sigh. "It's been torture. At some moments, I'm convinced that he's still out there somewhere and I just need to keep praying and hoping. At other times, I think I just need to accept the fact that he is dead and move on with my life. I don't know what to do."

"That must be an emotional roller coaster for you!" you say.

"It is," Amanda affirms. "It really is. I'm in this holding pattern. I don't want to give up on him but I'm just waiting. Waiting for something that may never happen."

"You mean, waiting for clear evidence that he is either dead or alive?" you ask.

"Exactly," she says. "And sometimes…this sounds horrible…but sometimes I find myself hoping for news of his death. It's not that I want him to be dead, it's just that not knowing is killing me."

"I don't think that is horrible at all, Amanda," you reassure her. "I think many people in your situation feel the same way. If you knew he was dead you could get on with your grieving. Not knowing really keeps you stuck."

"Yes, I feel really stuck. I don't know who I am or where I'm going with my life. I don't even know if I'm still married or not! If I'm ever going to have children and a family, which is something I'd like to do, I can't wait for years and years. I'm already 32 years old!"

"It really makes it hard for you to take any steps to plan a future, doesn't it?" you validate.

"Yes, it does. And then I feel so guilty for even thinking about that. John's parents are still hoping beyond hope that he will be found alive. When I think I should just let go and accept that he's dead, I feel like I'm giving up on him. What if he's out there somewhere just trying to get back home? I would feel so disloyal to move on with my life without him. John's parents haven't given up on him."

"I can see why that would be hard. And I'm not sure that comparing yourself with John's parents is a fair comparison," you suggest. "Losing a child and losing a spouse are very different experiences, and you are in a very different stage of life than John's parents."

"Maybe so," Amanda considers.

"And I don't believe, Amanda," you continue, "that you are a bad person for wanting to move on with your life. I think that is a very natural feeling. Are you in contact with John's parents often?"

"Not as much as we used to be. After a while I had to distance myself from them a little bit. Whenever I would spend time with them, I would leave feeling very anxious and confused."

"What do you think made you feel that way?" you ask.

"I guess it was hard seeing how painful it was for them and how their life pretty much revolves around memories and hopes about John now. It scares me to think that I could be stuck with this for the rest of my life."

"Yes, I can see why that would be hard. Let's pretend for a moment that you don't have to worry about the reactions from other people and that regardless of the decision you make, you get complete and absolute approval from everyone in your community. What do you think you would want to do? Would you want to get married again?"

"It depends on what day you ask me," Amanda says with a tone of frustration. "Today, I would probably say yes, but it changes all the time. Next week I might tell you something completely different. What I really want is John. I want my husband back. But how long do I wait?"

"I wish there was a concrete answer for you, Amanda," you say. "There is really no standard etiquette that society has outlined for people dealing with this kind of loss. You don't benefit from the guidelines that help people who are grieving a death." Amanda seems to be watching you closely and is very attentive to what you are saying. You continue, "The kind of loss you are experiencing is called an 'ambiguous loss' because it is so unclear. Ambiguous losses are extremely difficult to manage for the very reasons you have been describing."

"I'm glad to know there's a name for it," Amanda says. "I just wish I could figure out how to deal with it!"

"Yes, I'm sure this is very distressing for you. Tell me more about how it has affected you, your life, your health, how you spend your time," you suggest.

Amanda explains that outside of work she spends most of her time at home alone watching TV, usually with a glass of wine. She reported that her relationships with other military wives, which were once strong, have pretty much become non-existent. She also said that her sleep is often troubled with bad dreams and frequent night awakenings.

"Do you have any support? Friends or family you can talk to?" you ask.

"My parents are very supportive. They live across the country, but we talk regularly. They worry about me. I also have a good relationship with my brother but he's got young kids and is busy with his family, so I don't like to bother him." You also learn that Amanda enjoys her job and has a good work environment, though she seems to refrain from opening up too much to her co-workers.

"Tell me more about John," you prompt.

Amanda says they had been married for about six years prior to when he went missing and that they were planning to start a family when he returned from being deployed. They often talked about their plans for the future, how they would raise their kids, and places they wanted to travel.

"And for the last two years, you have been stuck in limbo. Does that seem to fit?"

"Mm-hm," she nods. "Limbo is a good word for it."

You ask Amanda about the emotions she has surrounding the loss and she struggles to name them. "At first it was just devastating, you know? But we had hope. We kept thinking we'd learn something. But now…I'm not sure what to do with myself." For the first time, you notice tears in her eyes and you wonder if she has become accustomed to numbing her emotions.

You ask, "Do you think you have let yourself grieve John, Amanda?"

"I was just sitting here wondering that as we were talking. I don't know that I have. I know I've cried about it. I know I've missed him. But I'm not sure I've really grieved or if I'm even *supposed* to grieve. I kind of just feel…frozen," she says.

You nod in understanding. "You know, for many of us, when something really difficult happens we try to avoid thinking about it or letting ourselves have feelings about it. It may feel better in the short run but it tends to catch up with us. It would be understandable if that was what you were doing since in this case there is also no clear path forward. Do you think that fits for you at all?"

"Maybe," Amanda considers. "You think that's why I feel frozen? That I'm avoiding facing this?"

"That could be part of it. Granted, I've known you for less than an hour now so I may be completely off base," you caution. "But I also think this situation is a very complex one. Not because of how *you* are dealing with it, Amanda, but because the situation itself is so ill defined. It may be that some level of avoidance is the only way to get through this while you try to live with the unknown about your husband. Does that make sense?"

"I think so," she says. "I hadn't really thought about it that way until now." You and Amanda discuss the difficult tension between grieving which she feels would mean letting go of John and her need to continue a life without him.

"I'm curious, Amanda. What made you decide to come in now?" you inquire.

"Well, there's a girl where I work. She's a few years younger than me. She got married a few months ago and she's already pregnant. She's always talking about her husband, their plans for the baby, the house they are building, on and on. She's really sweet, but," Amanda leans forward and whispers, "I can't stand her. I get so angry when she's around. And for no reason. She's done nothing wrong. She's never treated me unkindly or anything like that. I think I'm jealous. So, I figured it might be time to talk to someone."

You validate Amanda's feelings of jealousy, explaining how her co-worker's experience is highlighting all the losses she is trying to sort through.

"Obviously, there is a lot more to discuss, Amanda, but I feel very hopeful that our work together could benefit you. What do you think? Would you like to come in again?"

"Yes, I think I would," Amanda says. "I think I've been needing to do this for a long time. You've already given me a lot to think about and I think I need someone objective to help me with this."

7.5-1. What are Amanda's strengths?

7.5-2. Based on this first session, what are your initial thoughts about how Amanda is dealing with her husband's absence and what led to those impressions?

7.5-3. What additional information would be useful to obtain as you work with Amanda?

7.5-4. Outline a possible intervention plan for your work with Amanda.

7.5-5. What specific coping skills do you think Amanda could benefit from learning?

7.5-6. Per Boss's recommendation, brainstorm some possible dialectical statements that may help Amanda navigate the loss of John.

REFERENCES

Adrian, J. A., & Stitt, A. (2017). Pet loss, complicated grief, and post-traumatic stress disorder in Hawaii. *Anthrozoös*, *30*(1), 123–133. https://doi.org/10.1080/08927936.2017.1270598

Aho, A. L., Malmisuo, J., & Kaunonen, M. (2018). The effects of peer support on post-traumatic stress reactions in bereaved parents. *Scandinavian Journal of Caring Sciences*, *32*(1), 326–334. https://doi.org/10.1111/scs.12465

Albuquerque, S., Narciso, I., & Pereira, M. (2018). Posttraumatic growth in bereaved parents: A multidimensional model of associated factors. *Psychological Trauma: Theory, Research, Practice, and Policy*, *10*(2), 199–207. https://doi.org/10.1037/tra0000305

American Veterinary Medical Association. (2017–2018). *Pet ownership and demographics sourcebook* [PDF]. www.avma.org/sites/default/files/resources/AVMA-Pet-Demographics-Executive-Summary.pdf

Bartolomei, J., Baeriswyl-Cottin, R., Framorando, D., Kasina, F., Premand, N., Eytan, A., & Khazaal, Y. (2016). What are the barriers to access to mental healthcare and the primary needs of asylum seekers? A survey of mental health caregivers and primary care workers. *BMC Psychiatry*, *16*(1), 336.

Black, B., Wright, P., & Limbo, R. (2015). *Perinatal and pediatric bereavement*. Springer Publishing Company.

Boss, P. (2016). The context and process of theory development: The story of ambiguous loss. *Journal of Family Theory & Review*, *8*(3), 269–286. https://doi.org/10.1111/jftr.12152

Boss, P., & Ishii, C. (2015). Trauma and ambiguous loss: The lingering presence of the physically absent. In K. E. Cherry (Ed.), *Traumatic stress and long-term recovery: Coping with disasters and other negative life events* (pp. 271–289). Springer.

Bowlby, J. (1980). *Attachment and loss: Loss, sadness and depression* (Vol. 3). Basic Books.

Bryant, R. A., Edwards, B., Creamer, M., O'Donnell, M., Forbes, D., Felmingham, K. L., Silove, D., Steel, Z., McFarlane, A. C., Van Hooff, M., Nickerson, A., & Hadzi-Pavlovic, D. (2020). A population study of prolonged grief in refugees. *Epidemiology and Psychiatric Sciences*, *29*. https://doi.org/10.1017/s2045796019000386

Casey, L. S., Reisner, S. L., Findling, M. G., Blendon, R. J., Benson, J. M., Sayde, J. M., & Miller, C. (2019). Discrimination in the United States: Experiences of lesbian, gay, bisexual, transgender, and queer Americans. *Health Services Research*, *54*(52), 1454–1466. https://doi.org/10.1111/1475-6773.13229

Charney, M. E., Bui, E., Sager, J. C., Ohye, B. Y., Goetter, E. M., & Simon, N. M. (2018). Complicated grief among military service members and veterans who served after September 11, 2001. *Journal of Traumatic Stress*, *31*(1), 157–162. https://doi.org/10.1002/jts.22254

Cheung, D. S., Ho, K. H., Cheung, T. F., Lam, S. C., & Tse, M. M. (2018). Anticipatory grief of spousal and adult children caregivers of people with dementia. *BMC Palliative Care*, *17*(1). https://doi.org/10.1186/s12904-018-0376-3

Clute, M. A. (2015). Living disconnected: Building a grounded theory view of bereavement for adults with intellectual disabilities. *OMEGA – Journal of Death and Dying*, *76*(1), 15–34. https://doi.org/10.1177/0030222815575017

Coelho, A., De Brito, M., & Barbosa, A. (2018). Caregiver anticipatory grief. *Current Opinion in Supportive and Palliative Care*, *12*(1), 52–57. https://doi.org/10.1097/spc.0000000000000321

Coelho, A., De Brito, M., Teixeira, P., Frade, P., Barros, L., & Barbosa, A. (2020). Family caregivers' anticipatory grief: A conceptual framework for understanding its multiple challenges. *Qualitative Health Research*, *30*(5), 693–703. https://doi.org/10.1177/1049732319873330

Cozza, S. J., Fisher, J. E., Zhou, J., Harrington-LaMorie, J., La Flair, L., Fullerton, C. S., & Ursano, R. J. (2017). Bereaved military dependent spouses and children: Those left behind in a decade of war (2001–2011). *Military Medicine*, *182*(3), e1684–e1690. https://doi.org/10.7205/milmed-d-16-00101

Cozza, S. J., Hefner, K. R., Fisher, J. E., Zhou, J., Fullerton, C. S., Ursano, R. J., & Shear, M. K. (2020). Mental health conditions in bereaved military service widows: A prospective, case-controlled, and longitudinal study. *Depression and Anxiety*, *37*(1), 45–53. https://doi.org/10.1002/da.22971

Department of Defense. (2014). *Department of defense suicide event report*. www.dspo.mil/Portals/113/Documents/CY%202014%20DoDSER%20Annual%20Report%20-%20Final.pdf

Diamond, D. J., & Diamond, M. O. (2014). Understanding and treating the psychosocial consequences of pregnancy loss. *Oxford Handbooks Online*. https://doi.org/10.1093/oxfordhb/9780199778072.013.30

Doka, K. J. (1989). Disenfranchised grief. In K. J. Doka (Ed.), *Disenfranchised grief: Recognizing hidden sorrow* (pp. 3–23). Lexington Books.

Dooley, C. M., Carroll, B., Fry, L. E., Seamon-Lahiff, G., & Bartone, P. T. (2019). A model for supporting grief recovery following traumatic loss: The tragedy assistance program for survivors (TAPS). *Military Medicine*, *184*(7–8), 166–170. https://doi.org/10.1093/milmed/usz084

Harrington-LaMorie, J., Jordan, J. R., Ruocco, K., & Cerel, J. (2018). Surviving families of military suicide loss: Exploring postvention peer support. *Death Studies*, *42*(3), 143–154. https://doi.org/10.1080/07481187.2017.1370789

Hidalgo, I. M. (2017) The effects of children's spiritual coping after parent, grandparent or sibling death on children's grief, personal growth, and mental health (Doctoral dissertation). https://digitalcommons.fiu.edu/etd/3467

Holloway, K. (2009). A name for a parent whose child has died. *Duke Today*. https://today.duke.edu/2009/05/holloway_oped.html

Ingham, C. F., Eccles, F. J., Armitage, J. R., & Murray, C. D. (2016). Same-sex partner bereavement in older women: An interpretative phenomenological analysis. *Aging & Mental Health*, *21*(9), 917–925. https://doi.org/10.1080/13607863.2016.1181712

Iraq and Afghanistan Veterans of America. (2017). *IAVA 2017 annual member survey: A look into the lives of post-9/11 veterans*. https://iava.org/wp-content/uploads/2016/05/IAVA_Survey_2017_v11update.pdf

Jacoby, V. M., Hale, W., Dillon, K., Dondanville, K. A., Wachen, J. S., Yarvis, J. S., Litz, B. T., Mintz, J., Young-McCaughan, S., Peterson, A. L., & Resick, P. A. (2019). Depression suppresses treatment response for traumatic loss–related posttraumatic stress disorder in active duty military personnel. *Journal of Traumatic Stress*, *32*(5), 774–783. https://doi.org/10.1002/jts.22441

Killikelly, C., Bauer, S., & Maercker, A. (2018). The assessment of grief in refugees and post-conflict survivors: A narrative review of etic and emic research. *Frontiers in Psychology*, *9*. https://doi.org/10.3389/fpsyg.2018.01957

Kim, M. A., Yi, J., Sang, J., & Jung, D. (2019). A photovoice study on the bereavement experience of mothers after the death of a child. *Death Studies*, 1–15. https://doi.org/10.1080/07481187.2019.1648333

Koenig Kellas, J., Castle, K., Johnson, A., & Cohen, M. (2017). Communicatively constructing the bright and dark sides of hope: Family caregivers' experiences during end of life cancer care. *Behavioral Sciences*, *7*(4), 33. https://doi.org/10.3390/bs7020033

Kokou-Kpolou, C. K., Moukouta, C. S., Masson, J., Bernoussi, A., Cénat, J. M., & Bacqué, M. (2020). Correlates of grief-related disorders and mental health outcomes among adult refugees exposed to trauma and bereavement: A systematic review and future research directions. *Journal of Affective Disorders*, *267*, 171–184. https://doi.org/10.1016/j.jad.2020.02.026

Krosch, D. J., & Shakespeare-Finch, J. (2017). Grief, traumatic stress, and posttraumatic growth in women who have experienced pregnancy loss. *Psychological Trauma: Theory, Research, Practice, and Policy*, *9*(4), 425–433. https://doi.org/10.1037/tra0000183

Lacour, O., Morina, N., Spaaij, J., Nickerson, A., Schnyder, U., Von Känel, R., Bryant, R. A., & Schick, M. (2020). Prolonged grief disorder among refugees in psychological treatment—Association with self-efficacy and emotion regulation. *Frontiers in Psychiatry*, *11*. https://doi.org/10.3389/fpsyt.2020.00526

Leon, I. G. (2017). Reproductive loss and its impact on the next pregnancy. In M. Muzik & K. L. Rosenblum (Eds.), *Motherhood in the face of trauma: Pathways towards healing and growth* (pp. 69–83). Springer.

Lindstrom, C. M., Cann, A., Calhoun, L. G., & Tedeschi, R. G. (2013). The relationship of core belief challenge, rumination, disclosure, and sociocultural elements to posttraumatic growth. *Psychological Trauma: Theory, Research, Practice, and Policy*, *5*(1), 50–55.

Litz, B. T., Contractor, A. A., Rhodes, C., Dondanville, K. A., Jordan, A. H., Resick, P. A., Foa, E. B., Young-McCaughan, S., Mintz, J., Yarvis, J. S., & Peterson, A. L. (2018). Distinct trauma types in military service members seeking treatment for posttraumatic stress disorder. *Journal of Traumatic Stress*, *31*(2), 286–295. https://doi.org/10.1002/jts.22276

Lubens, P., & Silver, R. C. (2019). U.S. combat veterans' responses to suicide and combat deaths: A mixed-methods study. *Social Science & Medicine*, *236*, 112341. https://doi.org/10.1016/j.socscimed.2019.05.046

Markin, R. D., & Zilcha-Mano, S. (2018). Cultural processes in psychotherapy for perinatal loss: Breaking the cultural taboo against perinatal grief. *Psychotherapy*, *55*(1), 20–26. https://doi.org/10.1037/pst0000122

Mason-Angelow, V. A. (2017). *Bereavement support for adults with learning disabilities: An inclusive participatory study* (Doctoral dissertation). https://research-information.bris.ac.uk/en/studentTheses/bereavement-support-for-adults-with-learning-disabilities-an-incl

Messam, L. L., & Hart, L. A. (2019). Persons experiencing prolonged grief after the loss of a pet. *Clinician's Guide to Treating Companion Animal Issues*, 267–280. https://doi.org/10.1016/b978-0-12-812962-3.00015-0

Moon, P. J. (2016). Anticipatory grief: A mere concept? *American Journal of Hospice and Palliative Medicine*, *33*(5), 417–420. https://doi.org/10.1177/1049909115574262

Morris, S., Fletcher, K., & Goldstein, R. (2019). The grief of parents after the death of a young child. *Journal of Clinical Psychology in Medical Settings*, *26*(3), 321–338. https://doi.org/10.1007/s10880-018-9590-7

Nocon, A., Eberle-Sejari, R., Unterhitzenberger, J., & Rosner, R. (2017). The effectiveness of psychosocial interventions in war-traumatized refugee and internally displaced minors: Systematic review and meta-analysis. *European Journal of Psychotraumatology*, *8*(2), 1388709. https://doi.org/10.1080/20008198.2017.1388709

Nolan, R., Kirkland, C., & Davis, R. (2019). LGBT* after loss: A mixed-method analysis on the effect of partner bereavement on interpersonal relationships and subsequent partnerships. *OMEGA – Journal of Death and Dying*. https://doi.org/10.1177/0030222819831524

October, T., Dryden-Palmer, K., Copnell, B., & Meert, K. L. (2018). Caring for parents after the death of a child. *Pediatric Critical Care Medicine*, *19*, S61–S68. https://doi.org/10.1097/pcc.0000000000001466

O'Leary, R. (2019). Equal bereavement for same sex partners. *Bereavement Care*, *38*(2–3), 129–132. https://doi.org/10.1080/02682621.2019.1679473

Otani, H., Yoshida, S., Morita, T., Aoyama, M., Kizawa, Y., Shima, Y., Tsuneto, S., & Miyashita, M. (2017). Meaningful communication before death, but not present at the time of death itself, is associated with better outcomes on measures of depression and complicated grief among bereaved family members of cancer patients. *Journal of Pain and Symptom Management*, *54*(3), 273–279. https://doi.org/10.1016/j.jpainsymman.2017.07.010

Powell, J. (2019). Loss and grief in people with intellectual disability. In F. Timmins & S. Caldeira (Eds.), *Spirituality in healthcare: Perspectives for innovative practice*. Springer.

Salakari, A., Kaunonen, M., & Aho, A. L. (2014). Negative changes in a couple's relationship after a child's death. *Interpersona: An International Journal on Personal Relationships*, *8*(2), 193–209. https://doi.org/10.5964/ijpr.v8i2.166

Silove, D., Ventevogel, P., & Rees, S. (2017). The contemporary refugee crisis: An overview of mental health challenges. *World Psychiatry*, *16*(2), 130–139. https://doi.org/10.1002/wps.20438

Simon, N. M., O'Day, E. B., Hellberg, S. N., Hoeppner, S. S., Charney, M. E., Robinaugh, D. J., Bui, E., Goetter, E. M., Baker, A. W., Rogers, A. H., Nadal-Vicens, M., Venners, M. R., Kim, H. M., & Rauch, S. A. (2018). The loss of a fellow service member: Complicated grief in post-9/11 service members and veterans with combat-related posttraumatic stress disorder. *Journal of Neuroscience Research*, *96*(1), 5–15. https://doi.org/10.1002/jnr.24094

Spain, B., O'Dwyer, L., & Moston, S. (2019). Pet loss: Understanding disenfranchised grief, memorial use, and posttraumatic growth. *Anthrozoös*, *32*(4), 555–568. https://doi.org/10.1080/08927936.2019.1621545

Steen, S. E. (2019). Raising the bar: Development of a perinatal bereavement programme. *International Journal of Palliative Nursing*, *25*(12), 578–586. https://doi.org/10.12968/ijpn.2019.25.12.578

Steil, R., Gutermann, J., Harrison, O., Starck, A., Schwartzkopff, L., Schouler-Ocak, M., & Stangier, U. (2019). Prevalence of prolonged grief disorder in a sample of female refugees. *BMC Psychiatry*, *19*(1). https://doi.org/10.1186/s12888-019-2136-1

Testoni, I., De Cataldo, L., Ronconi, L., & Zamperini, A. (2017). Pet loss and representations of death, attachment, depression, and euthanasia. *Anthrozoös*, *30*(1), 135–148. https://doi.org/10.1080/08927936.2017.1270599

Thorp, N., Stedmon, J., & Lloyd, H. (2018). "I carry her in my heart": An exploration of the experience of bereavement for people with learning disability. *British Journal of Learning Disabilities*, *46*(1), 45–53. https://doi.org/10.1111/bld.12212

Triplett, K. N., Tedeschi, R. G., Cann, A., Calhoun, L. G., & Reeve, C. L. (2012). Posttraumatic growth, meaning in life, and life satisfaction in response to trauma. *Psychological Trauma: Theory, Research, Practice, and Policy*, *4*(4), 400–410.

United Nations High Commissioner for Refugees. (2020, June 18). *Figures at a glance*. UNHCR. Retrieved June 26, 2020, from www.unhcr.org/en-us/figures-at-a-glance.html

Vegsund, H. K., Reinfjell, T., Moksnes, U. K., Wallin, A. E., Hjemdal, O., & Eilertsen, M. B. (2019). Resilience as a predictive factor towards a healthy adjustment to grief after the loss of a child to cancer. *PLOS ONE*, *14*(3), e0214138. https://doi.org/10.1371/journal.pone.0214138

Weiss, E. L., Hino, D., Canfield, J., & Albright, D. L. (2017). Military families: Strengths and concerns: Reintegration and beyond. In J. Beder (Ed.), *Caring for the military: A guide for helping professionals* (pp. 72–92). Routledge.

Whittle, S., & Turner, L. (2007). *Bereavement: A guide for transsexual, transgender people and their loved ones* [PDF]. United Kingdom National Health Service. www.scottishtrans.org/wp-content/uploads/2013/06/NHS-Bereavement-A-guide-for-Transsexual-Transgender-people-and-their-loved-ones.pdf

Wong, P. W., Lau, K. C., Liu, L. L., Yuen, G. S., & Wing-Lok, P. (2017). Beyond recovery: Understanding the postbereavement growth from companion animal loss. *OMEGA – Journal of Death and Dying*, *75*(2), 103–123. https://doi.org/10.1177/0030222815612603

Worden, J. W. (2018). *Grief counseling and grief therapy: A handbook for the mental health practitioner* (5th ed.). Springer Publishing Company.

Yarvis, J. S., Byren, G. N., & Stryker-Thomas, H. (2017). Treating co-occurring conditions in the returning warrior. In J. Beder (Ed.), *Caring for the military: A guide for helping professionals* (pp. 191–201). Routledge.

Young, H. (2016). Conceptualising bereavement in profound and multiple learning disabilities. *Tizard Learning Disability Review*, *21*(4), 186–198. https://doi.org/10.1108/tldr-09-2015-0035

Young, H. (2017). Overcoming barriers to grief: Supporting bereaved people with profound intellectual and multiple disabilities. *International Journal of Developmental Disabilities*, *63*(3), 131–137. https://doi.org/10.1080/20473869.2016.1158511

Zetumer, S., Young, I., Shear, M. K., Skritskaya, N., Lebowitz, B., Simon, N., Reynolds, C., Mauro, C., & Zisook, S. (2015). The impact of losing a child on the clinical presentation of complicated grief. *Journal of Affective Disorders*, *170*, 15–21. https://doi.org/10.1016/j.jad.2014.08.021

CHAPTER 8

Practice Implications for the Professional

Working with bereaved individuals is a powerful and moving experience. It can be an incredibly rewarding and meaningful endeavor because of the profound impact it has on individuals when they are at a vulnerable time in their lives. It also involves challenging moments which might cause workers to feel drained, discouraged, frustrated, sad, overwhelmed, and unmoored. Despite adherence to professional boundaries between client and counselor, the act of being emotionally present for someone who is mourning a loved one touches the practitioner personally. This may be in part because of the practitioner's personal experience with loss. However, even practitioners who have not grieved a loved one's death may find that working with the bereaved can at times be a draining and overwhelming experience. Additionally, providing grief counseling involves regular and intimate contact with the prevalence, probability, and impact of death (their own and their loved ones), a reality that is uncomfortable to confront. The impact that grief counseling has on practitioners is further heightened when the loss is traumatic in nature. Being in close relationship with a trauma survivor and hearing the details of their pain can cause practitioners to confront their vulnerability to the randomness of tragedy and loss and thereby influence their felt sense of safety and security.

Attention to how the counseling process affects the practitioner is essential to competent and ethical practice with bereaved and traumatically bereaved clients. This chapter will discuss vicarious trauma and burnout in addition to the role of self-awareness, self-care, supervision and consultation, and continued education in mitigating the negative impact of this work on practitioners.

VICARIOUS TRAUMA

Practitioners who work with a high volume of traumatically bereaved clients must be alert to the possibility of developing vicarious trauma (VT). Sometimes used interchangeably with the terms compassion fatigue, secondary trauma, and trauma exposure response, VT refers to the internal adverse changes that can happen to therapists who empathically engage with traumatized individuals. VT results in significant alterations to the therapist's core self, beliefs about others, and assumptive worldviews about trust, safety, and intimacy (Flint, 2018). The condition develops over a period of

DOI: 10.4324/9780429053634-8

time as the interactions with clients' trauma narratives accumulate (Hernandez-Wolfe, 2018). Symptoms of VT resemble those of PTSD and may include hyperarousal, intrusive images gleaned from hearing about their clients' experiences, memory problems, dissociation, nightmares, and depression (Flint, 2018; Hazen et al., 2020). It is also common for therapists' personal relationships to be negatively affected in addition to their overall physical, mental, emotional, and spiritual health (Hazen et al., 2020).

If not addressed, VT can encroach on the work of practitioners by adversely impacting their motivation and feelings of self-efficacy which can be a precursor to burnout (Sartor, 2016). Of equal concern is the effect that VT has on the interactions between therapists and those they serve. Practitioners impacted by VT often find it difficult to empathize with their clients and they may struggle to stay present while listening to their traumatic experiences (Boulanger, 2018). Often unconsciously, therapists may steer discussions away from disturbing material as a way to protect themselves from the impact of hearing it. They are also more likely to blur boundaries with clients and assume unprofessional roles, thus placing them at risk for acting unethically (Hazen et al., 2020). Factors believed to contribute to the development of VT include:

- A large number of traumatized clients in one's caseload (Sartor, 2016)
- Inability to obtain consultation or supervision
- Failure of the practitioner to obtain therapy for themselves
- Little specialized education and training in trauma and grief and loss
- The therapist's coping style (Iqbal, 2015).

Fortunately, healing from VT is possible, and there are several actions that can mitigate against its development. These include self-awareness, regular practice of self-care, supportive supervision, education, and training. These elements, which are discussed in greater detail, are fundamental to maintaining healthy boundaries, ethical practice, and practitioner well-being in all helping professions. The high stress involved in working with traumatized clients means these practices are of paramount importance. In addition, a culture comprised of supportive colleagues is tremendously beneficial and mitigates any self-blame practitioners may have for being adversely affected by their work experience (Iqbal, 2015). In their book, *Trauma Stewardship: An Everyday Guide to Caring for Self while Caring for Others*, Lipsky and Burk (2009) provide an excellent discussion for understanding the effects of trauma exposure along with practical guidance for healing.

BOX 8.1 THE 16 WARNING SIGNS OF TRAUMA EXPOSURE RESPONSE

- Feeling Helpless and Hopeless
- A Sense that One Can Never Do Enough
- Hypervigilance
- Diminished Creativity
- Inability to Embrace Complexity

- Minimizing
- Chronic Exhaustion/Physical Ailments
- Inability to Listen/Deliberate Avoidance
- Dissociative Moments
- Sense of Persecution – feeling a profound lack of efficacy in one's life
- Guilt
- Fear
- Anger and Cynicism
- Inability to Empathize/Numbing
- Addictions
- Grandiosity: An Inflated Sense of Importance Related to One's Work

Source: Lipsky and Burk, 2009, pp. 47–113

Vicarious Resilience

A new concept, vicarious resilience, emerged from the study of mental health professionals who work with survivors of torture. Vicarious resilience is born out of the reciprocal relationship between client and therapist and refers to the ways practitioners can be positively affected by their work with trauma survivors. As clinicians empathically connect with clients who have experienced trauma, they sit face to face with unthinkable stories of powerlessness, in addition to inspiring testimonies of resourcefulness and adaptation. In the joint endeavor of helping clients make sense of and find meaning in their experience, therapists often develop great admiration for their clients and learn from their adversity. They may experience greater appreciation for their internal and environmental strengths, enhanced clarity on their goals and priorities, heightened confidence in their professional skillfulness, and an augmented capacity for compassion and empathy (Iqbal, 2015).

Three interrelated dynamics must be present for therapists to benefit from vicarious resilience: a willingness to be affected by clients, a recognition of how the client's multiple social identities shape their experiences, and conscious acknowledgment of the practitioner's own relationship with power, privilege, or marginalization. When these elements are aligned the therapist is in a position to truly understand their client's journey and learn from their hardship (Hernandez-Wolfe, 2018). The increased self-awareness and learning that develop via vicarious resilience lend themselves to supporting active self-care and ethical practice among practitioners (Hernandez-Wolfe, 2018). Vicarious resilience is congruent with a strengths-based approach in that it emphasizes fortitude and positive growth in the face of tragedy.

BURNOUT

As with all who work in situations of high intensity, working with the bereaved and traumatically bereaved can make practitioners vulnerable to developing a sense of burnout. Maslach and Leiter (2016) define burnout as a psychological condition caused by extended exposure to persistent interpersonal stressors at work. They contend that burnout is characterized by three central features: "overwhelming exhaustion, feelings of cynicism and detachment from the job, and a sense of ineffectiveness and lack of accomplishment" (Maslach & Leiter, 2016, p. 103). Exhaustion may be experienced as fatigue, a sense of apathy about the work, and feeling too depleted to attend to clients. Cynicism and detachment involve disparaging attitudes toward clients, irritability, pessimism, and emotional distancing from clients and co-workers. A reduced sense of effectiveness is reflected in decreased productivity, insufficient capacity to cope, and beliefs that one's work is not valued by others. These symptom clusters highlight the environmental conditions that contribute to burnout and the ways it impacts one's perception of both self and others (Maslach & Leiter, 2016). Burnout develops gradually over a period of time and, if unaddressed, can result in the practitioner leaving the profession.

The risk of developing burnout increases when one's place of employment has a dearth of supportive resources, oppressive policies, when workers have high caseloads and feel a lack of control in the workplace (Lee & Miller, 2013; Maslach & Leiter, 2016). In addition, professionals with a history of trauma, personality disorders, unaddressed anxiety, depression, or addictions are at elevated risk for experiencing burnout (Skinner, 2015). Beginning practitioners who are new to the profession are more apt to experience increased stress in the initial years of their career as they struggle to find a healthy work–life balance and adjust to more realistic expectations for the profession. Insufficient support and supervision also place practitioners at increased risk of developing burnout (Skinner, 2015). Burnout, however, is not an inevitable condition and can be prevented by cultivating self-awareness and practicing self-care.

SELF-AWARENESS

The delivery of quality services to clients is grounded not only in knowledge and skills but in the practitioner's capacity for self-reflection and self-awareness. Self-awareness refers to the ability to recognize one's own thoughts, feelings, attitudes, beliefs, and relationships; to be able to distinguish these from those of the client; and to appreciate the role that these factors play in the helping relationship (Urdang, 2010). Self-awareness evolves with practice, supervision, the ability to acknowledge mistakes, and a desire to learn. It also involves an openness to growing and stepping away from what is familiar and comfortable as new thoughts, feelings, and experiences take their place among formerly held beliefs and attitudes. Self-awareness helps to safeguard practitioners from boundary violations, burnout, and extensive work-related stress (Urdang, 2010).

In addition, there is a notable correlation between self-awareness and the ability to practice cultural humility with clients. Taking time to reflect on and become aware of one's identities, beliefs, biases, and differences allows us to learn how we come to view things the way we do. It also opens us to experiencing conflicts and inconsistencies in our beliefs that force us to question our assumptions and widen how we interpret the behaviors of others. In this regard, practitioners must not only be aware of the intersecting social groups with which they identify including race, ethnicity, gender, sexuality, and social class but to also be cognizant of where they fit in the broader socio-political hierarchy as a result of these identities (Garran & Werkmeister Rozas, 2013). Only by understanding their own relationship with power and privilege can practitioners have a fuller understanding of their reactions to clients as well as the ways that their clients' lives are shaped by these elements. As Garran and Werkmeister Rozas (2013) explain,

> In order to better comprehend certain feelings, inclinations, reactions, and proclivities to one's group one must recognize the role of power and privilege, and how they rule the social order. Locating oneself in the social order is not enough, though. One has to be apprised of the myriad threads of power and privilege which do or do not inhabit his or her identities.
>
> (p. 103)

We all operate in ways that reflect automatic behaviors and responses derived from a combination of individual characteristics and previous life experiences. Ethical practice dictates that clinicians ceaselessly strive for increased insight into their internal responses and the behaviors they generate so that they do not inadvertently impair their interactions with clients. Responses that carry a heightened emotional charge often originate from personal vulnerabilities and past emotional wounds. These sensitivities can easily create "blind spots" in the practitioner's awareness, perception, and judgment and as a result may negatively affect their work with clients (Pomeroy & Garcia, 2018).

While interacting with clients, practitioner self-awareness includes attending to what the client is expressing while simultaneously observing their own thoughts, feelings, and physical sensations. As defined by Fogel (2020), embodied self-awareness is "the present-moment experiencing of sensations that arise from within our bodies, including our emotions" and is considered essential to effectively working with clients, particularly those who are survivors of trauma (p. 39). The concept is based on knowledge of how neural networks process information from the external environment resulting in changes to the autonomic, cardiovascular, respiratory, digestive, hormonal, and immune systems (Fogel, 2020). Though clients are often helped by learning to be mindful of their physical sensations, the therapist's use of embodied self-awareness is also critical to being attuned with those they serve, and thus makes the therapeutic work more productive.

For example, James is meeting with a traumatically bereaved client, Odette, whom he has been seeing for several weeks. During the session, Odette is discussing her feelings of abandonment and becomes very distressed. As she begins sobbing loudly, James notices that he is feeling repulsed by her. He is aware that his jaw has tightened, and he is feeling "put upon" by having to listen to her. He realizes he had the thought of "how can I cheer her up?" which then led to an awareness that he would like to avoid being present to her strong emotions. As he continues to non-judgmentally observe his reaction, he becomes aware that his current feelings toward Odette are similar to those he experiences with his mother who is often dramatic and demanding of James's attention and assistance. This awareness enables James to remind himself that Odette is not his mother and that his role with her is as a professional with defined boundaries. He also recalls a conversation with his supervisor who stressed that being present and attentive with clients who are in great distress is paramount to trying to "fix" their grief. This internal check-in allows James to respond to the client in a manner that is accepting of her intense emotional expression and present to her pain.

Improving Self-Awareness

Practitioners can mitigate the degree to which their personal issues influence their work with clients by using supervision, education, and training to cultivate non-judgmental self-awareness. In addition, acquiring therapy for themselves supports the development of enhanced self-awareness, increased insight, and improved mental and emotional health.

Knapp et al. (2017) recommend the following questions and corresponding actions as an avenue for practitioners to enhance their self-awareness:

- **Am I cognizant of my automatic emotional responses?** Before and after sessions, therapists can be mindful of their "emotional temperature" or review the sentiments their client expressed in the session and recall their internal responses.
- **Am I correct in how I assess my knowledge and expertise?** To guard against the common tendency to overestimate their abilities, practitioners can obtain collegial support, participate in professional study groups, and obtain supervision to more accurately assess what constitutes quality work. They can also request that their clients complete evidence-based evaluations on the services they received.
- **Do I accept that I possess unconscious preconceived biases?** While it is not comfortable to admit to having prejudices, it is an inherent part of being human. Because rebuke usually only encourages denial or avoidance, it is far more effective to accept this fact with compassion, which can then lead to honest reflection and productive learning. While being non-judgmental with clients is the desired result, a more attainable goal would be to *manage* the judgments we carry, a practice that is grounded in self-awareness.
- **Am I completely aware of my personal and professional values?** Clinicians must know themselves and be mindful of how their beliefs guide their actions. This helps them more easily recognize value conflicts within themselves and with their clients. A written list of values or objects that symbolize these values can serve as visible reminders.

SELF-CARE

An essential element of being self-aware involves the ability to acknowledge one's physical, mental, emotional, and spiritual needs and limitations. Working with the bereaved and survivors of trauma is a very demanding endeavor focused on serving others. On top of this, many helping professionals carry large caseloads, must meet numerous bureaucratic requirements, and work in organizations that are continually expecting them to do more with less. Practitioners can easily become stretched so thin that they have no reserves left for caring for themselves or lose sight of what their needs are altogether. When continually pouring from an empty cup, practitioners are left with an inadequate supply of the internal physical and psychological energy needed to stay professionally effective. These are prime conditions for developing physical and mental health problems, vicarious trauma, and burnout, and when unaddressed can negatively impact clients. Hence, practicing self-care is indispensable to providing quality services to clients and thus is considered an ethical obligation and required behavior of practitioners (Flint, 2018).

In addition to mitigating work-related stress, self-care "can serve as a means of empowerment that enables practitioners to proactively and intentionally negotiate their overall health, well-being, and resilience" (Lee & Miller, 2013, p. 96). A lifestyle that includes regular self-care practices helps practitioners maintain professional effectiveness, enjoy their work, and sustain a lengthy career in the profession (Flint, 2018). Self-care can be categorized into two distinct but tacitly intertwined processes: personal self-care and professional self-care. Personal self-care focuses on nurturing and replenishing one's self outside of the professional role assumed in the work environment (Skinner, 2015). Professional self-care entails practices that enhance the "effective and appropriate use of the self in the professional role" (Lee & Miller, 2013, p. 98).

Lee and Miller (2013) suggest that self-care practices can be grouped into separate structures of support for personal and professional self-care. Using these structures of support, practitioners can create a personalized self-care plan that addresses their unique needs and is suitable to their personality and environment. Structures of support for personal self-care direct attention to the following domains: physical, psychological and emotional, social, spiritual, and leisure. Structures of support for professional self-care include managing the amount of work and effective use of time, providing support to one's role as a professional, being mindful of one's behavior and attitudes about work, spending time with supportive colleagues, advocating for one's work role or profession, and continuing education (Lee & Miller, 2013, p. 100).

Self-care practices can take many forms and are unique to the individual. Playing with dogs, for example, may feel restorative for one worker but draining to another. Some examples of personal self-care behaviors include the following:

- Attending to the body's cues to eat, sleep, hydrate, and use the bathroom
- Eating nutritious foods
- Exercising
- Expressing emotions in healthy ways such as with journaling or therapy
- Nurturing personal relationships
- Spending time with family and friends
- Engaging in enjoyable activities
- Making time for relaxation
- Spending time in nature
- Participating in a community of positive and supportive people
- Attending to one's need for purpose, meaning, creativity, and hope
- Engaging in art forms such as music, dance, painting, or theater
- Meditating
- Participating in a faith community.

Some examples of professional self-care include the following:

- Taking breaks from work
- Planning one's tasks for the day
- Being organized
- Arriving and leaving work on schedule
- Attending relevant meetings on time
- Developing efficient systems for accomplishing tasks
- Participating in supervision and consultation
- Collaborating with colleagues
- Getting additional education and training
- Expressing workplace needs and concerns to management
- Advocating for the profession.

An intentional and active commitment to self-care practices and the use of readily available coping strategies are key to sustaining a vibrant personal and professional life. All practitioners need to develop strategies to care for their personal and professional needs and be attuned to what self-care entails for them. In addition, practitioners should know their personal warning signs that may signal the need for increased attention to self-care. The Self-Care Awareness exercise at the end of this chapter can guide practitioners in becoming thoughtful and deliberate stewards of themselves.

While self-care is most commonly considered an individual endeavor, organizations also play an important role in supporting staff members' needs in culturally relevant ways (Pyles, 2020). This involves deliberately attending to the way that institutionalized practices influence counselor well-being. Elements to be considered include management and leadership style, discriminatory practices, caseload numbers and complexities, job descriptions, camaraderie among workers, and the availability of supervision (Flint, 2018). In addition, the organizational culture should be one that values the need for self-care and understands it is an expected and necessary aspect of sustaining quality services to clients (Cayir et al., 2020).

PROFESSIONAL SUPERVISION AND CONSULTATION

Supervision is an important component of competent practice and the delivery of quality services. In addition to providing the practitioner with objective and expert guidance, supervision can powerfully attenuate how clinicians are affected by their work (Knight, 2018). Although supervisors do not provide counseling on personal issues to their supervisees, they play an important role in helping supervisees recognize and make sense of how they respond to their work with clients, including the exposure to trauma and loss that is experienced. By legitimizing and normalizing their reactions, supervisors empower clinicians to select self-care strategies that will help them manage the ways the work impacts them (Knight, 2018). This is particularly important for grief counselors who are also grieving personal losses.

Just as trauma-informed care is recommended for use with clients (see Chapter 3), trauma-informed supervision is equally important for clinicians. Trauma-informed supervision, grounded in a relational approach, is characterized by kindness, compassion, and acceptance that fosters collaboration and teamwork between supervisor and supervisee. By creating an atmosphere of trust, supervisees have the safety to be open and vulnerable about clinical matters and concerns, and also reflect on the impact the work is having on them without fear of judgment or reprisal. Also, fundamental to trauma-informed supervision is well-defined boundaries and expectations along with frequent and reliable availability for consultation (Berger et al., 2018; Hazen et al., 2020; Knight, 2018).

While all practitioners benefit from this kind of supervision, it is of crucial importance for clinicians providing services to traumatically bereaved persons because it models the approach clinicians should use with their clients and enhances experiential learning. As is true when working with clients, the relationship is one of shared power in which the supervisee's viewpoints are heard respectfully and decisions are made jointly (Berger et al., 2018). The benefits of this approach are further amplified when combined with a strengths-based orientation. Like clients, practitioners are empowered through emphasizing their successes, highlighting their proficient use of skills, and acknowledging evidence of growth (Berger & Quiros, 2014).

Throughout one's career, continued consultation is highly recommended for both beginning and seasoned practitioners. Indeed, it is an ethical obligation for practitioners to obtain professional consultation and ensures competent practice with clients (Pomeroy & Garcia, 2018).

CONTINUING EDUCATION AND TRAINING

The knowledge base of mental health, grief and loss, and trauma is continually evolving. As emerging problems require study and new investigations are undertaken, practitioners are obligated to stay informed on research, theories, and methods for helping clients, and to obtain additional training to enhance their skills. Doing so enables professionals to honor their respective ethical codes, "practice within their area of competence and develop and enhance their professional expertise" (National Association of Social Workers [NASW], 2017). Certainly, clients are entitled to qualified and competent service (NASW, 2003). Continuing education also allows practitioners the ability to advance themselves in the field, enhance their career satisfaction, and buffer them from frustration and burnout.

Practitioners are encouraged to become life-long learners. More than simply training, continuing education is life-enhancing, motivating, and cultivates relationships with other professionals. Participating in educational seminars and workshops often results in a renewed sense of commitment and enthusiasm as well as recharging a practitioner's energy for practice.

PROFESSIONAL ETHICS AND VALUES IN GRIEF COUNSELING

While each professional counseling association has their own code of ethics regarding professional and ethical conduct of practice, we will focus on the National Association of Social Workers (NASW) Code of Ethics and apply it to work with bereaved and traumatically bereaved clients. The NASW Code of Ethics sets forth the mission and core values of the profession, the ethical standards as they relate to clients, and outlines the social worker's commitment to client well-being, self-determination, cultural sensitivity, confidentiality, and respect. In addition, the standards provide the social worker with a set of guidelines for providing informed consent, competent record keeping, fees for service, and other administrative duties for ethical practice. The standards provide guidelines, not rules, for conducting social work practice and set forth a set of core values on which social workers can base their ethical decision making. These core values include service, social justice, dignity and worth of the person, importance of human relationships, integrity, and competence. The code of ethics embodies the mission and responsibilities of social workers in a broad variety of practice milieus and is not meant to dictate daily activities of the social work profession. The complete code of ethics can be found on the NASW website at www.naswdc.org.

In addition, NASW has established specific ethical standards for palliative and end of life care, including bereavement and grief counseling. These standards suggest that social workers practicing in this specialized area should have an adequate knowledge base of the potential ethical issues and value conflicts that may arise. NASW has outlined 11 ethical standards as they relate to palliative and end of life care. The standards shown in Box 8.2 are discussed in detail in the NASW Standards for Palliative and End of Life Care (2004) which may be accessed at www.naswdc.org.

BOX 8.2 NASW STANDARDS FOR PALLIATIVE AND END OF LIFE CARE

Standard 1: Ethics and Values
Standard 2: Knowledge
Standard 3: Assessment
Standard 4: Intervention/Treatment Planning
Standard 5: Attitude/Self-Awareness
Standard 6: Empowerment and Advocacy
Standard 7: Documentation
Standard 8: Interdisciplinary Teamwork
Standard 9: Cultural Competence
Standard 10: Continuing Education
Standard 11: Supervision, Leadership, and Training

Source: NASW, 2004, pp. 4–5

These standards are an integral component of ethical grief counseling and permeate the process of assessment and intervention with bereaved clients. It is important that practitioners be familiar with their respective profession's code of ethics.

Self-Care Awareness Exercise:

1. Name three things that you enjoy doing outside of work.
2. What are some actions you can take to create a boundary between your work life and your personal life?
3. What are some thoughts or behaviors that can serve as signals to you that you may be in danger of developing vicarious trauma or are in need of self-care?
4. What are some potential triggers that could place you at risk for vicarious trauma?
5. What support systems do you have in place to help you cope both personally and professionally?

THE INVISIBLE SUITCASE ANALOGY

The Invisible Suitcase analogy offers a metaphor for understanding the impact of prior grief experiences on the practitioner and the dynamic interaction between client and counselor in the therapeutic relationship. Developed by Ian Woodroffe, the Invisible Suitcase analogy provides a method for uncovering those internal responses to grief that may be hidden from conscious awareness. This analogy is easy to understand and remember making it useful in practitioner training as well as in direct work with clients. Woodroffe explains the Invisible Suitcase analogy as follows:

When you were born, you were given an invisible suitcase. You cannot detach yourself from your suitcase, so it has been with you all your life regardless of how old you are! Two things you need to know about your invisible suitcase:

1. It packs itself – you have no control over the packing process.
2. It opens itself and usually you have no control over where and when your suitcase opens.

Since you were born, your suitcase has packed itself and for the sake of convenience, the material packed in your suitcase has been divided into three categories:

- **Category #1 – Facts**
  - Factual information has been packed in the suitcase (e.g. dates, these are "uncluttered facts")
  - *How many inches in a foot?*
  - *What is your mother's maiden name?*
  - *What is your birth date?*

- **Category #2 – Facts and Emotions**
  - These are facts that have emotions attached to the fact. The fact and the emotion are inseparable and as soon as the fact is recalled the emotions are instantly in the present.
  - *Perhaps it is an anniversary date?*
  - *The day you graduated from college?*
  - *What happened on 9/11?*
- **Category #3 – Emotions**
  - Packed in your suitcase may be some emotions that are not consciously attached to any fact or event. "Free Floating Emotions" may surface at any time without us being aware of why.
  - *Have you ever listened to music that suddenly brings you to tears?*

So your suitcase has packed itself with:

- Facts
- Facts and Emotions
- Emotions.

Your suitcase opens itself!

- Your suitcase opens itself and usually when you *least* expect it!
- The suitcase is opened by "triggers" – such as dates, sounds, smells, places, gestures, lookalikes, seasons, tastes, familiar words/phrases.

How the suitcase opens:

- This opening process is unconscious which is why we never know where or when the suitcase may open.
- Without thinking, suddenly it opens and the accompanying emotions are upon us.
- The opening process is timeless. Many, many years later the emotions from a past event can come to the surface just when we thought we had forgotten.

Your opened suitcase:

- What has been packed in your suitcase may come from your personal life or your work life.
- When the suitcase opens and powerful emotions surface from the past, there is always a purpose for the emotions to "come to light."
- It may be that some pressure needs to be released – that emotions at the time were "tidied away" and now wish to be expressed – that some "emotional healing" still needs to take place.

What do you do?

- When your suitcase opens, you have a choice. You can acknowledge what has happened or you can close your suitcase.

Uh oh, my suitcase just exploded!

- The best way of acknowledging your suitcase has opened is to share what has happened with someone who will not judge you or make fun of you.
- When you share your experience with another, you need someone who will listen without asking lots of questions, someone who will understand that you may be feeling pain and who will not try to "make it better."
- Sharing your experience will not remove it from your suitcase. It probably means that if this past emotion is triggered again in the future it will be less intense.
- You may choose to close your suitcase and there may be a very sound reason why you do this, e.g. public exposure, an inappropriate time, etc. You may close your suitcase because that is what you have always done.
- Constantly closing your suitcase may have consequences. Our physical body is connected to our emotional body. We have a sense of well-being when our physical and emotional/spiritual (if that is the word you would use) is in balance.
- This means that if our emotions are not expressed appropriately then we may become "out of balance." The unexpressed emotions may turn into physical symptoms or altered behaviors.
- Sometimes it is wise to think about our physical symptoms in light of what is happening to us in our emotional life.
- Sometimes we can attend to the physical symptoms, but miss being aware of the emotions.
- Constant closure of your suitcase can damage your health. Self-awareness can be the foundation of a sense of well-being. Awareness of other people's feelings is the foundation for support and care.
- Respect your suitcase as you journey through life. This is part of the experience of life, including grieving a loss.

With permission from Ian Woodroffe, "The Invisible Suitcase." No part of this metaphor may be reproduced without the written permission of the author. (ian@goldtraining.co.uk)

Invisible Suitcase Exercise:

1. Create a list of ten experiences that are packed in your suitcase.
2. List some emotions connected with these experiences.
3. List some triggers associated with these experiences and emotions.
4. Recall a time when your suitcase opened unexpectedly. Describe what happened and how you responded.
5. What client situations could potentially open your suitcase?
6. What would be appropriate steps to take if your suitcase opens?

CASES

CASE 8.1

Identifying Information:

Client Name: Veronica Maldonado
Age: 24 years old
Race/Ethnicity: Hispanic
Marital Status: In a relationship with a man
Educational Level: Master's degree
Occupation: Social worker

Background Information:

Veronica began working full-time in the bereavement department at a hospice nine months ago. Her primary job duty is to provide counseling to the families of the hospice's patients, in addition to bereaved persons in the wider community. She also leads a support group for people who have lost their mothers. The following is Veronica's first session with Anita Davenport, a therapist with over 15 years of experience.

Initial Interview:

ANITA: Tell me what brings you here, Veronica.

VERONICA: I just feel so stressed out all the time! I feel like I'm losing my mind. I just can't seem to keep it all together.

ANITA: Tell me what is stressing you out?

VERONICA: I don't know, exactly. That's part of the problem. It just seems to be this permanent state I'm in. I'm either really tense or completely exhausted or both.

ANITA: Tell me more about what you *feel* when you are stressed out? Are you anxious, afraid, sad, angry…?

VERONICA: It's anxiety, I guess. And I'm more irritable than I normally am. I seem to get frustrated very easily.

ANITA: What are some things that frustrate you?

VERONICA: Well, last weekend my boyfriend went out of town. He was supposed to be back by 2 p.m. on Sunday. Well, 2 o'clock came and went and I didn't hear from him. I kept calling him on his cell phone, but I guess he was out of range. He didn't get in until two hours later. I absolutely flipped out. I told him that if he was going to be late, he needed to call me and let me know!

ANITA: What specifically about your boyfriend being late and not calling upset you?

VERONICA: I was worried. What if something had happened to him? I kept having visions of him lying dead on the highway!

ANITA: I see. What are some other examples of times that you have felt frustrated or anxious?

VERONICA: Let's see.… Well, there is always work. I can't seem to get all my documentation done and I always have a list of clients that I need to call. By the time I get home, I'm completely wiped out. I practically fall into bed but then I can't get to sleep!

ANITA: What's happening that you can't sleep?

VERONICA: I just can't turn my mind off.

ANITA: What are you thinking about?

VERONICA: Work, usually – like all the stuff I need to do the next day. And my clients.

ANITA: What kinds of thoughts are you having about your clients?

VERONICA: I find myself playing the sessions over again in my head and thinking about what I said and what I might say in our next session. And sometimes I'm just imagining the stories they have told me. Actually, that is probably why I flipped out on my boyfriend. You see, I have a client right now who was in a car accident with her husband. She survived, but he died at the scene. It's been very traumatic for her and she has really come to depend on me to help her through it.

ANITA: So, do you think your reaction to your boyfriend being late was really a reaction to hearing such a traumatic story from your client?

VERONICA: Yeah, I guess so. I hadn't realized that until just now.

ANITA: It sounds like you are working during the day and at night! It's no wonder you are exhausted! And hearing intimate details of such sad and traumatic stories will certainly take a toll on you. Do you think that could be the source of your stress?

VERONICA: You are probably right. I do seem to carry all of my clients' stories around with me. I find that I think about them all the time.

ANITA: How is that for you?

VERONICA: It drains me. And if you stop to think about it, it's really unsettling how such tragic things happen to people every day and that it can happen to anyone at any time. I think it's been making me worry about my mom more lately. I see these people in my Loss of Mother group just agonizing over their mother's death. I imagine what that would be like for me, and it's just awful. I would be a mess if I lost her! Sometimes I feel like I'm just waiting for my mom to die. Not that I want her to! But I know that she will someday. When you do this kind of work you are constantly reminded of that. I've even had nightmares about it.

ANITA: I see that you are getting a little teary as you talk about this.

VERONICA: Yes, I guess I haven't realized the kind of impact my work has been having on me.

ANITA: It sounds like we need to help you find ways to take care of yourself while you are doing this kind of work. Tell me, what is your caseload like? How many clients are you seeing?

VERONICA: I see about 30 or so people per week and facilitate the support group.

ANITA: My goodness! That's a full load! What is your schedule like? Is it a 9 to 5 schedule?

VERONICA: My schedule is different every week. It varies depending on when the clients can meet with me. Sometimes I have a lot of morning appointments and sometimes I see more people in the evenings. And then some days I see clients in the morning and in the evening with gaps of time in between. I usually use that time to catch up on my documentation, though.

ANITA: You know, Veronica, if I had a work situation like yours, I think I would feel very stressed out. Not only are you working around the clock in some fashion or another, but you have a high caseload, some very tough and painful client situations, and it doesn't sound like you really have any time for yourself! Am I right? Do you feel like you have a life outside of your work?

VERONICA: No. You're right. Work is my life. And actually, my boyfriend snapped at me the other day and said, "Can we please talk about something besides your job?"

ANITA: So, work seems to be taking over your personal life and is even interfering with your relationship.

VERONICA: Yeah, I guess it is. But what am I supposed to do? My clients are vulnerable and in tremendous pain. They need me. How am I supposed to just cut them off?

ANITA: If you are working with bereaved persons you are certainly working with people who are in a great deal of pain and, yes, your clients are at a vulnerable place in their lives right now. Your dedication to your clients is outstanding, Veronica. But I'm concerned about how long you can keep this up and how effective you can be with your clients when you are so stressed out that you have become a client yourself.

VERONICA: I guess I thought I was just doing my job and being a dedicated social worker.

ANITA: All of that is true. And perhaps you have some unrealistic expectations about what your clients expect from you and what is realistic to expect from yourself. Very often when people are in a vulnerable, needy place, they will take everything you offer them. Our goal with clients, however, is not to create a dependence on us but to help them know how to help themselves. Does that make sense to you?

VERONICA: I think so.

ANITA: Also Veronica, remember that being a counselor does not make you superhuman. In fact, it's your humanity and your superb ability to have empathy for other people that makes your work so intense and personal for you.

VERONICA: Hmm...I think I understand what you mean.

ANITA: And as you well know, your relationship with your clients is everything. It's the foundation upon which you are able to be productive in your work with them. A healthy and productive client–therapist relationship begins with a healthy therapist. In other words, I am concerned not only about how all of this is affecting you but how it is affecting your clients.

VERONICA: Wow. I had never really looked at it that way.

ANITA: I am sure you tell your clients about the importance of self-care.

VERONICA: Yes, all the time.

ANITA: Are you practicing what you preach? Are you taking care of yourself?

VERONICA: Not really. I guess I figured that it didn't apply to me because I'm a counselor.

Anita and Veronica continue to talk about ways that Veronica could set boundaries at her work and implement a practice of self-care. Veronica schedules another appointment with Anita for the following week.

8.1-1. Do you think Veronica is at risk for developing vicarious trauma or burnout? Provide evidence to support your answer.

8.1-2. What perspectives does Veronica have about herself and her work that contribute to her stress?

8.1-3. What are some possible solutions to help Veronica manage the stress of her work?

8.1-4. How might Veronica use her therapy with Anita to help her cope with the work stresses in life-enhancing ways?

8.1-5. How does participation in outside activities ameliorate vicarious trauma?

CASE 8.2

Identifying Information:

Name: Jenny Jackson
Age: 30 years old
Race/Ethnicity: African American
Marital Status: Married
Educational Level: Master's degree
Occupation: Social worker

Consultation with Supervisor, Elizabeth Martin:

Jenny schedules an appointment with her supervisor to discuss the following family with whom she had an initial interview.

Background Information:

Gary, a 58-year-old Chief Financial Officer of a large corporation, sought counseling with his two young adult, unmarried children after his wife of 35 years died in a tragic boating accident. He stated that they have a house on the lake and over Labor Day, several boats full of people collided. His wife was the only person who died from the accident. Gary was primarily interested in getting counseling for his two children, Wendy and Michelle. He stated that although he misses his wife, he has found a new partner that he plans to marry. The children, both in their mid-20s, tell Jenny that it's not right; it's too soon after their mother's death; this woman is just after their father's money and home; and that she's 20 years younger than he is. They add that their mother only died five months ago and that they are furious with their father for jumping into another relationship without giving them a chance to resolve their own grief. They feel like he doesn't care about their feelings and that he didn't really care about their mother. It is clear that Gary wants counseling for his children so that they will accept his new fiancée. It is also clear that the children want Jenny to convince Gary of the egregious mistake he will make if he marries this new woman.

JENNY: So, that's the information I have, so far. I don't have any idea of what to do now.

ELIZABETH: Did you meet with the family together or with the father separately from the children?

JENNY: I met with all of them together. Do you think I need to meet with the children separately?

ELIZABETH: You might want to schedule an appointment with the children and the father separately since it sounds like there is a lot of tension between father and children. It would give all of them an opportunity to tell you how they are really feeling without filtering their feelings or information.

JENNY: Okay, that sounds like a good idea. But I'm also concerned about getting caught in the middle of this family battle.

ELIZABETH: Take a step back and look at the situation. What do you think is the major underlying theme that's going on with this family?

JENNY: I'm not sure. It seems like everyone is angry at everyone else. Those girls were absolutely furious with their father. And the father is not too happy with his children either.

ELIZABETH: Okay, so there is a lot of anger in the family. What else?

JENNY: Well, the two girls seem very defensive since they feel like an intruder has stepped into their lives. And Gary is being fairly self-centered right now, it seems.

ELIZABETH: So, it sounds like you might be siding with the girls?

JENNY: Hmmm, does it sound that way? I hadn't thought about it but maybe I am.

ELIZABETH: I think with family situations where there is conflict you have to be careful not to be triangulated into the family drama. You can become the third party that the other two parties can either side with or blame for everything that goes wrong. Does that make sense?

JENNY: Oh, yes, I can see how that could happen. I'm still wondering how to deal with Gary and the daughters.

ELIZABETH: Yes, let's get back to what is really going on in this family. Do you have any other thoughts about that?

JENNY: Well, I guess there's a lot of family conflict following the death of the mother/wife that needs to be worked out.

ELIZABETH: Yes, I agree and what is that conflict REALLY about?

JENNY: Oh, I see what you are getting at. The whole family is going through the grief process in different ways. Is that what you're talking about?

ELIZABETH: Yes, that's my take on it. Gary seems to either be in denial about his grief or is feeling very lonely without a partner and wants to fill that empty space in his life.

JENNY: His daughters, on the other hand, are still in the initial phases of grief and are feeling very attached to their mother. Their allegiance is with her and they can't tolerate the thought of her being replaced.

ELIZABETH: Quite a family dilemma, wouldn't you say?

JENNY: Yes, and I don't want to create a bigger problem by getting caught in the middle of this family's dilemma. Do you think I should just see Gary individually and then schedule a separate appointment for the daughters?

ELIZABETH: Jenny, as you know, grief isn't a black or white issue. In fact, most of the time, people who are going through the grief process are in a very gray area of their lives. Put yourself in Gary's place for a moment. He's 58 years old and just lost his wife in an accident. He's a very successful businessman and has his whole life ahead of him. What do you think he's thinking about?

JENNY: If I were in Gary's place, I'd be feeling very sad and lonely. I'd be thinking about my daughters who are grown and living their own lives and about being alone. Success doesn't mean much if you are all by yourself. Here's a man who was married for 35 years so he doesn't know how to be single. He probably hates being alone and wants company. This younger woman is attracted to him which makes him feel good and like he's being given another chance in life. Am I on the right track?

ELIZABETH: Your ideas are good possibilities. Now, put yourself in the daughters' place. What would you be thinking and feeling?

JENNY: You see it's easier for me to identify with the daughters since I'm female and closer to their ages. So I can imagine how traumatic it would be to lose my mother at such a young age and feel totally grief-stricken and lost. I would imagine they have been thinking about all the things that they will miss about having their mother around and all the future things she will not be a part of. They are probably grieving the fact that she won't be at their weddings, the births of their children, all the events that will happen in the future for them. It could take a long time before their grief begins to subside and it could take a lifetime before they feel there isn't a hole in their lives left by their mother. Does that make sense?

ELIZABETH: Yes, those issues are probably very real for the daughters right now. And, how do these two different cases make you feel?

JENNY: I guess I do empathize more with the daughters because of their gender and age. It's just easier for me to imagine. But, I can also see Gary's perspective and what his needs might be right now.

ELIZABETH: Yes, so let's look at some options. What are some ways that you could work effectively with this family?

JENNY: Well, one option would be to see them separately for one or two sessions and then try to get them to work out their differences together. Another option would be to just see the daughters separately from the father and let them process their grief reactions so that they can accept the fact that the mother is gone and that Gary is going to move on with his life.

Jenny pauses for a moment and then begins thinking out loud.

I wonder, though, if it would be an ethical issue for me to see the father and the daughters separately. Maybe I should refer either the father or the daughters to another therapist. Maybe it would be unethical for me to see the father individually and then the daughters separately. Maybe I can't be unbiased in this case or maybe I can't get caught in the middle of this conflict, so I need to refer someone to another therapist. I'm not sure what to do.

ELIZABETH: Jenny, you've come up with several options. I think it would be wise to see Gary individually for one session and the daughters individually for one session and I think you'll have much more assessment information upon which to base your decision. In the meantime, it might be good to read through the code of ethics and see if there are issues that resonate with this case that you need to consider. Once you've seen Gary and the daughters separately, let's meet again and discuss the next steps. How does that sound?

JENNY: That makes sense to me. I will schedule them for next week. Thanks.

8.2-1. List three new insights that Jenny had about this case as a result of supervision.
8.2-2. If you were Jenny, what questions would you want to ask the daughters in the next session?
8.2-3. If you were Jenny, what questions would you want to ask the father in the next session?
8.2-4. Read over the code of ethics of your profession and note the standards that relate to this ethical dilemma.
8.2-5. What do you think Jenny should do in this case?

CASE 8.3

A Day in the Life of a Grief Counselor:

Claire Harper is a licensed master social worker with seven years of clinical social work experience. For the last three years she has worked in the bereavement department of a hospice agency doing pre- and post-death bereavement counseling and grief support groups. A typical workday for Claire consists of the following:

Claire wakes in time to work out at the gym, dress, eat a good breakfast, and get into work by 9 a.m. She spends the first hour at her job checking voicemail messages, reading agency memos, making chit chat with other staff members, and catching up on client documentation. She sees her first client at 10 a.m. – Mr. Sanchez, an elderly man whose wife died of a long terminal illness. After this session, Claire has just enough time to complete the documentation for this client before seeing her next client, Jared, a young man whose girlfriend committed suicide. The session with Jared was pretty intense due to the traumatic nature of the death. Claire jotted down some notes to help her remember what she would need to document and took a few moments before her next session to stretch, get something to drink, and confirm her lunch plans with her co-worker, Deborah. Claire's noontime session was with Carlos, a very active and demanding 4-year-old boy whose father died in a work-related accident. This was Claire's third session with Carlos and she knows that his high energy level and short attention span often leave her feeling spent after their sessions. This is why she schedules Carlos right before lunch – she knows she will need the break before seeing clients again.

Claire thinks to herself, "Thank goodness I was able to persuade my supervisor to let me schedule my own clients. That little bit of self-advocacy has gone a long way toward keeping me sane in this job!" Just as she is about to leave her desk to go to lunch, her phone rings. "Sorry, folks," Claire says to herself. "I'm off duty!" She continues out the door and lets her voicemail get the call.

Claire and Deborah go to lunch together at a nearby cafeteria. Deborah works in the agency's marketing department. Claire and Deborah talk about some new policies that the agency has just issued and a lot about their personal lives. Claire enjoys spending time with Deborah because she is always able to make Claire laugh.

Every now and then, Claire calls Deborah and says, "I'm getting too serious! When can I get my next dose of Deborah?" Deborah and Claire have also committed to encouraging each other to exercise and eat well. Claire and Deborah finish lunch quickly so that they have some time to peruse their favorite shoe store, a delightful diversion from death and dying!

Upon returning to the agency, Claire returns a few phone calls, schedules a couple of sessions for the following week and begins her trek down the hallway, one she does several times a day, to retrieve her next client. Claire notices how she has come to use this time walking the hallway to transition back into her role as counselor. Thoughts of those shoes that caught her eye during lunch are filed away for consideration at another time. She takes deep breaths and deliberate steps. It's as if she is psychologically dressing herself for a special occasion.

Claire's next session is with Julia, a blind woman whose seeing eye dog died. For Claire, Julia's story is particularly sad, and she finds herself getting slightly tearful during the session. After the session, Claire adds Julia's name to the list of things she wants to discuss in her next supervision meeting. Though she couldn't articulate precisely what about this session moved her more than any other, especially at that moment with her next client waiting in the lobby, she senses that Julia's story "opened her suitcase" and thus will merit more attention from her.

Claire's next session is with Hannah, an 8-year-old girl whose father died of cancer. Claire has grown quite fond of Hannah during their three months of seeing each other and their work together seems to be the reason for Hannah's improvements. In fact, it may soon be time to start tapering off the frequency of Hannah's sessions, even though Claire will miss seeing her. Claire makes another note to ask her supervisor about this. Claire finds herself feeling quite proud that her work with Hannah has gone so well, and, she'll admit, a little surprised, too. Claire's experience working with children is not as extensive as her experience with adults. Those conferences she attended last year really helped her feel more confident and knowledgeable about how to work with children. "It's nice," she thinks, "to see that it paid off."

Claire's final work duty is attendance at a case staffing meeting in which staff members from other disciplines (nursing, home health, occupational therapy, etc.) meet to discuss the clients they are serving. Claire is attending this staffing because she has been working with the Aguilar family on issues related to anticipatory grief. It's insightful for Claire to hear of the interactions other staff members have had with Mrs. Aguilar and her son, Roberto, but she also feels disturbed by some of the comments she hears that imply criticism and judgment of the family. Claire takes a deep breath and says to herself, "Here I go!" before jumping into the conversation. Claire points out some of the family's strengths that are relevant to the discussion and does some educating about family dynamics associated with anticipatory grief. This seems to temper the staff members' judgmental attitudes and gives them a more compassionate way of thinking about the Aguilar family. "Whew!" she thinks. Though it always makes her a little nervous, Claire prides herself on her ability to advocate for her clients in a way that doesn't alienate the staff or raise their defenses.

With the termination of the case staffing, the end of Claire's day is in sight. She returns to her desk to finish up some client documentation, return phone calls, and make copies of the materials she wants to hand out in the support group she is facilitating later that week.

Claire can't help but sigh with pleasure as she leaves the agency building and feels the fresh air hit her face. She turns off the agency phone she is required to carry during work hours and begins her journey home, pondering the day's events and digesting the stories she has heard that day. Once home, Claire changes into some comfortable clothes. Though she does this for physical comfort and ease, this ritual has also become a metaphor for helping Claire separate herself from the stories, the facial expressions, the worries, and the tears of the clients she has seen that day. The fall of her worn work clothes as they sink into the laundry hamper signify the final act of separation. Now is Claire's time.

Claire's boyfriend, Lawrence, joins her for dinner after which they look at travel magazines and make vacation plans. As Claire flips through the pages of one magazine, her eyes land on an advertisement featuring a golden retriever.

"Oh," Claire says. "This dog reminds me of Lucy!"

"Who is Lucy?" Lawrence asks.

"She was the dog I had in my childhood," Claire answers. "My parents got her as a puppy when I was just a baby. We kind of grew up together."

Claire thinks to herself, "Maybe that's why Julia's story about losing her guide dog rattled me. I remember being devastated when Lucy died."

Claire goes on to share fond memories of Lucy with Lawrence. It somehow makes her feel a little better to remember Lucy out loud.

As evening approaches, Claire and Lawrence say goodnight and she prepares for bed. She cuddles up with a good book and loses herself in another world, one that has nothing to do with death and dying, until sleep is irresistible.

8.3-1. Identify the things Claire does to balance her work life with her personal life.

8.3-2. Identify the things Claire does that help her stay fresh and alert for her clients.

8.3-3. What are some methods that Claire uses to make the transition between her personal life and her work life?

8.3-4. How will Claire's self-awareness help her maintain her effectiveness with her clients? Write a short paragraph using the Suitcase Theory.

8.3-5. What did you like about the way Claire conducted her day? What would you change? Why?

8.3-6. In 150–300 words, describe your ideal job as a grief counselor. What are your hopes and fears? What do you perceive your strengths to be in your role as a grief counselor?

REFERENCES

Berger, R., & Quiros, L. (2014). Supervision for trauma-informed practice. *Traumatology*, *20*(4), 296–301. https://doi.org/10.1037/h0099835

Berger, R., Quiros, L., & Benavidez-Hatzis, J. R. (2018). The intersection of identities in supervision for trauma-informed practice: Challenges and strategies. *The Clinical Supervisor*, *37*(1), 122–141. https://doi.org/10.1080/07325223.2017.1376299

Boulanger, G. (2018). When is vicarious trauma a necessary therapeutic tool? *Psychoanalytic Psychology*, *35*(1), 60–69. https://doi.org/10.1037/pap0000089

Cayir, E., Spencer, M., Billings, D., Hilfinger Messias, D. K., Robillard, A., & Cunningham, T. (2020). "The only way we'll be successful": Organizational factors that influence psychosocial well-being and self-care among advocates working to address gender-based violence. *Journal of Interpersonal Violence*, 088626051989734. https://doi.org/10.1177/0886260519897340

Flint, S. M. (2018). Preventing vicarious trauma in counselors through the implementation of self-care practices. *The Alabama Counseling Association Journal*, *42*(1), 111–127.

Fogel, A. (2020). Three states of embodied self-awareness: The therapeutic vitality of restorative embodied self-awareness. *International Body Psychotherapy Journal*, *19*(1).

Garran, A. M., & Werkmeister Rozas, L. (2013). Cultural competence revisited. *Journal of Ethnic and Cultural Diversity in Social Work*, *22*(2), 97–111. https://doi.org/10.1080/15313204.2013.785337

Hazen, K. P., Carlson, M. W., Hatton-Bowers, H., Fessinger, M. B., Cole-Mossman, J., Bahm, J., Hauptman, K., Brank, E. M., & Gilkerson, L. (2020). Evaluating the facilitating attuned interactions (FAN) approach: Vicarious trauma, professional burnout, and reflective practice. *Children and Youth Services Review*, *112*, 104925. https://doi.org/10.1016/j.childyouth.2020.104925

Hernandez-Wolfe, P. (2018). Vicarious resilience: A comprehensive review. *Revista de Estudios Sociales*, (66), 9–17. https://doi.org/10.7440/res66.2018.02

Iqbal, A. (2015). The ethical considerations of counselling psychologists working with trauma: Is there a risk of vicarious traumatisation? *Counselling Psychology Review*, *30*(1), 44–51.

Knapp, S., Gottlieb, M. C., & Handelsman, M. M. (2017). Self-awareness questions for effective psychotherapists: Helping good psychotherapists become even better. *Practice Innovations*, *2*(4), 163–172. https://doi.org/10.1037/pri0000051

Knight, C. (2018). Trauma-informed supervision: Historical antecedents, current practice, and future directions. *The Clinical Supervisor*, *37*(1), 7–37. https://doi.org/10.1080/07325223.2017.1413607

Lee, J., & Miller, S. (2013). A self-care framework for social workers: Building a strong foundation for practice. *Families in Society: The Journal of Contemporary Social Services*, *94*(2), 96–103. https://doi.org/10.1606/1044-3894.4289

Lipsky, L. V., & Burk, C. (2009). *Trauma stewardship: An everyday guide to caring for self while caring for others*. Berrett-Koehler Publishers.

Maslach, C., & Leiter, M. P. (2016). Understanding the burnout experience: Recent research and its implications for psychiatry. *World Psychiatry*, *15*(2), 103–111. https://doi.org/10.1002/wps.20311

National Association of Social Workers [NASW]. (2003). *NASW standards for continuing professional education* [PDF]. www.socialworkers.org/LinkClick.aspx?fileticket=qrXmm_Wt7jU%3d&portalid=0

National Association of Social Workers [NASW]. (2004). *NASW standards for palliative and end of life care* [PDF]. www.socialworkers.org/LinkClick.aspx?fileticket=xBMd58VwEhk%3d&portalid=0

National Association of Social Workers [NASW]. (2017). *Code of ethics of the National Association of Social Workers*. www.socialworkers.org/About/Ethics/Code-of-Ethics/Code-of-Ethics-English

Pomeroy, E. C., & Garcia, R. B. (2018). *Direct practice skills for evidence-based social work: A strengths-based text and workbook*. Springer Publishing Company.

Pyles, L. (2020). Healing justice, transformative justice, and holistic self-care for social workers. *Social Work*, *65*(2), 178–187. https://doi.org/10.1093/sw/swaa013

Sartor, T. A. (2016). Vicarious trauma and its influence on self-efficacy. *VISTAS Online 2016*, 1–13.

Skinner, J. (2015). Social work practice and personal self-care. In K. Corcoran & A. R. Roberts (Eds.), *Social workers' desk reference* (3rd ed., pp. 130–139). Oxford University Press.

Urdang, E. (2010). Awareness of self—A critical tool. *Social Work Education*, *29*(5), 523–538. https://doi.org/10.1080/02615470903164950

Index

Locators in *italics* refer to figures. Locators in **bold** refer to tables.

For Product Safety Concerns and Information please contact our EU representative GPSR@taylorandfrancis.com
Taylor & Francis Verlag GmbH, Kaufingerstraße 24, 80331 München, Germany

www.ingramcontent.com/pod-product-compliance
Ingram Content Group UK Ltd.
Pitfield, Milton Keynes, MK11 3LW, UK
UKHW052053230926
475702UK00026B/1211
* 9 7 8 0 3 6 7 1 1 2 1 5 8 *